Foods for Special Dietary Regimens

Edited by

Elevina E. Pérez Sira

Instituto de Ciencia y Tecnología de Alimentos
Facultad de Ciencias Universidad Central de Venezuela
Venezuela

Foods for Special Dietary Regimens

Editor: Elevina E. Pérez Sira

ISBN (Online): 978-981-4998-06-2

ISBN (Print): 978-981-4998-07-9

ISBN (Paperback): 978-981-4998-08-6

©2021, Bentham Books imprint.

Published by Bentham Science Publishers Pte. Ltd. Singapore. All Rights Reserved.

need for a court order if at any point you breach any terms of this License Agreement. In no event will any delay or failure by Bentham Science Publishers in enforcing your compliance with this License Agreement constitute a waiver of any of its rights.

3. You acknowledge that you have read this License Agreement, and agree to be bound by its terms and conditions. To the extent that any other terms and conditions presented on any website of Bentham Science Publishers conflict with, or are inconsistent with, the terms and conditions set out in this License Agreement, you acknowledge that the terms and conditions set out in this License Agreement shall prevail.

Bentham Science Publishers Pte. Ltd.
80 Robinson Road #02-00
Singapore 068898
Singapore
Email: subscriptions@benthamscience.net

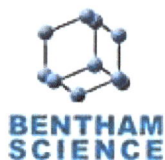

CONTENTS

PREFACE i

LIST OF CONTRIBUTORS ii

CHAPTER 1 SPECIAL DIETARY REGIMES: A GLANCE 1
Elevina E. Pérez Sira, Frederick Schroeder and *Mily Schroeder*
INTRODUCTION 1
CLASSIFICATION AND DESCRIPTION OF CONSUMERS 2
FOODS FOR SPECIAL DIETARY USES AND FUNCTIONAL FOODS 4
FOOD FUNCTIONS 5
DEFINITIONS ASSOCIATED TO THE BODY FUNCTION OF FOODS 5
MACRO AND MICRONUTRIENTS 6
    Macronutrients 6
    Micronutrients 12
SPECIAL DIETARY RAW MATERIAL 13
EFFECT OF THE TECHNOLOGICAL PROCESSES ON THE FOOD PROPERTIES 13
LABELING AND LEGISLATION 15
FOOD DEVELOPMENT FOR SPECIAL REGIMES 17
RECIPES 19
    Homemade Flour 19
    Homemade Passion Fruit Fluor 19
    Homemade Ginger Flour 20
CONSENT FOR PUBLICATION 20
CONFLICT OF INTEREST 20
ACKNOWLEDGEMENT 20
REFERENCES 20

CHAPTER 2 FOODS FOR VEGETARIANS 27
Elevina Pérez Sira
INTRODUCTION 27
NUTRITIONAL AND HEALTH IMPLICATIONS 29
TYPE OF VEGETARIAN CONSUMERS 31
FOOD-BASED DIETARY GUIDELINES AND VEGETARIAN FOOD PYRAMIDS 31
NUTRIENTS AND VEGETARIANS 34
    Macronutrients 35
    Micronutrients 35
VEGETARIAN DIETS THROUGH LIFE STAGES 37
PROCESSING FOOD FOR VEGETARIANS 40
RECIPES 41
    Veggie Rice Fried 41
    Vegan Mole Chilaquiles with Greens and Beans 42
    Ratatouille 46
    African Peanut Stew 47
    Roasted Kumara (Sweet Potato) Salad 48
    Aquafaba (Egg White Substitute) 49
    Vegan Mayonnaise 50
    Pasta and Vegan Meatballs 50
    Vegan Parmesan Cheese 52
    Bread Crumbs 52
    Vegan Yogurt 53
CONSENT FOR PUBLICATION 53

CONFLICT OF INTEREST 53

ACKNOWLEDGEMENT 53

REFERENCES 53

CHAPTER 3 FOODS FOR THE ELDERLY 58

Elevina Pérez Sira

INTRODUCTION 58

NUTRITION AND ELDERLY 59

ANOREXIA OF AGING 60

XEROSTOMIA, CHEW CAPACITY, AND PRESBYPHAGIA (DRY MOUTH, LOSS OF
CHEW CAPACITY, AND DIFFICULTY TO SWALLOW) 60

ANOSMIA OR HYPOSMIA (LOSS OF TASTE AND SMELL) 62

SARCOPENIA (INADEQUATE PROTEINS DIET) 64

HYPOTHYROIDISM (LOW IODINE DIET) 66

OSTEOPENIA/OSTEOPOROSIS 67

CONSTIPATION 68

FOOD FOR THE ELDERLY 68

RECIPES 70

    Breadfruit or Eggplant Purée from Pre-mix 70

    Mashed Beetroot-Cocoa from Pre-mix 71

CONSENT FOR PUBLICATION 74

CONFLICT OF INTEREST 74

ACKNOWLEDGEMENT 74

REFERENCES 74

CHAPTER 4 FOODS FOR ATHLETES 79

Elevina Pérez Sira, Frederick Schroeder and *Mily Schroeder*

INTRODUCTION 79

NUTRITION AND SPORT 80

MANAGING BODY COMPOSITION 81

SPECIAL REQUIREMENTS 82

ENERGY BALANCE AND AVAILABILITY 83

MACRO AND MICRONUTRIENTS 84

    Water 84

    Carbohydrates 85

    Proteins 86

    Fats 87

    Vitamins and Minerals 88

GOALS OF AN ADEQUATE SPORTS DIET 88

SUPPLEMENTS AND PERFORMANCE ENHANCERS 88

    What is a Supplement? 88

RECIPES 92

    Quick Energy Bite 92

    Avocado Cocoa Smoothie 92

    Protein Acai Bowl 93

    Pumpkin Cream 93

    Beetroot-Chocolate Chips Cookies 94

CONSENT FOR PUBLICATION 94

CONFLICT OF INTEREST 94

ACKNOWLEDGEMENT 95

REFERENCES 95

CHAPTER 5 FOODS FOR DIABETICS 100
Elevina Pérez Sira
   INTRODUCTION 100
   DIET AND DIABETES 104
   CONVENTIONAL AND NON-CONVENTIONAL RAW MATERIALS FOR DIABETIC FOOD 105
   SWEETENERS OVERVIEW 115
      Saccharides 116
      Non-saccharides 118
   DIETARY APPROACHES TO PRODUCE FOOD FOR DIABETIC CONSUMERS 124
   SOURCES OF FOODS WITH INSULIN SECRETING, INSULIN MIMETIC, AND INSULIN SENSITIZING PROPERTIES 125
   GLYCEMIC AND, INSULINIC INDEX AND GLYCEMIC LOAD 130
      Glycemic Index (GI) 130
      Glycemic Load (GL) 131
      Insulin Index (FII) 131
   RECIPES 132
      Eggplant Dip and Chips 132
      Grilled Eggplant 133
      Eggplant, Tomato and Passion Fruit Chutney 134
      Passion Fruit Jam 134
      Passion Fruit-Yogurt Ice Cream 135
      Plantain-Ginger Men Cookies 136
      Ginger/Mistletoe/Almond Biscuit 136
   CONSENT FOR PUBLICATION 137
   CONFLICT OF INTEREST 137
   ACKNOWLEDGEMENT 137
   REFERENCES 137

CHAPTER 6 FOOD FOR PHENYLKETONURIC CONSUMERS 152
Elevina Pérez Sira and *Antonieta Mahfoud*
   INTRODUCTION 152
   TREATMENT STRATEGIES 156
   INCIDENCE OF PKU 157
   NUTRITION AND PKU DIET 158
   DEVELOP AND INNOVATION OF FOOD FOR PKU 160
   RECIPES 165
      Peruvian Carrot Gnocchi in Spinach Sauce 165
      Beetroot and Carrot Cream 166
      Cassava-Chocolate Chips Cookies 166
      Cassava Bread 167
   CONSENT FOR PUBLICATION 168
   CONFLICT OF INTEREST 168
   ACKNOWLEDGEMENT 168
   REFERENCES 168

CHAPTER 7 FOODS FOR CELIAC AND AUTISTIC CONSUMERS 173
Elevina Pérez Sira
   INTRODUCTION 173
      Wheat Related Illnesses 173
      Gluten 177

CELIAC DISEASE DIAGNOSIS AND PATHOGENESIS 178
    Summary 182
GLUTEN-FREE DIET 183
SUBSTITUTES OF GLUTEN FLOUR 184
    Rice (*Oryza sativa*) 184
    Corn (*Zea mays*) 187
    Sorghum (*Sorghum bicolor M*) 188
    Potato (*Solanum tuberosum*) 189
    Non-convectional Sources 190
    Sweet potato (*Ipomoea batatas*) 191
    Yams (*Dioscorea* spp) 191
    Cassava (Manihot esculenta C) 191
    Carrot (Daucus carota S), and Beetroot (Beta vulgaris) 191
    Beans 192
    Pseudocereals 192
OTHER DIETETIC CONSIDERATIONS 192
GLUTEN-FREE BAKERY PRODUCTS AND PASTA 195
RECIPES 196
    Gluten-Free Pastas (Rigatoni and Fettuccini) 196
    Microwavable Cupcake 197
CONSENT FOR PUBLICATION 197
CONFLICT OF INTEREST 198
ACKNOWLEDGEMENT 198
REFERENCES 198

CHAPTER 8 DYSLIPIDEMIA AND FOODS 206
Elevina Pérez Sira
INTRODUCTION 206
HYPERCHOLESTEROLEMIA 207
    Cholesterol 207
    Lipoproteins 208
    Hypertriglyceridemia 210
    Hypotriglyceridemia 211
DYSLIPIDEMIA CAUSES 211
FATTY FOODS AND FATTY ACID PROFILE 213
ESSENTIAL FATTY ACIDS 214
    Avocado 218
    Nuts (Almonds, Hazelnuts, Peanuts, and Pecans) 219
    Fish (Such as Herring, Mackerel, Salmon, Trout, and Tuna) 220
    Other Foods 223
    Examples of Food with Saturated Fats 223
    Examples of Foods Trans Fats 224
FAT REPLACERS 224
PRACTICAL HINTS FOR FAT-FREE FOOD 226
    Dietary Fibers 226
    Sugars 228
RECIPES 229
    Zucchini Spaghetti 229
    Hawaiian Chicken Kabobs 230
    Homemade Beef Broth 230
    Broccoli/Green Beans Beef 231

      Salmon Avocado Salad 232

      Yacón/Fruit Salad 232

CONSENT FOR PUBLICATION 233

CONFLICT OF INTEREST 233

ACKNOWLEDGEMENT 233

REFERENCES 233

CHAPTER 9 COVID-19 AND FOOD: AN IMMUNOLOGICAL STRATEGY 239

Elevina Pérez Sira

INTRODUCTION 239

RECIPES 245

      Chicken Wing with Licorice Sauce 245

      Licorice Extract 246

      Licorice Syrup 246

      Chinese Yam with Star Anise, Ginger, and Lime 247

      Citrus Salad with Licorice Vinaigrette 247

      Dark Chocolate-Acai Chips Cookies 248

      Homemade Beet-Licorice Twizzles 248

      Beet-Licorice Ice Cream 249

CONSENT FOR PUBLICATION 250

CONFLICT OF INTEREST 250

ACKNOWLEDGEMENT 250

REFERENCES 250

SUBJECT INDEX 253

PREFACE

Good nutrition is a vital share of a healthy lifestyle. The diet combined with physical activity can help consumers to reach, and maintain a healthy weight, reducing the risk of chronic diseases, and promote overall health. From ancient times, the role of diet has been established in preventing disease enclosed in the Hippocrates of Cos (Greece, V century BC - IV century BC) aphorism: "Let food be your best medicine and your best medicine be your food. Hippocrates was driving the idea of preventive medicine with the diet as the main factor. These days, some consumers do not know or ignore the meaning of the relationship between diet and health, and there exists a gap among the consumers, food security, and food processor in regards to food for the prevention of consumers illness caused by life stages or styles. The market offers to conventional consumers a myriad of food developed, there is no food for special regimens, such as athletes, elderly, phenylketonuric, dyslipidemia, and diabetic, among others. Today, there is no commitment from the research sector and the food industry to fill this gap. The information given by the book must fill the preference of the audience of professionals who work in the areas of Food Science and Technology, Nutrition, Chemical Engineering, Agronomy, Nutrition/Medical, Medicine, Pharmacy. Moreover, general consumers, students (undergraduate, graduate) from different levels and areas, and specific consumers preferred conditions such as; diabetics, obese peoples, phenylketonuric, celiac, autistics, old people, vegetarians, and athletes. Good nutrition is a vital share of a healthy lifestyle. The diet combined with physical activity can help consumers to reach and maintain a healthy weight, reducing the risk of chronic diseases, and promote good overall health. This conception strengthens the concept of food security to professionals who work in the areas of Food Science and Technology, Nutrition, Chemical Engineering, Agronomy, Nutrition/Medical, Medicine, Pharmacy. As well as a preference by; general consumers, students (undergraduate, graduate) from different levels and areas, and specific consumers such as, diabetics, obese peoples, phenylketonuric, celiac, autistics, old peoples, vegetarians, athletes.

Elevina Pérez Sira
Instituto de Ciencia y Tecnología de Alimentos
Facultad de Ciencias Universidad Central de Venezuela
Venezuela

List of Contributors

Antonieta Mahfoud   Instituto de Estudios Avanzados IDEA, Unidad de Errores Innatos del Metabolismo, Venezuela

Elevina Pérez Sira   Instituto de Cienciay Tecnología de Alimentos, Facultad de Ciencias, Universidad Central de Venezuela, Caracas, Venezuela

Frederick Schroeder   University of Arizona, Bio-medical Engineer, Tucson, Arizona, Venezuela

Mily Schroeder   St. Mary University, Education and Leadership Department, Minneapolis, Minnesota, USA

CHAPTER 1

Special Dietary Regimes: A Glance

Elevina E. Pérez Sira[1,*], Frederick Schroeder[2] and **Mily Schroeder[3]**

[1] *Instituto de Ciencia y Tecnología de Alimentos, Facultad de Ciencias, Universidad Central de Venezuela, Caracas, Venezuela*

[2] *University of Arizona, Bio-medical Engineer, Tucson AZ, USA*

[3] *St. Mary University, Education and Leadership Department, Minneapolis, MN, USA*

Abstract: The relationship between foods and health and their influence on the prevention of diseases was established a long time ago. To corroborate this relationship and impact on consumer health; this chapter focuses on definitions associated with special dietarian regimes, classifying and describing different types of consumers, and defining the types of special foods. It also describes the food functions and definitions associated with its function on the body. The macro and micronutrients, special dietary raw material, and the effect of the technological processes on food properties are addressed. The labeling and its legislation, steps for food development, and recipes to produce nonconventional flour are also discussed.

Keywords: Consumers, Food development, Food labeling, Functional foods, Medical foods, Nutrients, Special dietary regimes.

INTRODUCTION

Hippocrates of Cos in Greece, 500-400 BC, working on preventive medicine had the first clue; from his observations of illness causes [1]. Hippocrates emphasized, that the type of diet, besides the lifestyle of the consumers, drives the differences in their health state [2]. He hypothesized a good selection of food for diet should be one of the answers to the upcoming healthy state of consumers [2]. According to the Hippocrates postulate, a good choice of foods in the diet should be the solution to the future health of any consumer.

Special dietary regimens are a pre-requisite for preventive medicine as a state security strategy. Therefore, the effort of the food industry must be focused on this area.

* **Corresponding author Elevina Pérez Sira:** Instituto de Ciencia y Tecnología de Alimentos, Facultad de Ciencias, Universidad Central de Venezuela, Caracas, Venezuela; Tel: +58.212.751 4403; Fax: + 58.212.751.3871; E-mail: elevina07@gmail.com

From the definition of the Codex Alimentarius in 2009 [3], a special regimen of alimentation is any diet that includes products expressly elaborated to cover necessities of food which are vital by physical or physiological conditions, or specific disorders. In this context, the identification of the conditions is necessary to be able to choose the right foods, which allows the design of the special regimen diet. Depending on the need, the foods for special regimens can be classified as follows:

Products for healthy people under special conditions include; fortified or enriched foods, foods for infants and children, and food without animal proteins.

Products for people with physiological and metabolic disorders such as; food modified in its energy value, low sugar food, food altered in its protein and/or lipid content, low sodium foods, and gluten-free foods.

A balanced and enough quantities of foods are an essential requirement for the optimal health of the human. By definition "Foods" is any diet constituent for human consumption, which can be processed, semi-processed or raw and includes beverages, chewing gum, and Ingredients. The ingredient is a substance used in food processing. Food definition does not include cosmetics or tobacco or substances used only as drugs [4, 5].

Foods are formed by macro (water, proteins, carbohydrates, and fats), micronutrients (vitamins and minerals), and traces of bioactive and flavor components. Each food has a peculiar color, odor, taste, and texture characteristics. The individual sensorial quality of the foods is defined by color, appearance, flavor (taste and aroma), and texture.

CLASSIFICATION AND DESCRIPTION OF CONSUMERS

Despite the advances in the industry, there are few choices of healthy foods in the markets. Besides, several processed foods could be non-nutritive, affecting consumers' health. Usually, consumers with special diets regimes do not have an adequate option at the market for foods. Hence, food processors and distributors must support these groups of consumers by producing types of foods adequate to their condition or style of life.

The production of these types of food must be handled by stimulating the consumption of healthy foods and improving strategy space and location in the supermarket to be easily found by the consumers. Furthermore, these groups recurrently must be considered as regular and essential groups, when defining food safety regulations.

Based on the food for special regimens classification, and in the context of food, security, and marketing, it should define two types of consumers:1) traditional consumers and 2) consumers with special food regimes [6 - 10].

1. Traditional consumers have two subclassifications: conventional and conservative consumers:

1a. Conventional consumers are those who respond to a biological need, and all food availability, attending to society's customs, aspirations, and expectations. Usually, they do not choose the foods, and consequently, they could reach the 2b categorization (consumers with physiological or metabolic disorders, who need special foods).

1b. Conservative consumers are those, who choose healthy foods, and read food labels and healthy food literature. Moreover, they are also aware of the impact of the foods on the ambient.

2. Consumers with special dietary regimes also have two subclassifications: those with a specific lifestyle or state condition, and consumers suffering disorders controlled or prevented with special foods.

2a. Consumers with a specific lifestyle or state condition. They have a cultural or religious conditions lifestyle (vegetarian, athletes) or age state condition (infant, elderly) that need special food regimes. These consumers must choose healthy foods, read food labels, and healthy food literature, and also must be aware of the impact of the foods on the ambient. They must consider in their diets all healthy information, before eating the foods.

2b. Consumers suffering physiological and metabolic disorders that can be controlled or prevented with special food regimes. These disorders are among the non-communicable diseases (NCDs), which are diseases of long duration resulting from a combination of genetic, physiological, environmental, and behavioral factors [11, 12].

NCDs are connected to vulnerable consumers living in non-developed countries where rapid unplanned urbanization and unhealthy lifestyle have prevalence. However, many people from developed countries have a chance to suffer this physiological or metabolic disorder due to their lifestyle. All of them are susceptible to have metabolic risk factors, which can cause cardiovascular sickness and probably premature death [11, 13, 14]. Much of these indicators (risk factors) are associated with the consumer's nutrition [15].

Several diseases are from unhealthy or inadequate food intake as; cardiovascular, hypertension, Diabetes Mellitus, mental disorders, obesity, dyslipidemia, celiac, phenylketonuric, cancer, osteoporosis, intolerance to carbohydrates (lactose) or protein (gluten, peanut protein). Further chapters of the book will discuss the relationship between food/nutrition/health associated with some of these diseases.

FOODS FOR SPECIAL DIETARY USES AND FUNCTIONAL FOODS

The relationship between health and food is recognized by the different institutions of the world food security [14, 15]. Therefore, the food industry is modifying food formulation to offer the consumers' foods adequate to their needs. In this context, purposes and functional foods are classified as follows: Foods for Special Dietary Uses (FDUS), Foods for Special Medical Purposes (FSMP), and Functional Foods (FF).

According to the Foods Codex Stan, 146-2009 [14] Special Dietary Uses (FDUS) are foods mainly processed or formulated to satisfy particular dietary requirements, which exist because of a particular physical or physiological condition and specific diseases and disorders, presented as such. The composition of these foodstuffs must differ significantly from the composition of ordinary foods of comparable nature if such ordinary foods exist. The definition of Foods for Special Dietary Uses (FSDU) has been restricted to foods that (a) furnish a particular dietary requirement that exists because of a physical or physiological condition, such as convalescence, pregnancy, lactation, infancy, and specific diseases and disorders; (b) supply a vitamin, mineral, or other dietary property to supplement the diet by increasing total dietary intake; (c) meet a special dietary need when such foods are the sole item of the daily diet [16, 17].

On the other hand, Foods for Special Medical Purposes (FSMP) was defined by Codex Stan 180-1991 [18] as a category of foods for special dietary uses, which are specially processed or formulated and presented for the dietary management of patients and may be used only under medical supervision.

A functional food (FF) is or appears like, conventional food. It is part of a standard diet and is consumed regularly in normal quantities. It has proven health benefits that reduce the risk of specific chronic diseases or beneficially affect target functions beyond its essential nutritional function [19, 20].

Another associated definition is bioactive components; they are compounds with biological activity promising as medications to the disease treatments; among these are several phytochemicals from plants. All these sources are available in nature for the production of FSDU, FSMP, and FF.

FOOD FUNCTIONS

Due to the world demographic explosion researcher have implemented procedures and techniques for better uses of the raw material to develop foods, which could cover special dietary needs. For better applications of the development, the functions of the food must be considered.

According to Mudambi and Rajagopal [5], there are three foods function: physiological, social, and psychological.

- Physiological functions: Food is the source of energy that comes from its macro and micronutrient components. Foods are ingested and transformed into usable nutrients in the body, to grow, keep warm, and built it.
- Social functions. Food is a part of human's social existence, and it is offered in homes and churches. Foods are an expression of love, friendship, and social acceptance.
- Psychological functions: In addition to satisfying physiological and social needs, food satisfies particular emotional needs and makes people feel secure.

DEFINITIONS ASSOCIATED TO THE BODY FUNCTION OF FOODS

There are several important definitions of the food functions associated with the body [5] such as:

• *Nutritional Status:* Nutritional status is the body state resulting from the food intake and its use by the body. It can be good or poor. Signs of a good nutritional status are good-natured personality, body with firm and developed muscles, weight and height correlated, healthy hair, skin, eyelids, and membranes of the mouth, clear eyes, and good appetite. Contrary, a poor nutritional status is characterized by an apathetic or irritable personality, undersized poorly developed body, abnormal body weight (too thin or fat and flabby body), muscles small and flabby, pale or sallow skin, too little or too much subcutaneous fat, dull or reddened eyes, lusterless and rough hair, poor appetite, lack of vigor and endurance for work and susceptibility to infections.

• *Nutrition:* is associated with several terms, which are as follows: malnutrition that can be undernutrition and overnutrition. Both of them are associated with a deficiency, excess, or imbalance of nutrients in the diets.

• *Diet:* it is referred to as the amount and types of food eaten.

• *Nutritional Care*: It refers to the planning, preparing, and improving acceptably and attractive meals to feed persons, through the valuation of the current meal patterns.

Other definitions are essential to mention:

• *Health:* The WHO [21] defined health as the state of complete physical, mental, and social well-being and not merely the absence of disease or infirmity. Food Nutrients are substances that provide nourishment essential for growth and the maintenance of life [22, 23].

• *Food Security*: is a condition that exists when all people, always, have physical, social, and economic access to enough, safe, and nutritious food that meets their dietary needs and food preferences for an active and healthy life [24].

• *Food Quality* of is the combination of characteristics that differentiate an individual from other of the same species determining the degree of acceptability for the user [25].

MACRO AND MICRONUTRIENTS

The essential components of food referred to as proximate composition includes moisture, ash, lipid, protein, and carbohydrate contents. Besides energy values (kcal), all of them are summarized into food composition tables at national and international levels [26]. National tables describe the composition of the internal and inherent foods of a country. International tables describe food composition through the Codex Alimentarius, which refers to all foods from the world. The tables are quite important for product development, quality control (QC), or regulatory purposes. They are expressed as the percentual content (%) in the food. The sum of these essential components is equal to 100% and represents the total weight of the food [27].

On the other hand, the whole set of nutritionally essential components of foods that provide values for energy and nutrients are classified as macro and micronutrients. Macronutrients are referred to as the nutrient that uses in gram ranges (water, protein, carbohydrates, and fats), while micronutrients are need in the micrograms range (vitamins, and minerals).

Macronutrients

Energy as calories is essential for the body's physiological development in the life process.

Water is considered as a macronutrient for several authors [28 - 31], due it is entirely essential for the body's metabolism as a lubricant and shock absorber. About 60% of body weight is made of water. The exigencies of the amount of water by the body are higher as compared with the other nutrients. Water's function in the body is as a solvent, a reaction medium, a reactant, and a reaction product [29].

Carbohydrates are an important source of energy in the diet, supplying 4 cal/g [30, 31]. The Institute of Medicine recommends that 45–65% of the total calories of diet should come from carbohydrates [32 - 35].

For completing a balanced diet, the consumption of carbohydrate-rich foods, including vegetables, fruits, grains, nuts, seeds, and dairy products, is suggested. Carbohydrates occur for body uses in three forms: sugar, starch, and fiber.

Sugars are natural sweetening, used in different functional applications in food processing. Nutritionally, it has been related to overweight and obesity. However, available data show no direct link between moderate consumption of sugars and serious diseases or obesity, and the concern is more about the overconsumption of sugars, which can be a problem with any food or nutrient [36, 37].

Sugars are found naturally in fruits, vegetables, and dairy products, honey, molasses, and maple syrup. The sugars term includes sucrose (table sugar), fructose, galactose, glucose, lactose, and maltose. The sources of sugars are corn, beetroot, and cane.

Starch is the plant's reserve food supply. Once isolated from the botanical source, starch is a white odorless dry powder with inherent functional properties depending on its botanical source. This functional diversity makes starch appropriate for diverse food applications. Additionally, physical, chemical, and enzymatic modifications on starch structure transform and improve its functional properties and facilitating its utilization for different purposes [38].

Historically, in addition to its caloric contribution, most of the uses of starch as a functional ingredient focus on the improvement of appearance, taste, mouthfeel, and stability of the products. Nutritionally the starch provides most of the calories eaten by consumers, due that the starchy raw materials and ingredients are usually available in enough amounts in most diets.

On the other hand, starch bioavailability is an issue of much nutritional concern. The starch structure is broken down, during metabolism into simple sugars, which are absorbed by the body. One of the physiological properties of the starch in the body is to produce the sense of feeling full for a longer period, due it transformation into sugar in the body is longer and its absorption for hence need more time than simple sugars. The recommendations suggest high inclusion as much as possible in the diet of unrefined food because during starchy foods refining several nutrients are loses [39, 40].

Advances in the understanding of the digestive physiology of dietary carbohydrates have confirmed a kind of resistant starch *in vitro* to the hydrolysis of the enzyme amylase. Other studies have shown starch that resisted digestion in the stomach and small intestine of healthy subjects. Further analysis has revealed the presence of fermented starches in the large intestine *in vivo*. Resistant starch (RS) is the term used to describe these starches [41].

RS has nutritional importance as dietary fiber and in the prevention of illness. The nutritional label in some countries includes RS in the term 'Dietary fiber'. Recently international food institutions agreed on a legal inclusion of RS in the dietary fiber composition through its definition, and analysis procedure [42].

The term 'Dietary Fiber' (DF) was first introduced in the 1950s, referring to plant cell wall materials; later it was used to describe a class of plant-originated polysaccharides, which cannot be digested and absorbed in the gastrointestinal tract [43]. This non-digestible material is nutritionally very important in the digestive tract, cleaning it during its transit by the body, absorbing water, and eliminating waste products.

As a function of its water solubility, there are two fiber types; soluble and insoluble with specific functional properties for good health. Fiber may help to prevent certain diseases such as heart disease, cancer, and diabetes. While not eating enough fiber can cause constipation and other intestinal problems, overeating, fiber can cause nutrients to pass through the system too quickly to be absorbed [40]. It is suggested consumption of 25 g of dietary fiber daily. On the other hand, it is important not to confuse dietary fiber with crude fiber, since they are nutritionally and illness preventive very different terms [44, 45].

Other nutritional differentiation of dietary fiber includes, as pointed out by Căpriță *et al.* [46], the fiber naturally occurring in foods, and the functional fibers. Functional fibers are those isolated fibers, which have a positive physiological effect.

The food industry uses several hydrocolloids as thickeners, texturizers, stabilizers, and emulsifiers. The hydrocolloids use are based on their technological functionality and high palatability. Many of them, categorized as dietary fiber, have the capacity to enhanced health.

Fats and their derivatives, collectively known as lipids are one of the major organic molecules that influence in quantity and quality the body physiology [47 - 49]. In the body lipids are used to build steroids and hormones and as solvents for hormones and fat-soluble vitamins. The main biological functions of the lipids are to form part of the structure of the biological membrane and to store energy for the cell. They are significant components of the nervous system [50 - 52].

Lipids have the highest caloric content compared to carbohydrates and proteins, providing 9 calories per gram. Extra fat stored in adipose tissue is burnt when the body has run out of carbohydrates. The term lipid besides fats and oils also includes waxes and their derived compounds (such as; complex lipids, hormones, steroids, vitamins, and pigments lipophilic). The main difference between fat and oil is in its chemical structure; fats contain saturated fatty acids in a high proportion making them in a solid state at room temperature. In contrast, oils contain mainly unsaturated fatty acids, making them a viscous liquid state at room temperature.

The fatty acid structure focus on three aspects:

Chemically, the triglyceride molecule is the basis of all fats (lard, shortening) and oils. This structure means that one fat molecule is formed for three molecules of fatty acids combined with a molecule of glycerol. This combination of long chains of fatty acids can be unsaturated or saturated. Fatty acids are molecules formed by long straight-chain aliphatic carboxylic acids. They usually have are C4 to C22, with C18 most common [53].

Nutritionally and chemically the fatty acids are aliphatic straight-chain molecules, which have a methyl group at one end of the molecule and a carboxyl group (Δ) at the other end (Fig. **1**) [54]. The carbon atom next to the carboxyl group is the alfa (α) carbon, and the subsequent one the beta (ß) carbon. The carbon omega (ω) position indicates the double bond closest to the methyl end.

E.g., α-linolenic acid (ALA), which shorter name is $18:3^{\Delta 9, \, 12, \, 15}$

CH3-(CH3)--CH2-CH2-COOH ω ß α; $CH_3\text{-}(CH_3)_n\text{-}CH_2\text{-}CH_2\text{-}$ COOH ω ß α

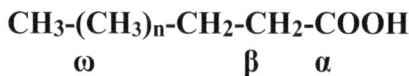

$$\textbf{CH}_3\textbf{-(CH}_3\textbf{)}_n\textbf{-CH}_2\textbf{-CH}_2\textbf{-COOH}$$
$$\omega \qquad\qquad\qquad \beta \quad\ \alpha$$

Fig. (1). Nomenclature for PUFA omega-3 [54].

Nutritionally and functionally fatty acids are saturated, mono and polyunsaturated, and Trans. Saturated are those fats, which contain fatty acids (from the natural or processed origin) chains having all or mostly single covalent bonds. In unsaturated fats, the fatty acid chains have natural or by the effect of the process, all or predominantly multiple double bonds. They are represented by monounsaturated fatty acids (MUFA; one double bond), polyunsaturated fatty acids (PUFA; more than one double bond), and trans fatty acids (TFA).

Lipid's type and amount of intake define the risk of coronary heart disease. A high intake of lipids (over 35 percent of calories) induces high-fat saturated ingestion. Contrarily, a low intake of lipids (below 20 percent of calories) increases the risk of inadequate intake of vitamin E and essential fatty acids [55].

Nowadays, it is recognized that omega-3 and 6 fatty acids are essential for body normal development, playing an important effect on disease prevention and treatment [56]. Its adequate intake must be a function of the omega-6/omega -3 ratio. It has been suggested that the relative amount of linoleic acid (omega 6 or ω-6) and alfa-linolenic acid (omega 3 or ω-3) must be below a 10:1 ratio, due to its competitive and biological essentials and different functions [57 - 59].

The natural chemical configuration of fatty acids molecules is the stable cis configuration; however, many foods also contain monounsaturated Trans fatty acids (TFA). Usually, TFA occurring in food are a product of the procedure of hydrogenation of fats, to increase their melting point, making them stables, resistant to oxidation, and with long shell life [60, 61].

The high intake of TFA fatty acids has been associated with several diseases. However, according to Dhaka *et al*. [62], considering banning all TFA from the diet would be detrimental as this would include banning *Trans* fats such as vaccenic acid (VA), which could be positive for health. Vaccenic acid is a natural fat of ruminants and in human milk. Therefore, it is occurring in dairy products such as milk, butter, and yogurt [63, 64].Proteins have an important development role in the body (functional, structural, metabolic, and developmental), and provide 4 calories per gram. Adequate dietary protein is essential for overall human health, with recommendations differing throughout the human life span [65]. Therefore, it is imperative the recommendations of the adequate amount of high-quality protein intake stimulate ideal health, and do not merely meet needs to prevent protein deficiency [66]. The adequate requirement of protein is this that satisfies the metabolic demand and complete nitrogen equilibrium in the body. Since there are not proteins body store, an inadequate intake of protein leads to a negative protein balance, resulting in muscle atrophy, impaired muscle growth or regrowth, and functional decline [65].

The essential amino acids are leucine, isoleucine, valine, lysine, threonine, tryptophan, methionine, phenylalanine, and histidine. Histidine has been established as an essential amino acid, because of the detrimental effects observed on body hemoglobin concentrations when individuals eat a histidine-free diet [67, 68].

According to Lacey [67], the amino acid glutamine becomes "conditionally essential" in critical illness. The author pointed out that glutamine is a unique amino acid that has many functions, such as respiratory fuel, balance acid-base regulator, nitrogen carrier, and nucleic acids, nucleotides, amino sugars, and proteins.

On the other hand, Laidlaw and Kopple (1987) and Reeds (2009) [68, 69] have proposed a classification of the indispensability of amino acids based on clinical and therapeutic considerations, considering arginine, citrulline, ornithine, cysteine, and tyrosine as essential amino acids. They also had arguments about the relationship that has of the non-essential and conditionally essential amino acids with physiological function (Table **1**).

Table 1. Amino acids to make all types of protein source [69].

Non-Essential or Dispensable	Essential or Indispensables	Conditionally Indispensable
Alanine	Leucine	Arginine
Arginine	Isoleucine	Cysteine
Aspartic acid	Valine	Glutamine
Cysteine	Threonine	Glycine
Glutamic acid	Tryptophan	Proline
Glutamine	Methionine	Serine
Glycine	Phenylalanine	Tyrosine
Proline	Histidine	Asparagine
Serine	-	-
Tyrosine	-	-
Asparagine	-	-
Alanine	-	-

It has been pointed out that ingestion of essential amino acids offers more efficient nutritional functionality to enhance muscle protein synthesis as compared with the ingestion of intact protein [70]. The amino acid proportionality pattern, digestibility, and bioavailability of amino acids are the most critical determinants of protein quality [65, 71].

The protein quality refers to its ability to complete a metabolic action, as a function of the matrix in which protein is consumed, and the protein amount demanded by the body [71]. Therefore, the quality of protein is determined by the equilibrium between metabolic demand and the dietary requirement [72], denoting that the Dietary requirement = Metabolic demand.

The dietary requirement is the amount of protein or its constituent amino acids or both, that must be supplied in the diet to satisfy the metabolic demand and achieve nitrogen equilibrium, and the metabolic demand for amino acids and protein is the flow of amino acids through those pathways that together maintain the structure and function of the body, thus the protein Efficiency of Utilization is calculated from:

$$\text{Dietary Requirement} = \frac{\text{Metabolic Demand}}{\text{Efficiency of Utilization)}}$$

On the other hand, protein digestibility is the balance of amino acids across the small intestine (mouth to terminal ileum: ileal digestibility), or the entire intestine (mouth to anus: fecal digestibility). It is the difference between intake and losses, and it provides a measure of the extent of digestion and absorption of food protein such as amino acids by the gastrointestinal tract [72].

The amino acid proportionality pattern, digestibility, and the bioavailability of amino acids are the most critical determinants of protein quality [65, 71].

Pomeranz and Meloan [51] defined ash as the inorganic residue from the incineration of organic matter. Food type and the analytical procedure are determinants for the amount and composition of ash. In spite that the mineral content is a precise measure of the amount of specific inorganic components present within a food, such as Ca, Na, K, and Cl [73], the ash content is an indirect measure of mineral content in food. The mineral content is nutritionally crucial. It is mandatory; that the nutritional labeling report the concentration and type of some specific minerals present in food. In a quality context, many foods depend on the concentration and type of minerals they contain, including their taste, appearance, texture, and stability.

Micronutrients

Micronutrients are essential elements required by the body in minor quantities for completing its physiological functions and maintain health [74].

Vitamins required by the body in microgram or milligram amounts are classified as water-soluble and fat-soluble vitamins. The water-soluble vitamins include folate, folic acid, thiamin (B_1), riboflavin (B_2), niacin o nicotinic acid (B_3), pantothenic acid (B_5), pyridoxine (B_6), biotin (B_7), cyanocobalamin (B_{12}). And the fat-soluble vitamins include vitamins A, C, D, K, and E. They act in the body as cofactors in the conversion of food in energy, metabolism, the formation of cells, hormonal production, energy storage, systems nervous, immune, and digestive, growth and development, vision, antioxidant, blood pressure regulation, wound healing, blood clotting, and strong bones [74].

Minerals are inorganic substances occurring naturally in soil and water. Since living organisms do not synthesize them, humans and animals must consume fourteen of these elements from the foods. They are calcium, chloride, chromium, copper, iodine, iron, magnesium, manganese, molybdenum, phosphorus, potassium, selenium, sodium, and zinc. The functions on the body of the minerals are in blood clotting, bone-teeth formation, constriction and relaxation of blood vessels, hormone secretion and function, muscle contraction, nervous, immune, and digestive system function, acid/base balance, fluid balance, metabolism, antioxidant, cell, and tissue formation, reproduction, blood pressure and sugar regulation, cardiac heart rhythm, wound healing, muscle contraction, taste and smell, wound healing [74].

SPECIAL DIETARY RAW MATERIAL

Raw materials (ingredients, processing aids, and packaging materials) in the food industry are materials or substances used in the primary production or manufacturing of finished food products. As such, they must meet regulatory requirements (safe and legal for your intended use) and characteristic specifications (contribute to the functionality and quality of your process and product) [75]. There are numerous non-conventional ingredients obtained from plants to produce food for special regimes. In this context, it can be made flour with vegetables and fruit such as; eggplant, cocoa, and passion fruit peel, ginger rhizomes, curcumin, *etc*. These raw materials have bioactive compounds (phytochemicals) that made them quite valuable for foods of regimes special. Several tropical and Andean roots and tubers and fruits as the *Musaceae* genus are useful to produce gluten-free flour by using conventional dehydration techniques [76 - 84]. Legumes are also valuable to produce flour just using milling and sieve procedures or elaborating concentrates and isolate from it. Phenylalanine-free glycomacropeptides from whey and bean *of Erythrina edulis* [84] and the uses of natural sweeteners such as stevia [85] are another alternative.

EFFECT OF THE TECHNOLOGICAL PROCESSES ON THE FOOD PROPERTIES

Since a healthy diet is a financial and nutritional investment, it is necessary to retain the highest dietary portions during the preparation. Therefore, it is necessary to be aware of the numerous factors that, during food processing, influence the stability and losses of the food's nutritional composition. It can be mentioned among them; plant or animal genetic origin, climate condition, postharvest procedures, and the processing, conservation, packing, and storage condition [86, 87].

Almost all foods must be processed by different procedures before they are eaten. The main nutritional and commercial reasons for processing foods are to make them digestible, safe, and shelf-stable. Only a few foods need minimal processing, but most foods need different treatments to be preserved and for increasing the digestibility and availability of their nutrients. However, the preparation and preservation of food involve processes that influence negatively its nutritional value.

Foods have nutrient losses or changes produced for the application of thermal processes (bleaching, retorting, pasteurization, dehydration extrusion, and freezing) such as; lixiviation, isomerization *Trans* to *Cis*, oxidation, nonenzymatic brown reaction, interactions, and formation of toxic substances [86, 88 - 92].

Processing methods, such as milling, fermentation, germination (sprouting), extrusion, also alter the nutrients of the food.

The impact of the treatment on a nutrient depends on its sensitivity to the processing conditions (heat, oxygen, pH, and light). Exposure to them will alter sensible nutrients, such as vitamins and pigments [86, 89].

Heat, for example, could destroy some thermolabile nutrients in some condition, but in others could maintain its nutritive value by inactivating enzymes, liberating nutrient from the unusable food matrix, and enhancing nutrient bioavailability [88]. Examples as: the phytic acid, which is a natural blocker of the bioavailability of several minerals (Zn, Fe), the cooking procedure reduces its action by 50% in grains products. The reduction of phytohemaglutinin (PHG), or reducing the action of the egg proteins (conalbumin and avidin) natural binder and for hence blockers of iron and vitamin B are other examples [86, 87, 90].

The procedure of sprout grain minimizes the mineral-blocking effect of phytic acid and maximizes the mineral availability [87].

Processing with water reduces the amounts of nutrients as these get lixiviate out and leave behind. Blanching, for example, results in leaching losses of vitamins and minerals. Also, milling and extrusion can cause the physical removal of minerals during processing. The bioavailability of crucial minerals, such as iron, zinc, and calcium, is significantly affected by the fiber, phytic acid, and tannin content of foods. The time and temperature of processing, product composition, and storage are all factors that substantially impact the vitamin status of the foods [89].

During frozen storage, some factors influence nutrient stability. They are the temperature of the freezing unit and its range of fluctuation, the length of storage, the size of the cut, the thawing method, and the packaging method.

The refrigeration and freezing procedures could induce nutrients losses, especially of vitamins and minerals. Temperature, storage length, humidity, and light are important factors that need to be monitored during cool storage. Interruption of the frozen temperature could produce thaw drip, with consequence losses of soluble proteins, vitamins, and minerals. Some vegetables are more sensitive than others to loss of vitamins under refrigerated storage (broccoli more sensitive than and green beans). Fresh fruits are not stable for long periods in the refrigerator and will deteriorate rapidly. Milk may undergo vitamin loss during refrigerated storage, mainly because of its exposure to light and oxygen. In milk, some vitamins, such as riboflavin, are severely affected by the light. Riboflavin converted to lumichrome and lumiflavin, catalyze the inactivation of ascorbic acid.

Processing food alters the nutrient quality, but industrial procedures have handled technological innovation to minimize them. Moreover, consumers should be conscious that losses in the poor nutritional quality of foods may result from improper use of cooking and storage techniques available at home [93].

LABELING AND LEGISLATION

The flow of information through adequate food labels and advertising is important in the marketplace. Labels are particularly pertinent in regards to food products. Labels are mandatory because of their impacts on food choices. Food labeling laws make sure consumers get vital information about the foods they consume [94, 95]. Food labeling contains data provided by food processors that informs the consumer about the food they buy. It helps consumers to make informed choices and allows consumers to store and use the food safely [96]. All countries and regulatory bodies in the world must be responsible for the labeling and standards policy on issues of food safety and nutrition. In this context, there exist mandatory information that must be in labels. According to the FSA [96], there are twelve mandatory items of information that must be in the label as follow:

1. The name of the food. It is illegal for food to have false or misleading names or descriptions.

2. List of ingredients. The list of ingredients on a food label must have a heading that includes the word 'ingredients'. Ingredients must be listed in descending order of weight when the product was prepared.

3. Quantitative Ingredient Declaration (QUID). When ingredients are emphasized on the label to categorize the food, the quantities of these ingredients should be shown to make sure that consumers are not misled. This is the QUID.

It should be used where:

• The ingredient is in the name of the food or is usually associated with that name.

• The ingredient is emphasized on the labeling in words, pictures, or graphics.

• The ingredient is essential to characterize food and to distinguish it from another product that it could be confused with.

• The minimum percentage of the ingredient in the food must be given either next to the name of the food or in the ingredients list.

4. Net quantity: This is the weight or volume of the product without the packaging. It must be provided in metric units (kilos and grams or liters, centiliters, and milliliters).

5. Instructions for use: These are the manufacturer's instructions for preparing the food.

6. Indication of minimum durability: This information is about the storage and use of food, which aims to help consumers to use food safely and reduce waste. There are two main types of date marks required:

• Best before – This date mark appears on most pre-packaged foods.

• Consumers can use the food after this date, but it may not be the best quality

7. Storage conditions and/or conditions for use. It must be regarding the storage type uses: Dry, fridge, or freezing.

Following these instructions makes sure the food will last if the date is shown if it hasn't been opened, or that it remains safe after opening.

8. The name or business name and address of the food business operator. The label should contain the name or business name and address of the food business operator. If a consumer is not satisfied with how food is labeled, they should contact the food business operator.

9. Country of origin or place of provenance.

10. Food allergens: Food allergy, food intolerance, and celiac disease can cause

some people to become ill. Food labels must help people with a food allergy, food intolerance, or celiac disease to make safe food choices.

There are 14 food allergens (including derivatives) that by law must be emphasized in the ingredients list on the label if they are deliberately added [96]: peanut, nuts, cereals containing gluten (wheat, barley, rye, oats, spelt, and kamut), eggs, milk, fish, lupin, mustard, sesame seeds, mollusks (such as mussels and oysters), crustaceans (such as lobster and crab), soybeans, celery, Sulphur dioxides and sulphites (in beverages).

11. Nutrition information: If a nutrition or health claim is made about a food *e.g.* high fiber or low in fat, nutrition information must be provided. Nutrition labeling will become a mandatory requirement from 13 December 2016. If a business is voluntarily providing a nutrition panel on its label it must comply with the requirements of the Food Information Regulation from 13 December 2014 [96].

12. Alcohol strength. Alcohol strength must be provided if a drink contains more than 1.2% alcohol.

FOOD DEVELOPMENT FOR SPECIAL REGIMES

Food development is a methodic and technological procedure conceived with researches on the new or modified formulation, or process flowchart, which induce to obtain products to satisfying a known or supposed consumer need. Therefore, product development offers original products, product improvements, product modifications, and new brands, and development activities [97].

The development and commerce of foods for special regimes are rather multifaceted, expensive, and risky due to the special requirement of these foods. Besides the potential technological obstacles and legislative aspects, the consumer physiological requirements must be also attended to when developing these foods.

The success key factor in negotiating market opportunities is consumer acceptance. Similarly, to the development of conventional products is carried out, the team working on the development of foods for special regimes must go through the same steps such as generation and screening of the ideas, market research, product specification, feasibility study, production process development, development of the prototype, and sensory test [97].

A generation and screening of the ideas proceed to the market research. Its production is the methodical search for new products from internal and external ideas. The internal ideas come from personnel at all levels, as well as business programs of the corporation, and the external come from outside of the corporation (customers, competitors, distributors, suppliers, and outside design companies or external developers). The screening technique is to reduce the lots of ideas that have been generated from a topic or product, seeking good ideas and discards bad ones by using the technique of sieving, systemic approach, and costprofit [97].

Market research is the scientific investigation of a potential market by collecting, analyzing, and interpreting the data from the past, present, or future of the products and services offered by this market, and their potential consumers. Data recollects information of the characteristics, spending habits, location, and needs of the business's target market, the industry, and the competitors faced.

The product design specification requests all information available from the prototypes developed in the 'ballpark' experiments [98]. The aim 'ballpark' study is to set, by a factorial design, the limits of the raw materials and the processing variables, which give acceptable product qualities as judged by the consumer [99]. Three factors determine the quality of design: a deep understanding of customer requirements, translation of these requirements into a product, and continuous improvement of the design process. Close cooperation among marketing, research, and development, and engineering improves the design process [98].

Feasibility study. It is a controlled process for identifying problems and opportunities, determining objectives, describing the situation, defining successful outcomes, and assessing the range of cost and benefits associated with several alternatives for solving problems [100].

Process development links product design. In this context, there are three aspects of the study: 1. Unit operations are categorized as separation, assembling, conversion, and preserving operations (heating, pasteurization, sterilization, freezing, chilling, drying, mixing, emulsifying, tumbling, pumping, conveying, and packing). 2. Unit processes that are the chemical, biological, and microbiological changes (gelatinization, hydrolysis, oxidation, browning, protein denaturation, vitamin destruction, destruction and growth of microorganisms, fruit ripening, and meat tenderizing). 3. Processing limits (maximum and minimum). These can be temperatures, rates of increase/decrease in temperature, viscosities, mixing speeds, shear rates, and pH, as well as processing times, availability, and cost of equipment and services such as water quantity and steam pressures.

Sensory test after the prototyping, sensory evaluation is the final tool for concept development and proof. There are several techniques to taste the final products. They are discriminative and descriptive. Whatever is the method, each of them has a specific function to be successfully launching the product. However, before launching the new product, it is necessary to perform the marketing studies, which comprise the offer, demand, price, and marketing analysis. Conclusively, there is an interrelationship among the design implementation before it is launching that goes through the prototyping, analysis, and sensory evaluation.

RECIPES

Homemade Flour

(Banana, Beetroot, Breadfruit, Cassava, Carrot, Eggplants, Peruvian Carrot, Spinach, and Sweet Potato Flour).

Ingredients (~ 500g of each flour)

2.5kg	Bananas (unripe) green	2.5kg	Peruvian carrot
2.5kg	Beetroots	2.5kg	Spinach
2.5kg	Breadfruits	2.5kg	Sweet potato
2.5kg	Cassava roots	-	-
2.5kg	Carrot	-	-
2.5kg	Eggplants	-	-

Preparation

Except for the bananas, cut in 0.5-inch sized slices, the cleaned and peeled ingredients. Previous to dehydration; the green bananas (grade I in maturity) with shells are blanched (20 minutes at 98°C), and the unripe bananas unshelled are sunk in a solution of 0.5% citric acid. The eggplants are previously sliced, microwaved for 1-minute. The spinach leaves are carefully separated from the stems and cleaned before dehydration. The dehydration is at 45 °C, by putting the sliced raw materials separately on the trays of the digital home food dehydrator previously heated. The raw material was dehydrated separately during a time of 24 hours. Ground and sieve the dehydrated pieces by using a home mill and a colander. Pack hermetically in plastic bags or glass containers (labeled) at room temperature for later uses.

Homemade Passion Fruit Fluor

Ingredients.

3.5kg	Passion fruit
1.5 liter	Water
80ml	Lemon juice

Preparation

Cut by half the passion fruits. Remove pulp from it, and do not discard it. Freeze the pulp and reserve; it could be used for several recipes later. Place skins in a large saucepan, add water and lemon juice, cover it, and bring to boil, reduce heat, simmer, and cover 10 minutes. Drain the liquid. Carefully with a knife cut all outer-pigmented skin (exocarp) of each half and discard it. Transfer all the passion fruit halves to the oven at 120°F (50°C) for 8 hours or until it is dried. Elaborate the flour by mixing in a blender and passing it through a fine colander. Store in an airtight container and put it at room temperature. Take 2 tablespoons daily of the flour by dissolving it into juice, salad, or meal. Flour also can be used to elaborate baked goods, flan, and gelatin, among others.

Homemade Ginger Flour

Ingredients

900g	Ginger rhizomes large

Preparation

Clean the fresh ginger thoroughly with plenty of potable water and sliced it. Transfer the slices to the oven at 165°F (75 °C) during the first 90 min, and ended at 131 °F (55°C) to reach an equilibrium moisture content of 12% or until it is dried. Elaborate the flour by mixing in a blender and passing it through a fine colander. Store in an airtight container and put it at room temperature.

CONSENT FOR PUBLICATION

Not Applicable.

CONFLICT OF INTEREST

The author confirms that this chapter contents have no conflict of interest.

ACKNOWLEDGEMENT

Declared none.

REFERENCES

[1]   Grammaticos PC, Diamantis A. Useful known and unknown views of the father of modern medicine, Hippocrates and his teacher Democritus. Hell J Nucl Med 2008; 11(1): 2-4.
       [PMID: 18392218]

[2]   Microsoft Encarta Online Encyclopedia. 2006. http://www.webcitation.org/query?id=12570078419

24009

[3]   CODEX STAN. Norma general para el etiquetado y declaración de propiedades de alimentos preenvasados para regímenes especiales146-2009 2009. http://www.fao.org

[4]   Food and Drug Administration/World Health Organization (FAO/WHO). 2010. www.fao.org

[5]   Mudambi SR, Rajagopal MV. Fundamentals of foods, nutrition, and diet therapy New Age International. New Delhi, India: Ltd Publisher 2012; pp. 3-9.

[6]   Williams HH. Differences between cow's and human milk. JAMA 1961; 175(2): 104-7.
[http://dx.doi.org/10.1001/jama.1961.63040020005006a] [PMID: 13785439]

[7]   World Health Organization WHO. Infant and young child nutrition. Geneva, Switzerland: WHO 2003.

[8]   Johnston M, Landers S, Noble L, Szucs K, Viehmann L. Section on Breastfeeding. Breastfeeding and the use of human milk. Pediatrics 2012; 129(3): e827-41.
[http://dx.doi.org/10.1542/peds.2011-3552] [PMID: 22371471]

[9]   Greer FR. American Academy of Pediatrics Committee on Nutrition. Reimbursement for foods for special dietary use. Pediatrics 2003; 111(5 Pt 1): 1117-9.
[PMID: 12728102]

[10]   American Academy of Pediatrics Policy. Statement section on breastfeeding. Breastfeeding and the use of human milk. Pediatr 2012; 129(3): e827-41.
[http://dx.doi.org/10.1542/peds.2011-3552]

[11]   World Health Organization WHO. Noncommunicable diseases 2017. http://www.who.int/mediacentre/factsheets/fs355/en/

[12]   World Cancer Research Fund International. NDC Alliance 2017. http://www.wcrf.org

[13]   NOM-086-SSA1. Norma Oficial Mexicana Bienes y Servicios Alimentos y Bebidas no Alcohólicas con modificaciones en su composición. Especificaciones Nutrimentales 1994.

[14]   2009. http://www.fao.org/fao-who-codexalimentarius/standards/list-standards/es/

[15]   World Health Organization WHO. World Health Organization 2015. http://www.who.int/gho/ncd/mortality_morbidity/en/ b

[16]   Chopra JG. Current regulatory status of foods for special dietary uses. Am J Public Health 1976; 66(4): 351-3.
[http://dx.doi.org/10.2105/AJPH.66.4.351] [PMID: 1267078]

[17]   Food and Drug Administration (FDA). Title 21- Chapter I-Food and Drugs. Department of Health and Human Services. Subchapter B--Food for human consumption. Part 105-Foods for special dietary use. [Code of Federal Regulations]. [Title 21, Vol. 2]. 2018.

[18]   Codex Alimentarius. CODEX STAN 180-1991. Norma general para el etiquetado y declaración de propiedades. Codex Standard for the labeling of and claims for foods for special medical purposes 1991.

[19]   Ross S. Functional foods: the Food and Drug Administration perspective. Am J Clin Nutr 2000; 71(6) (Suppl.): 1735S-8S.
[http://dx.doi.org/10.1093/ajcn/71.6.1735S] [PMID: 10837331]

[20]   Doyon M. Functional foods: A conceptual definition. Br Food J 2008; 110(11): 1133-49.
[http://dx.doi.org/10.1108/00070700810918036]

[21]   World Health Organization (WHO). Official Records of the World Health Organization N° 2. 1946; p. 100.

[22]   Kirkby E. Introduction, definition, and classification of nutrients.Marschner's mineral nutrition of higher plants. 3rd ed. New York: Academic Press 2012; pp. 3-5.
[http://dx.doi.org/10.1016/B978-0-12-384905-2.00001-7]

[23]   English Oxford Living Dictionary. 2019. https://en.oxforddictionaries.com

[24]   Food and Drug Administration (FAO). 2002. http://www.fao.org

[25]   Barrett DM, Beaulieu JC, Shewfelt R. Color, flavor, texture, and nutritional quality of fresh-cut fruits and vegetables: desirable levels, instrumental and sensory measurement, and the effects of processing. Crit Rev Food Sci Nutr 2010; 50(5): 369-89.
[http://dx.doi.org/10.1080/10408391003626322] [PMID: 20373184]

[26]   National Agricultural Library. 2019.United States Department of Agriculture https://ndb.nal.usda.gov

[27]   Codex Alimentarius International Food Standard. Codex Alimentarius Commission (CAC). 2020. http://www.fao.org/fao-who-codexalimentarius/committees/cac/about/en/

[28]   Nielsen S. Proximate assays in food analysis.Food analysis. 5th ed. Boston, MA: Springer 2017; pp. 17-34.
[http://dx.doi.org/10.1007/978-3-319-45776-5_2]

[29]   Boeckner L. Water the nutrient 2009. http://extensionpublications.unl.edu

[30]   Jéquier E, Constant F. Water as an essential nutrient: the physiological basis of hydration. Eur J Clin Nutr 2010; 64(2): 115-23.
[http://dx.doi.org/10.1038/ejcn.2009.111] [PMID: 19724292]

[31]   Food and Drug Administration (FAO). Eating well for good health 2018. www.fao.org

[32]   Food Pyramid caring for your health. The 6 essential nutrients. 2018. [cited: 28th June 2020] Available from: www.foodpyramid.com/6-essential

[33]   Institute of Medicine. Food and Nutrition Board Dietary reference intakes: energy, carbohydrates, fiber, fat, fatty acids, cholesterol, protein, and amino acids. Washington, DC: National Academies Press 2002.

[34]   Institute of Medicine. Dietary Reference Intakes (DRIs): The essential guide to nutrient requirements. Washington, DC: National Academies of Sciences 2006; pp. 110-21.

[35]   Coleman E. What is the AMDR recommendation for carbohydrates? 2018. http://healthyeating.sfgate.com

[36]   Schorin M, Sollid K, Edge MS, Bouchoux A. The Science of sugars, Part I: A closer look at sugars. Nutr Today 2012; 47(3): 96-101.
[http://dx.doi.org/10.1097/NT.0b013e3182435de8]

[37]   Schorin M, Sollid K, Edge MS, Bouchoux A. The science of sugars, Part 2: Sugars and a healthful diet. Nutr Today 2012; 47(4): 175-82.
[http://dx.doi.org/10.1097/NT.0b013e3182441ffb]

[38]   Jane J. Starch Properties, Modifications, and Applications. J Macromol Sci A 1995; 32(4): 751-7.
[http://dx.doi.org/10.1080/10601329508010286]

[39]   Jenkins DJ, Wolever TM, Taylor RH, *et al.* Glycemic index of foods: a physiological basis for carbohydrate exchange. Am J Clin Nutr 1981; 34(3): 362-6.
[http://dx.doi.org/10.1093/ajcn/34.3.362] [PMID: 6259925]

[40]   Jenkins DJ, Jenkins AL, Wolever TM, Collier GR, Rao AV, Thompson LU. Starchy foods and fiber: reduced rate of digestion and improved carbohydrate metabolism. Scand J Gastroenterol Suppl 1987; 129: 132-41.
[http://dx.doi.org/10.3109/00365528709095867] [PMID: 2820027]

[41]   Englyst H, Wiggins HS, Cummings JH. Determination of the non-starch polysaccharides in plant foods by gas-liquid chromatography of constituent sugars as alditol acetates. Analyst (Lond) 1982; 107(1272): 307-18.
[http://dx.doi.org/10.1039/an9820700307] [PMID: 6283946]

[42]   Nugent AP. Review. Health properties of resistant starch. FNB 2005; 30: 27-54.

[43]   Jones JM. CODEX-aligned dietary fiber definitions help to bridge the 'fiber gap'. Nutr J 2014; 13: 34.
[http://dx.doi.org/10.1186/1475-2891-13-34] [PMID: 24725724]

[44]   Cummings JH. Dietary fibre. Gut 1973; 14(1): 69-81.
[http://dx.doi.org/10.1136/gut.14.1.69] [PMID: 4571071]

[45]   Trowell H, Burkitt D, Heaton K. Definitions of dietary fibre and fibre-depleted foods and disease. London: Academic 1985; pp. 21-30.

[46]   Căpriţă A, Căpriţă R, Gianet Simulescu VO, Drehe R-M. Dietary fiber: Chemical and functional properties. J Agroaliment Processes Technol 2010; 16(4): 406-16.

[47]   Food and Agriculture Organization of the United Nations (FAO). Food and Nutrition Paper 91. Fats and fatty acids in human nutrition Report of an expert consultation. Genève. 2008.

[48]   Valenzuela BR, Valenzuela BA. Overview about lipid structure 2013.http://cdn.intechopen.com
[http://dx.doi.org/10.5772/52306]

[49]   Tuscany Diet. Lipids: Definition, classification and functions. 2018. http://www.tuscany-diet.net

[50]   Christie WW. Lipid analysis. Oxford: Pergamon Press 1982.

[51]   Pomeranz Y, Meloan CL. Food Analysis Theory and Practice. 4th ed. Westport, Connecticut: AVI 1994; pp. 678-732.

[52]   Akoh CC, Min DB. Food lipids: Chemistry, Nutrition, and Biotechnology. 4th ed., Boca Ratón, FL, USA: CRC Press 2017.
[http://dx.doi.org/10.1201/9781315151854]

[53]   Shahidi F, Ed. 65 Scrimgeour C.Bailey's industrial oil and fat products. 6th ed., New York: John Wiley & Sons, Inc 2005.

[54]   Rustan AC, Drevon CA. Fatty Acids: Structures and Properties Encyclopedia of Life Sciences. New York: John Wiley & Sons, Ltd 2005; pp. 1-7.

[55]   Dietary Guideline for American. 2005.https://health.gov

[56]   Ros E, López-Miranda J, Picó C, Rubi MA, Babio N, Sala-Vila A, *et al.* Consenso sobre las grasas y aceites en la alimentación de la población española adulta; postura de la Federación Española de Sociedades de Alimentación, Nutrición y Dietética (FESNAD). Nutr Hosp 2015; 32(2): 435-77.
[PMID: 26268073]

[57]   Simopoulos AP. The importance of the ratio of omega-6/omega-3 essential fatty acids. Biomed Pharmacother 2002; 56(8): 365-79.
[http://dx.doi.org/10.1016/S0753-3322(02)00253-6] [PMID: 12442909]

[58]   Gago-Dominguez M, Yuan J-M, Sun C-L, Lee H-P, Yu MC. Opposing effects of dietary n-3 and n-6 fatty acids on mammary carcinogenesis: The Singapore Chinese Health Study. Br J Cancer 2003; 89(9): 1686-92.
[http://dx.doi.org/10.1038/sj.bjc.6601340] [PMID: 14583770]

[59]   Kelly OJ, Gilman JC, Kim Y, Ilich JZ, Ilich JK. Long-chain polyunsaturated fatty acids may mutually benefit both obesity and osteoporosis. Nutr Res 2013; 33(7): 521-33.
[http://dx.doi.org/10.1016/j.nutres.2013.04.012] [PMID: 23827126]

[60]   Ascherio A, Willett WC. Health effects of trans fatty acids. Am J Clin Nutr 1997; 66(4) (Suppl.): 1006S-10S.
[http://dx.doi.org/10.1093/ajcn/66.4.1006S] [PMID: 9322581]

[61]   Jones A, Fetter D, Zidenberg-Cherr S. 2016. http://nutrition.ucdavis.edu

[62] Dhaka V, Gulia N, Ahlawat KS, Khatkar BS. Trans fats-sources, health risks and alternative approach - A review. J Food Sci Technol 2011; 48(5): 534-41.
[http://dx.doi.org/10.1007/s13197-010-0225-8] [PMID: 23572785]

[63] Field CJ, Blewett HH, Proctor S, Vine D. Human health benefits of vaccenic acid. Appl Physiol Nutr Metab 2009; 34(5): 979-91.
[http://dx.doi.org/10.1139/H09-079] [PMID: 19935865]

[64] Gebauer SK, Destaillats F, Dionisi F, Krauss RM, Baer DJ. Vaccenic acid and *trans* fatty acid isomers from partially hydrogenated oil both adversely affect LDL cholesterol: a double-blind, randomized controlled trial. Am J Clin Nutr 2015; 102(6): 1339-46.
[http://dx.doi.org/10.3945/ajcn.115.116129] [PMID: 26561632]

[65] Thalacker-Mercer AE, Drummond MJ. The importance of dietary protein for muscle health in inactive, hospitalized older adults. Ann N Y Acad Sci 2014; 1328: 1-9.
[http://dx.doi.org/10.1111/nyas.12509] [PMID: 25118148]

[66] McNeill S, Monroe A. Diet/Health/nutrition 2008; 19-21. Available from: http://www.beefnutrition.org

[67] Lacey JM, Wilmore DW. Is glutamine a conditionally essential amino acid? Nutr Rev 1990; 48(8): 297-309.
[http://dx.doi.org/10.1111/j.1753-4887.1990.tb02967.x] [PMID: 2080048]

[68] Laidlaw SA, Kopple JD. Newer concepts of the indispensable amino acids. Am J Clin Nutr 1987; 46(4): 593-605.
[http://dx.doi.org/10.1093/ajcn/46.4.593] [PMID: 3310600]

[69] Reeds PJ. Dispensable and indispensable amino acids for humans. J Nutr 2000; 130(7): 1835S-40S.
[http://dx.doi.org/10.1093/jn/130.7.1835S] [PMID: 10867060]

[70] Landi F, Calvani R, Tosato M, *et al.* Review. Protein intake and muscle health in old age: from biological plausibility to clinical evidence. Nutrients 2016; 8(5): 295.
[http://dx.doi.org/10.3390/nu8050295] [PMID: 27187465]

[71] Millward DJ, Layman DK, Tomé D, Schaafsma G. Protein quality assessment: impact of expanding understanding of protein and amino acid needs for optimal health. Am J Clin Nutr 2008; 87(5) (Suppl.): 1576S-81S.
[http://dx.doi.org/10.1093/ajcn/87.5.1576S] [PMID: 18469291]

[72] WHO/FAO/UNU Expert Consultation Protein and amino acid requirements in human nutrition Report of a Joint WHO Technical Report Series 935 Geneva, Switzerland. 2002.

[73] McClements J. Food Chemistry (Food Science 541). Available from: Food Biopolymers and Colloids Research Laboratory 2020.

[74] 86 Food and Drug Administration (FDA). Vitamin and Mineral Chart. 2019. Available from: www.fda.gov

[75] Amsbary R. Quality assurance & food safety 2013. https://www.qualityassurancemag.com

[76] Pérez Sira EE, *et al.* Raíces y Tubérculos.De tales harinas, tales panes Granos harinas y productos de panificación en Iberoamérica Programa Iberoamericano de Ciencia y Tecnología para el Desarrollo. Córdoba, Argentina: CYTED 2007; pp. 363-401.http://agro.unc.edu.ar

[77] Sívoli L, Vera K, Gahon D, *et al.* Evaluación de la harina de plátano (*Musa paradisíaca* L.) en ratones (*M. musculus*) fenilcetonúricos. Rev Cient Fac Cien V 2013; 54(2): 108-15.

[78] Pérez EE, Mahfoud A, Domínguez CL, Guzmán R. Roots, tubers, grains and bananas; flours and starches. Utilization in the development of foods for conventional, celiac, and phenylketonuric consumers. Food Processing Techno 2013; 4(3): 1-6.

[79]   Pérez EE, Faks J, Cira LE, Schroeder M, Diez N. Estimation of the dioscorin extracted from cultivars of yams (*Dioscorea* genus) growing in the Venezuelan Amazonas. Acta Hortic 2014; (1016): 53-60. [ISHS].
        [http://dx.doi.org/10.17660/ActaHortic.2014.1016.5]

[80]   Sívoli LJ, Ciarfella AT, Pérez EE. Functional and nutritional characterization of cassava flours for industrial applications.Cassava: Production, Nutritional Properties, and Health Effects. New York: Nova Publishers 2014; pp. 25-50.

[81]   Ciarfella AT, Sívoli LJ, Pérez EE. Food products developed using cassava roots and its derivatives: A review.Cassava: Production, Nutritional Properties, and Health Effects. New York: Nova Publishers 2014; pp. 161-76.

[82]   Pérez E, Sivoli L, Cueto D, Pérez L. Cassava flour an alternative to producing gluten-free baked goods and pasta.Cassava: Production, Consumption, and Potential Uses Plant Science Research and Practice. New York: NOVA Science Publisher 2017; pp. 87-104.

[83]   Anchundia MA, Pérez E. Nutritional characteristics and sensory evaluation of a drink made with sweet potato flour for people with phenylketonuria Agroindustrial Sci 2018; 8(1): 15-9.

[84]   Pérez E, Pérez L, Requena L, Mahfoud A, Domínguez CL, Rangel A, *et al.* Preparation of low-phenylalanine macro peptides and estimation of its phenylalanine content by fluorometric technique. J Nutr Ther 2013; 2(3): 145-53.
        [http://dx.doi.org/10.6000/1929-5634.2013.02.03.2]

[85]   González C, Tapia M, Pérez E, Pallet D, Dornier M. Main properties of steviol-glycosides and their potential in the food industry: A review. Fruits 2014; 69(2): 127-41.
        [http://dx.doi.org/10.1051/fruits/2014003]

[86]   Morris A, Barnett A, Burrows OA. Effect of processing on nutrient content of foods. CFNI 2004; 37(3): 160-4.

[87]   Tyagi SB, Kharkwal M, Saxena T. Impact of cooking on nutritional content of food. DU JURI 2015; 1(3): 180-6.

[88]   Bender AE. Nutritional effects of food processing. IJFST 1996; 1(4): 261-89.

[89]   Reddy MB, Love M. The impact of food processing on the nutritional quality of vitamins and minerals. Adv Exp Med Biol 1999; 459: 99-106.
        [http://dx.doi.org/10.1007/978-1-4615-4853-9_7] [PMID: 10335371]

[90]   Lee K, Clydesdale FM. Effect of thermal processing on endogenous and added iron in canned spinach. J Food Sci 1981; 46: 1064-7.
        [http://dx.doi.org/10.1111/j.1365-2621.1981.tb02992.x]

[91]   Friedman M. Review. Food browning and its prevention: An overview. J Agric Food Chem 1996; 44(3): 631-53.
        [http://dx.doi.org/10.1021/jf950394r]

[92]   Satyanarayana S, Kumar Pindi P, Singh A, Dattatreya A, Aditya G. Potential impacts of food and its processing on global sustainable health. J Food Process Technol 2012; 3: 2.
        [http://dx.doi.org/10.4172/2157-7110.1000143]

[93]   Severi S, Bedogni G, Manzieri AM, Poli M, Battistini N. Effects of cooking and storage methods on the micronutrient content of foods. Eur J Cancer Prev 1997; 6 (Suppl. 1): S21-4.
        [http://dx.doi.org/10.1097/00008469-199703001-00005] [PMID: 9167134]

[94]   Mathios AD. The importance of nutrition labeling and health claim regulation on product choice: An analysis of the cooking oils market. ARER 1998; 27(2): 159-68.
        [http://dx.doi.org/10.1017/S1068280500006481]

[95] Food and Agriculture Organization of the United Nations/World Health Organization (FAO/WHO). Food Standards Programa, Secretariat of the CODEXAlimentarius Commission. CODEX Alimentarius. Guidelines on Nutrition Labelling CAC/GL 2–1985 as Last Amended 2010. Rome.. 2010.

[96] Food Standard Agency (FSA) in Northern Ireland. 2019. https://www.food.gov.uk

[97] Winger R, Wall G. Agricultural and Food Engineering Working Document. 2006.

[98] Karničar Šenk M, Metlikovič P, Maletič M, Gomišček B. Development of New Product/Process Development Procedure for SMEs. Organizacija 2010; 43(2): 76-86.
[http://dx.doi.org/10.2478/v10051-010-0009-y]

[99] NZIFST. Creating new foods, the product developer's guide 2018. http://www.nzifst.org.nz

[100] Thompson A. Business feasibility study online 2005. http://bestentrepreneur.murdoch.edu.au

CHAPTER 2

Foods for Vegetarians

Elevina Pérez Sira[1,*]

[1] *Instituto de Ciencia y Tecnología de Alimentos, Facultad de Ciencias, Universidad Central de Venezuela, Caracas, Venezuela*

Abstract: Since the vegetarian diet is gaining increasing interest, in this chapter, there is a brief discussion of the compilation of the vegetarian's nutritional and health implications. The discussion focuses on the type of vegetarian consumers, the guidelines for a vegetarian diet, and the vegetarian food pyramids published. It also discusses the vegetarian diets through life stages and some processed food for vegetarians, including some home recipes.

Keywords: Foods for vegetarians, Health, Vegetarians, Vegetarian's pyramids, Vegetarian types.

INTRODUCTION

Due to the consensus about the beneficial effects of vegetable diets, this diet type has been gaining interest among various people. Vegetables have been considered essential foods in the world especially, in the Eastern regions for a long time ago. The interest in the vegetarian diet from consumers of the western side of the word is relatively recent and many of them adopt the vegetarian diet for several reasons, among these are health, inhuman handling of the animal, and the environmental impact. Whatever the limitations or barriers are these populations must be recognized by the food industry [1 - 5].

In literature, there is valuable information in regards to differences in omnivorous diets as compared with vegetables-based ones [6].These differences remark the importance of proteins as the most important dietary component to support life [7]. Proteins are essential for good health and are used for growth, health, and body maintenance. Hormones, antibodies, and other vital substances are composed of protein, and a high proportion of body weight (muscles) comes from proteins.

[*] **Corresponding author Elevina Pérez Sira:** Instituto de Ciencia y Tecnología de Alimentos, Facultad de Ciencias, Universidad Central de Venezuela, Caracas, Venezuela; Tel: +58.212.751.4403; Fax: +58.212.751.3871; E-mail: elevina07@gmail.com

There is a nutritional consensus that proteins from the animal source have a relevant role in these functions. Thus, the main concern among vegetarians is the quantity and quality of the proteins provided by a diet based solely on vegetables.

The protein quality of any diet can be classified into two groups as it is processed and used by our body: with low or with high physiological value. Those proteins that have not essential amino acids are considered as proteins with low quality (low physiological value). Contrarily proteins which contain a good balance in its content of essential amino acids are considered as protein of high quality (high biological value).

Proteins of animal origin are 90% most absorbable and digestible than those from vegetal sources (60-70%) [8, 9] and have the amino acid balance that the body needs; whereas vegetable proteins do not. Examples of animal proteins with a good balance are dairy products, eggs, meats, fish, and poultry contain a higher quality protein than the ones found in pasta, rice, fruits, and vegetable. However, both sources (animal and vegetal) can provide the necessary amino acids for protein synthesis and energy production [9]. Vegetarians need to ensure that their diet is well balanced. They should get the proteins found in animal foods, from different vegetal sources. As reported by Hever and Cronise in 2017 [10] legumes (beans, lentils, peas, and peanuts), nuts, seeds, soy foods (tempeh, tofu) provide high-quality proteins.

Other concerns in vegetarian diets are the intake of essential fatty acids, vitamins (D and B_{12}), and minerals (calcium, iron, zinc, and iodine). However, they can be supplied from several natural or processed vegetables, such as [10] greens, spinach, almonds, soybeans, calcium-fortified orange juice, fortified cereal, fortified soymilk, and tofu provide calcium. Whole grains, nuts, and legumes are good sources of zinc. Vitamin supplements, fortified foods (breakfast cereals, soy beverages, nutritional yeast) provide the needed vitamin B_{12}. Fortified dairy products, egg yolks, and fatty fish are rich in vitamin D. Also, breakfast cereals, with soymilk are to be considered in the diet. The omega-3 fatty acids can be consumed from fish in walnuts and ground flaxseeds. For iodine, the sources are seaweeds, cod, dairy, and iodized salt and iron come from dried or fortified beans and cereals, spinach, chard, and dried fruit.

People become vegetarians by economic, religious, or geographic [11]. Also, consumers prefer a vegetal diet because eating vegetables is healthier and vegetable cultivation produces lesser environmental impact as compared to foods from animals. Regarding the nutritional implication, much remains to be understood. However, it seems clear that vegetarians experience less coronary heart disease than meat-eaters [12].

By consensus, consumer vegetarians eat only vegetal foods, with the absence of meats. Some vegetarians do not eat animal products at all, and some can eat some animal sub-products but rely more on vegetables. There is not a single type of vegetarian diet. Further chapters discuss technical generalities about these consumers.

NUTRITIONAL AND HEALTH IMPLICATIONS

Vegetarianism has become a new trend and lifestyle because vegetarian diets provide important health benefits. This trend is creating a need for food developments in this business in recent times [13]. Vegetarian diets often provide plenty of fiber and less saturated fat, because they include more fruits, vegetables, whole grains, and legumes. The content and type of dietary fiber from vegetables contribute: to improve the bowel movement and lower cholesterol, to the balance of the concentration of glucose and transport on its matrix several phytochemicals and minerals through the human gut [13]. Regular consumption of a vegetablerich diet has undeniable positive effects on health since phytochemicals from vegetables can protect the human body from several types of chronic diseases [14].

Oxidative stress on the human being occurs naturally by the effect of diet, lifestyle, and environmental factors (contamination and emission), and plays a role in the aging process. Oxidative stress is the excessive production of cellular oxygen which surpasses the cell's antioxidant capacity, limiting the response capacity from the antioxidant and enzymatic cellular defense mechanism (such as, tocopherols, ascorbic acid, and glutathione, catalase, peroxidase, and superoxide dismutase). This oxidative stress, or cell oxidation, progressively produces degeneration on cells of its proteins, lipids, and, DNA inducing and illness in the human body. Proliferation of these damaged cells leads to cytotoxicity, genotoxicity, and even carcinogenesis [13, 15 - 22].

Various antioxidants phytochemicals (external) neutralize them by giving electrons to the free radicals. They indirectly participate in the cell signaling pathways sensitive to redox balance. Indeed, antioxidants (internal and external) scavenge free radicals, especially the reactive oxygen species inhibiting their production and the metabolic activation of carcinogens to alter the intracellular redox potential. Redox state, in turn, regulates the activity of many cellular transcription factors [14 - 16]. Therefore, a vegetable-rich diet has a high positive correlation with good health. The health benefit of vegetables should not be linked to only one compound or one type of vegetable, but a group of vegetables that provide better protection against certain chronic diseases. Hence, regular consumption of a vegetable-rich diet has undeniable positive effects on health since phyto nutraceuticals of vegetables can protect the human body from several types of chronic disease [14]. Vegetables in the daily diet have been strongly associated with overall good health, improvement of gastrointestinal health and vision, reduced risk for some forms of cancer, heart disease, stroke, diabetes, anemia, gastric ulcer, rheumatoid arthritis, and other chronic diseases [23, 24].

Hung *et al.* [25] conclusions pointed out that increased fruit and vegetable consumption is associated with a light, although a not statistically significant reduction in the development of the major chronic disease. The benefits appeared to be primarily for cardiovascular disease and not for cancer. Additionally, other authors have provided evidence that consuming more than 5 daily servings of fruit and vegetables shall reduce coronary heart disease. Moreover, consumers could obtain the best benefits when eating seven portion portions daily [26, 27]. On the other hand, Oyebode [28] has reported an inverse correlation between fruit and vegetable consumption and mortality. Later in 2018, a review on native fruits from sub-Saharan Africa shows that increasing their consumption keeps people healthy [29]. There, people believe that eating more fruits and vegetables can prevent and even cure several diseases among all the different populations [29]. The dietary guidelines in the United States [30] recommend eating several servings of fruits, vegetables, whole grains, beans, nuts, and lean meat daily because they can reduce the incidence of chronic illnesses such as obesity, heart disease, and diabetes. However, findings of a survey performed by IFIC in 2018 in the USA [31] report that on average, Americans consume fewer fruits/vegetables and more protein, than the amount recommended by the experts. The top two reasons for this: price and lack of access to good quality fruits and vegetables. The World Cancer Research Fund International [32], the American Chemical Society [33], and American Heart Association [34] recommend consuming a diet high in fruits and vegetables.

Kim *et al.* [35], results suggest that dietary patterns that are relatively higher in plant foods and relatively lower in animal foods may confer benefits for cardiovascular health. However as postulated by Phillips [6], more research is needed to establish whether vegetarianism has a role to play in protection against a range of other diseases that are less prevalent amongst vegetarian populations; lifestyle, as well as nutritional differences, will need to be taken into consideration. Following a vegetarian diet does not automatically equate to being healthier; vegetarians and meat-eaters alike need to be mindful of making appropriate dietary and lifestyle choices. A vegetarian person must make good food choices and follow a healthy lifestyle. A vegetarian diet low in nutrients or with an excess of fat and salt can be very harmful to health [35]. The same applies to people on a non-vegetarian diet.

TYPE OF VEGETARIAN CONSUMERS

Although the diet "vegetarian" implies eating habits with an emphasis on vegetables, in practice, it has been traditionally viewed as a diet with the absence of meat. The "vegetarian" word describes a range of dietary patterns, some being more restrictive than others. In a vegetarian diet, the nutrients must be the function of the selected foods; for instance, consumers with lactose intolerance cannot be Lacto-vegetarians. Some vegetarians can consume meat derivatives or fish. Phillips [6] describe the differences among vegetarians in Table **1**.

Table 1. Types of vegetarian diets [6].

Diet type	Description of Dietary Pattern
Semi-vegetarian (flexitarians)	Occasionally eats meat/poultry/fish.
Pesco-vegetarian (Pescatarian)	Exclude meat and poultry but includes fish (and possible other seafood). May include dairy products and eggs.
Lacto-ovo-vegetarian	Exclude all flesh foods. Include dairy products and eggs.
Ovo-vegetarian	Exclude all flesh foods and dairy products. Include eggs.
Lacto-vegetarian	Exclude all flesh foods and eggs. Include dairy products.
Vegan	Avoids all foods of animal original or different diets, increasing restrictions.
Macrobiotic	Usually vegetarian but may eat meat or fish if wild/hunted in the lowest or least restricted dietary regimens. Diet is usually based on brown rice with some fruit, vegetables, and pulses. The final stage of the diet consists of whole grains and limited liquids.
Fruitarian	Diet is usually based on fresh and dried fruits, nuts, seeds, and a few vegetables. The diet generally consists only of foods that do not kill the plant of origin.

FOOD-BASED DIETARY GUIDELINES AND VEGETARIAN FOOD PYRAMIDS

Food-based dietary guidelines must offer support to vegetarian people. Indeed, the Vegetarians Food Guides (VFGs) is a product of the revisions of the conventional food guides nutrient and its adaptation to the vegetarian dietary patterns [36, 37]. Although the recommendations from these guidelines can be similar, the food group composition and, more relevant, the potentially critical nutrients for vegetarians are quite different.

Although the recommendations from these guidelines can be similar, the food aggrupation and, the specific nutrients for vegetarians are quite different. VFGs must guide that recommends food for vegetarians considering their precise nutritional requirements VFGs need to offer confident instruction, which meets the most updated standards of quality and security of the vegetarian diet. These guides must include all plant foods, of preferment unprocessed, individual's calorie requirements, the addition of small amounts of foods of animal origin (dairy/eggs) in optimal concentrations; when need and the potential critical nutrients [38].

Therefore, the vegetarian food guidelines should be explicitly written for vegetarian people, by an expert in vegetarian nutrition, who is aware of the required need for the different types of vegetarian consumers and the effect of the on their health of excess/defect ratio. This guide should be a useful tool for planning diets for vegetarians, but also to offer food type and quantity which cover the requirement of all need nutrients and how to reach them.

According to Baroni [39], the modern basic principles of a healthy vegetarian diet are:

1. To consume large amounts and a variety of plant foods, emphasizing the intake of unrefined or minimally processed foods.
2. The consumption of dairy products and eggs is optional.
3. To choose carefully and limit vegetable fats, and to consume good sources of omega-3 fatty acids.
4. To consume adequate amounts of calcium and pay attention to vitamin D status.
5. To consume adequate amounts of vitamin B_{12}.
6. To consume generous amounts of water and other fluids.
7. To remember to pay attention to other healthy lifestyle factors.

Gomes Silva in 2015 [36] to complete and balance these modern basic principles have included the following food groups:

• Fruits
• Vegetables
• Dairy products (or plant-origin alternatives), milk*, vegetable beverages, yogurt*, cheese* (or its plant-origin alternatives), fermented milk*
• Legumes and derivatives, algae, legumes (beans, chickpeas, peas, lentils, broad beans), derivatives (tofu, miso), algae
• Cereals and tubers: rice, wheat, rye, corn, quinoa, oat, and derivative products (bread, toast, biscuits, pasta, cereal flakes) preferably whole meal, and potato
• Oleaginous fruits and seeds, peanuts, oleaginous fruits (whole nuts, almonds, cashew), oleaginous

• Fruits shortening (peanut and almond butter), seeds (chia, linseed, poppy, sesame)
• Fats–vegetable oils, vegetable shortening, and butter*
• Egg*-egg, egg white, egg yolk, egg products, and eggs of other species. Not included in the vegan diet.

Graphic illustrations, such as food pyramids can help visualize easy dietary intake, healthy patterns that are not only adequate but promote optimal health. For that reason, during the third international congress on vegetarian nutrition in 1997, an organizer subcommittee began a process that led to the development of a pyramid-shaped graphic illustration to guide vegetarians to make better choices [37, 38]. There are several food pyramids for vegetarians, and they are continually reviewed and made more reliable each time. The vegetarian pyramid is the fourth pyramid developed by the public health implications of traditional diets, sponsored by old ways (a nonprofit food and nutrition organization) and the Harvard School of Public Health. They, on different occasions, reviewed diverse dietary traditions around the world [40, 41].

Old ways' other pyramids focus on traditional diets found in specific geographic regions, including the Mediterranean, Latin America, and Asia. Old ways determined that it was time to update their 1997 version of the vegetarian and vegan diet pyramid. As with the other old ways of diet pyramids, the new pyramid was subject to revision considering the ongoing nutrition researching. This updated version combines both, vegetarian and vegan diets, in one pyramid, because these diets are complementary [37, 38, 40, 41].

The number of consumers who turn to more plant-based lifestyles is steadily increasing, and a vegetarian and vegan market is developing accordingly. The gastronomy sector is also increasingly catering to the demand from vegans and vegetarians. Food producers, food trading companies, and caterers have recognized this market, and commercial chains have begun to label own-brand products, in some cases, with self-developed logos [42].

To create a reliable label and following the EU Food Information Regulation, the European Vegetarian Union (EVU) [42] have proposed the following definitions with some regulations:

1. Vegetarian Foods

Foods that are not products of animal origin, and in the manufacture, preparation, or treatment of which no ingredients (including additives, carriers, flavorings, enzymes, and substances that are not additives but used in the same way and with the same purpose as processing aids) or processing aids of animal origin (processed or unprocessed) have been added or used intentionally, except for milk, colostrum, birds eggs, beeswax, honey and propolis, their constituents and products derived from them.

2. Vegan Foods

Foods that are not products of animal origin, and in the manufacture, preparation, or treatment of which no ingredients (including additives, carriers, flavorings, enzymes, and substances that are not additives but used in the same way and with the same purpose as processing aids) or processing aids of animal origin (processed or unprocessed) have been added or used intentionally.

3. Manufacturing

In the manufacture, preparation, treatment, or placing on the market of foods that are labeled as vegetarian or vegan, appropriate precautions must be taken, to avoid cross-contamination with products that do not comply with the requirements of paragraphs 1 and 2. However, the presence of this cross-contamination shall be allowed in foods that are labeled as vegetarian or vegan, provided that despite appropriate precautions such presence is technically unavoidable under good hygiene practice.

4. Indications or Symbols

If indications or symbols are used on foods that are likely to have the same meaning for the consumer as vegetarian or vegan, paragraphs 1 to 3 shall apply accordingly. Directly visible and reliable clarity is currently offered only by the *V-label of the EVU*, which labels both vegan and vegetarian products. International vegan and vegetarian organizations accept the criteria.

The increasing dissemination of the V-label testifies both to the trust consumers put in it and to the advantages that traders and producers gain from its deployment. More than 400 firms in Europe currently use the V label on thousands of products. Notable licensing partners include Aldi, Alpro, Coop, Friesland Campina, Griesson de Beukelaer, Migros, Spar, and Unilever [42]. Food producers, food trading companies, and caterers have recognized these tendencies and are increasingly bringing to the market vegetarian and vegan products that are directly recognizable as such for the consumer [42].

NUTRIENTS AND VEGETARIANS

The Appendix of the Gomes Silva *et al.* [36], manual, reports important recommendations of acceptable macronutrient distribution ranges, recommended intakes, and tolerable upper intake levels of micronutrients as follows:

Macronutrients

Vegetarians have not increased carbohydrates' needs, and they usually consume a higher quantity of fiber. The energy in a vegetarian diet is easily achieved from food with high-fat content and carbohydrates.

Vegetarians could suffer from protein deficiency when their diet is rich in highenergy-density foods. Protein and essential amino acids can be obtained from some cereals and legumes because they assure proteins like that in meat. A mix of cereals and legumes provides all essential amino acids because their profile is different and complementary among them. Therefore, its combination is a good choice. For example, lysine and threonine are deficient in cereals, contrary legumes contain less methionine, but they have more lysine and threonine than cereals, and vice versa. Among products with a high content of essential amino, therefore with a high biological value, are soy, quinoa, and amaranth, tempeh, tofu, lentils, pumpkin seeds, almonds, split peas, garbanzo beans (chickpeas), hemp seeds, millet. Matters to consider when processing these plant foods are protein digestibility (low in vegetables), and the presence of anti-nutritional factors that diminish protein digestibility (fiber, phytates, trypsin inhibitors, and hemagglutinins) [43].

Gomes Silva *et al.*, in 2015 [36] has pointed out that despite the vegetarian diets have low levels of fat and saturated fat, they are high in polyunsaturated fatty acids. Some vegetarians have restrictions on the amount of omega-3 intake. However, they could get an adequate omega-6/omega-3 ratio from some vegetable staple foods and avoid the consumption of hydrogenated and Trans fats present in processed food. Food like flax seeds and their oil contribute to a better n-6: n-3 balance, given that the proportion is about 1:5 [44]. As pointed out by Simopoulos 2002 [44] a lower ratio of omega- 6/omega-3 fatty acids is desirable in reducing the risk of many of the more prevalent chronic diseases.

Micronutrients

The vegetarian population may be at risk of vitamin B_{12} deficiency because its active form is only present in animal-origin and fortified foodstuffs. However, the Lacto-ovo vegetarians take the vitamin from eggs and dairy products. Another alternative is algae, which is rich in vitamin B_{12}, but, they have chemical forms with low bioavailability that make them difficult to absorb. Therefore, additional care is needed when selecting food sources with vitamins B_{12} and B_{12} supplements. Vegetarians, old people, children, pregnant women, and infants, as well as individuals suffering from acid-related diseases, can also benefit from vitamin B_{12}supplementation [44]. On the other hand, vegetarian food pattern is usually rich in folic acid, which may lead to misdiagnosing anemia caused by vitamin B_{12} deficiency [36].

Vitamin D deficiency comes from sun non-exposure, sun radiation is the central stimulus for producing vitamin D in the human body. In not tropical regions deficiencies of vitamin D are pandemic, then vitamin D dosage recommendations are usually not achieved by vegetarians or by non-vegetarians living in these regions. Therefore, there are recommendations for the consumption of vitamin D supplements, and vitamin D fortified foods in some regions of the world, especially in wintertime [44].

Vitamin D_2 supplements are of plant origin, and vitamin D_3 supplements are usually of animal origin [45]. Some food products such as milk, vegetable beverages, and margarine are vitamin D fortified, generally in the form of ergocalciferol [46].

According to Heaney *et al.* [47], vitamin D_3 is approximately 87% more potent in raising and maintaining serum 25(OH)D concentrations and produces 2- to 3-fold greater storage of vitamin D than does equimolar D_2. They suggest that given its greater potency and lower cost, D_3 should be the preferred treatment option when correcting vitamin D deficiency. The unique source of vitamin D for vegetarians is from plants. For instance, new cholecalciferol (Vitamin D_3) supplements are produced from lichens and mushrooms exposed to ultraviolet radiation [48, 49].

The consumption of vitamin A as retinol equivalents (from carotenoids), is increased in vegetarian diets. Although in diets with very low-fat levels, the absorption of carotenoids by the body may be compromised because they are liposoluble [36].

Vitamins E, K, and C, folates, riboflavin (B_2), and thiamin (B_1) are adequate in vegetarian dietary regimes [36].

One of the common concerns in the nutritional status of consumers is iron lack or insufficiency. Women, children, and strict vegetarian are among consumers with iron deficit risk. Due to that the iron bioavailability by the human body comes from the heme form and the iron from food of plant origin only contain non-heme iron, which has lower bioavailability, then iron recommended Daily Intake must be increased by 80% in the vegetarian population. People with iron deficiency or pregnant women, who need high iron dosages have a physiological adaptation, increasing absorption and decreasing excretion, making non-heme iron almost as well absorbed as heme iron. Contrary to phytate, polyphenol, or calcium, vitamin C is the most important facilitating factor in iron absorption, which is no problem for vegetarian consumers [36].

Among good sources of zinc are eggs, dairy products, bread, cereals, legumes, oleaginous fruits, and seeds It is recommendable to increase 50% the zinc level in a vegetarian diet because its bioavailability is committed by the phytate, fiber, and calcium present in food from plant. However, amino acids sulfured and organic acids improve their absorption [36].

Vegetarians obtain the necessary calcium through plant-origin food products. Lacto-ovo vegetarians benefit from excellent sources of calcium, such as milk, cheese, and yogurt. Maintaining vitamin D adequate levels and limiting consumption of caffeine are beneficial aspects regarding calcium levels maintenance [36].

There are a variety of foodstuffs with natural or fortified iodine content (algae, iodized salt, or supplements). However, its incorporation in the diet must be calculated to not exceed the maximum recommended doses. Vegetarians usually eat less selenium quantity but still meet the recommendations and their diets frequently provide the potassium need. Vegetarians usually eat less selenium quantity but still meet the recommendations and their diets frequently provide the potassium need. High magnesium levels found in vegetarian diets compensate for the lower bioavailability by diminution due to its bound with fiber and phytate [36].

Even though the phosphorous bioavailability is potentially low; its concentration is usually higher than the recommended, is the occurrence of deficiency improbable. Vegetarian's sodium consumption is usually low as compared with its non-vegetarians. Contents of manganese, chlorine, fluorine, and molybdenum are usually adequate in vegetarian diets [36].

In-plant seeds, phosphate, and inositol are storage as phytate. Phytate forms complexes with dietary minerals, especially iron and zinc, and causes a mineralrelated deficiency in humans. It also negatively impacts protein and lipid utilization. Some food processing methods such as cooking, soaking germinating, fermentation, and canning, improves absorption of those minerals by decreasing the phytate action [50].

VEGETARIAN DIETS THROUGH LIFE STAGES

Specific subgroups in the vegetarian population may be more at risk of nutrient deficiencies resulting from poor dietary intakes, or because of their high intake requirements. Vegetarians should take extra care to ensure that the nutrients needed meeting at the most vulnerable times in their life cycle, and more restricted diets containing minimal or no animal-derived foods require particularly careful planning [6].

It is the position of the American Dietetic Association [22], that appropriately planned vegetarian diets, including total vegetarian or vegan diets, must be healthful, nutritionally adequate, and provide health benefits in the prevention and treatment of certain diseases. Well-planned vegetarian diets are appropriate for individuals during all stages of the life cycle, including pregnancy, lactation, infancy, childhood, and adolescence, as well as for athletes.

According to several authors, a well-balanced vegetarian diet can provide for the needs of babies, children, and adolescents [51, 52]. However, it must ensure appropriate caloric intake and growth monitored.

It should pay attention to adequate protein intake and sources of essential fatty acids, iron, zinc, calcium, and vitamin B_{12}, and if sun exposure is not adequate vitamin D supplementation may be required in cases of strict vegan diets, with no intake of any animal products.

Furthermore, including good sources of the ω-3 fatty acid (linolenic acid) should be emphasized to enhance the synthesis of the long-chain fatty acid docosahexaenoic acid. It should appropriately advise pregnantly and nursing mothers to ensure that the nutritional needs of the fetus and infant meet adequately.

Breastfed vegan infants may need supplements of vitamin B_{12} if the maternal diet is inadequate, and older infants may need zinc supplements and reliable sources of iron and vitamins D and B_{12}. Also, there is a recommendation for the timing of solid food introduction for non-vegetarians. Tofu, dried beans, and meat analogs are protein sources for babies of around 7-8 months.

Vegan diet plans must be nutritionally adequate and support growth for infants. It should screen diets to avoid eating disorders in adolescents on restricted vegetarian or other such diets. Evidence from well-designed studies has concluded that babies, children, and adolescents grow and develop well when they consume a well-balanced vegetarian diet that includes the appropriate supplements [53].

A woman's nutritional health directly affects pregnancy outcomes and the quality of breast milk after birth. Vitamin D and calcium status in vegetarian women may be low, resulting in maternal bone demineralization.

Specker [54] reported that vitamin B_{12} deficiency results in neurologic damage in infants of vegetarian women. Vegetarian and vegan diets, defined as an eating style that avoids meat, fish, and poultry, can be healthful and nutritionally adequate for a pregnant woman. Critical nutrients for vegetarian pregnancy include protein, iron, zinc, calcium, vitamin D, vitamin B_{12}, iodine, and omega-3 fatty acids [54]. Concerning the ratio of linoleic acid to α-linolenic acid, it is vital to recommend diets with a ratio between 4:1 and 10:1 in vegetarians and recommend avoiding excessive intakes of linoleic acid [55].

According to Specker [54] vegetarian or vegan diet can meet the requirements for the nutrients, as mentioned above, although, in some instances, fortified foods or supplements can be especially useful in meeting the recommendations. However, pregnant vegetarians need to know the nutrient content of supplements targeted to make particular nutrient needs met. The specific, immediate health advantages of many vegetarian diets for pregnant women are the higher fiber content can help to alleviate constipation that commonly occurs in pregnancy.

Pregnant vegetarians tend to take higher doses of both folate and magnesium than do non-vegetarians. One small study has shown a marked reduction in the risk of preeclampsia in vegans compared to the general population. However, another study did not find similar results of this reduced risk [56]. Vegan children may also have fewer problems with allergies and digestive problems. Breastfeeding is best for your baby during the first year of life and is exclusively recommended for the first 4-6 months by the American Academy of Pediatrics [57]. All exclusively breastfed babies should also receive a vitamin D supplement since it is significant for bone health and development [58].

According to the American Heart Association [34], the plant-based diet is generally healthier, regardless of age. As people age, they need fewer calories, but the requirement for certain nutrients, such as protein, calcium, and vitamins D and B_6 increases as the senses of smell and taste start to decline. The intake of minerals, vitamins, and phytochemicals by older vegetarians and vegans helps them to keep their body weight in optimal conditions.

Because seniors have trouble chewing and swallowing food, especially fresh vegetables, they usually must cut, braise, mash, it is necessary to blend or liquefy them to soften the food and make it easier to swallow. Drinking enough water also helps older adults swallow. Seniors living alone are facing yet another problem, which is the loss of motivation to cook. Therefore, fixing ready-to-eat foods seems to be a solution. Vegan diets usually cost less than diets that contain meat. For a retiree on a fixed income, that can be appealing.

Athletes can also be vegetarians, but because of the potential inadequacies of a vegetarian diet, athletes may require a protein and vitamin/mineral supplement to ensure the diet is complete. The number of athletes becoming vegetarians of different types is increasing, so the health and fitness industry is warning about it. Up to these days, there is little information that discusses how to manage vegan diets for athletes. Except for the lack of meat, a vegetarian diet for athletes is not all that different from a regular healthy diet. Some vegetarian and vegan athletes choose raw and gluten-free diets, looking for greater energy gains.

According to Rogerson [59], a vegan diet can satisfactorily fulfill the needs of most athletes through the proper selection and management of food choices and with special attention to getting adequate levels of energy, following the macro and micronutrient recommendations along with appropriate supplementation. The author also concluded that supplementation with creatine and β-alanine might contribute to augmented performance-enhancing effects in vegans, who experience pre-existing low levels of these substances. Rogerson [59] also emphasized that further research is needed to elucidate the performance enhancing effects of these substances in vegan populations.

PROCESSING FOOD FOR VEGETARIANS

Vegetarians prefer to eat unprocessed foods even though there are several brands of processed food for vegetarians in the markets. Vegetarians have many concerns regarding processed foods. Rule number 21 from the eater's manual of Poland in 2011 [60] described as follows: "if it came from a plant, eat it; if it was made in a plant, don't." These rules indicate that processed foods such as vegan "meats" and "cheeses", processed oils, and sweets must be avoided.

Usually, to preserve the quality of processed foods, several additives and ingredients are used during manufacturing. These ingredients and additives are questioned because they should not be used in vegetarian diets. Among these ingredients are beeswax, honey, casein or milk by-products, confectionary glaze or candy, gelatin, and gelatin products, isinglass in beer and wine, L-cysteine in bread products, whey in bread and sweets, concentrate and hydrolyzed protein, among others. For example, the confectionery glaze used for candy contains about 35% of shellac. Shellac is an organic substance obtained from the resinous secretion of a small red insect called the lac insects or *Kerria lacca* [61].

Same with gelatin and its by-products, which come from collagen obtained from various animal body parts. The isinglass, a kind of gelatin obtained from fish, especially sturgeon, L-cysteine, which comes from poultry feathers, the "vegetable" or "vegetarian" L-cysteine that are produced by fermentation, using sugar beet.

Cheese whey is a liquid obtained after the precipitation of milk casein in the cheese-making process, it is of great importance in the dairy industry due to the large volume generated and its nutritional composition [62]. Protein concentrates usually contain additional ingredients that include fat, cholesterol, lactose, and gluten. And hydrolysates are the most expensive type of protein powder without an additional improvement in its digestibility.

However, there are circumstances when vegetarian foods must be processed; that is the case for senior vegetarians. As was before discussed, some senior has difficulty chewing and swallowing food, so they need to make that food adequate in size and texture for easy chewing and swallowing. When they are living alone, they may lose motivation to cook and probably need ready-to-eat vegetarian foods. Also, older adults usually lose the capacity to appreciate or taste different flavors in foods. All these facts drive older adults to lose appetite and, therefore, to suffer under nutrition.

Athletes are another example. Athletes that are far from home or college dining rooms need ready-to-cook foods that provide them the macro and micronutrients needed to ensure that their diets are complete and adequate for their sports requirements. They must have easy and fast means of getting reliable and nutritious foods.

Because the population of vegetarian athletes is increasing, the challenge of the food industry is to ensure the production of foods that meets their vegetarian diet requirements and do it without the use, as possible, of additives and derivatives from animals. The food industry must face this challenge that, aside from being a solution for food safety, has become quite a promissory business. There are already some different brands and types of these processed foods in the market, such as Morning Star Farms and Hellmann's.

RECIPES

Veggie Rice Fried

(https://www.dinneratthezoo.com/veggie-fried-rice/)

Ingredients.

14g	Sesame oil	75g	Peas
10g	Garlic, ground	87g	Corn, cooked
75g	Onion, chopped	150g	Eggs, whole
61g	Carrot, chopped	8g	Soy sauce
88g	Red Bell Pepper, chopped	750g	Rice, cooked
88g	Broccoli, chopped	-	-

Preparation

In a small bowl, beat the eggs and add salt to taste. Melt oil in a large skillet over medium-low heat. Add eggs and leave flat for 1 to 2 minutes. Remove eggs from skillet and cut into small pieces. Heat oil in the same skillet; add garlic, onion, and carrot and sauté until soft. Then add broccoli, peas, corn, rice, soy sauce, bell pepper. Stir fry together for about 5 minutes, then stir in egg. Serve hot.

Vegan Mole Chilaquiles with Greens and Beans

(https://www.pinterest.ie/dorastable/)

Vegan mole chilaquiles are tortilla chips covered in mole sauce and mixed with sautéed greens and black beans, then drizzled with almond cream and vegan queso cotija.

1. Tortillas

Ingredients for Corn Tortillas

24	Corn tortillas, cut into triangles (12ths) or (1 bag of corn chips)

Preparation

Preheat the oven to 400°F and place the tortilla triangle on two baking sheets lined with parchment, baking it for 15 to 20 minutes until crispy. Remove from the oven and set aside.

2. Greens and Beans

Ingredients for greens and beans.

2	Garlic cloves, minced	420g	Black beans, drained (1 can; 14 oz.)
250g	Spinach	-	-

Preparation

Heat a large sauté pan to medium heat and pour in ¼ cup of water. Add garlic and cook for 1 minute. Add spinach and mix. Once the spinach has cooked down (about 2 minutes), add black beans, seasoning with salt and pepper.

3. Vegetable Broth

Ingredients for homemade vegetable broth.

1liter	Water	100g	Carrots chopped
4g	Garlic cloves	3	Laurel leaves
100g	Onion (medium; cut in two-part)	15g	Parsley fresh chopped
100g	Celery chopped	15g	Thyme fresh chopped

Preparation

Place garlic, onions, celery, and carrots in a pot. Cook until softened, about 5 minutes, stirring often. Add the water, frozen vegetable scraps, bay leaves, parsley, and thyme. Reduce heat to low and simmer, partially covered, for 45 minutes.

4. Mole Poblano Homemade

Ingredients for homemade mole poblano

12	Guajillo Chiles, dried	70g	Almonds(skin-on)
6	Pasilla Chiles, dried	70g	Peanuts (raw shelled)
40g	Sesame seeds	35g	Pumpkin seeds (hulled)
20g	Aniseed (whole)	70g	Raisins
20g	Peppercorns black	2 slices	White Bread
5g	Cloves (whole)	2	Corn Tortillas, stale
5g	Thyme (dried)	100g	Onion, medium, thinly sliced
5g	Marjoram (dried)	30g	Garlic cloves, minced
3	Bay leaves; dried crumbled	50g	Tomatillos, husked, quartered
20g	Cinnamon stick, in pieces	100g	Tomato, large quartered
500g	Canola oil	200g	Dark Chocolate, chopped
1.8liter	Vegetable broth	60g	Sugar, plus more to taste
	Salt to taste	-	-

Preparation

Stem chiles and shake the seed transferring it's into a small bowl and set aside to roast. Tear the chiles into large pieces; set aside. Place 4 tablespoons of the reserved chile seeds and sesame seeds in a small cast-iron skillet set over medium heat.

Toast seeds, occasionally stirring, until they are lightly brown, about 2 minutes. Transfer seeds to a spice grinder. Add aniseed, peppercorns, and cloves to a nowempty skillet. Toast until fragrant, about 1 minute; transfer to the spice grinder with seeds. Add thyme, marjoram, bay leaves, and cinnamon to a spice grinder. Grind all seeds and spices into a fine powder. Transfer to a large bowl; set aside.

Heat oil in a medium skillet over medium-high heat to 350°F. Working in batches, fry chilies until slightly darkened, about 20 seconds per batch; transfer chilies to a paper towel-lined plate as each batch finish.

Remove skillet from heat and reserve. Transfer chilies to a large bowl and add boiling water to cover. Let stand for 30 minutes.

Strain the chiles, reserving soaking liquid. Working in 3 batches, place 1/3 of the chilies, 1/3 cup soaking liquid, and 1/4 cup vegetable broth into the blender and purée until as smooth as possible.

Set a fine-mesh strainer over a large bowl and strain chile mixture, using a rubber spatula to push through as much chile mixture as possible. Discard solids and set chile purée aside. Return skillet with oil to 350°F over medium-high heat. Fry almonds, peanuts, pumpkin seeds, and raisins until toasted (one at a time): About 1 minute for almonds, 45 seconds for peanuts, 20 seconds for pumpkin seeds, and 15 seconds for raisins. Transfer each batch to a paper towel-lined plate as done, transferring the almonds, peanuts, pumpkin seeds, and raisins to a bowl with spice mixture.

Frybread until golden brown, 1 to 2 minutes per side; transfer to a paper towellined plate. Fry tortillas until golden brown, about 1 minute per side; transfer to a paper towel-lined plate. Remove skillet from heat. Break bread and tortillas into small pieces and transfer to bowl with spice mixture.

Set a fine-mesh strainer over a small bowl and strain oil from the skillet.

Place 2 tablespoons of strained oil into a now-empty skillet. Heat over mediumhigh heat until shimmering. Add in onions and cook until browned, about 10 minutes, stirring occasionally.

Stir in garlic and cook until fragrant, about 1 minute. Transfer the onions and garlic to the bowl with spice mixture, leaving them as much oil in the pan as possible.

Return skillet to medium-high heat. When the oil is shimmering, add in tomatillos and tomatoes. Cook until softened, about 10 minutes, stirring occasionally. Transfer tomatillos and tomato to bowl with spice mixture. Add 2 1/2 cups of chicken broth to bowl with spice mixture.

Working in two batches, the purée spice mixture in a blender until as smooth as possible. Set a fine-mesh strainer over a large bowl and strain spice mixture, using a rubber spatula to push through as much spice mixture as possible. Discard solids and set the spice mixture aside.

In a large Dutch oven or pot, heat 3 tablespoons of reserved strained oil over medium-high heat until shimmering. Add in chile purée and cook, continually stirring until the mixture has thickened to the consistency of tomato paste, about 10 minutes.

Stir in the spice mixture, bring to a boil, and then reduce heat to low and simmer, frequently stirring, for 30 minutes. Stir in 4 cups vegetable broth and chocolate.

Simmer, partially covered, for 1 hour, stirring occasionally. Stir in sugar and season mole with salt and add sugar to taste.

Remove from heat, use immediately or transfer to airtight container and store in the refrigerator for up to a month.

5. Sauce

Ingredients for sauce.

215 ml	Mole Poblano
500 ml	Vegetable Broth

Preparation

Once the mole pastes dissolves, and the mixture starts simmering, add the second cup of vegetable broth. Bring to a simmer, stir, and remove from heat to reach thin cream soup consistency, adjust as necessary with vegetable stock.

Add chips, and the greens and beans into the pot with the mole.

Mix well to coat. Serve immediately and top with almond cream, vegan cheese Cotija, and onion.

Set a large pot to medium heat, add 1 cup of vegetable broth and mole paste. Stir.

6. Toppings

Ingredients for topping.

Dash	Almond Cream
Sprinkle	Vegan Queso Cotija
1	White Onion, cut into very thin rings

Ratatouille

(https://www.recetasdeescandalo.com/ratatouille-la-receta-de-la-películadeliciosas-verduras-al-horno/)

Ingredients

50g	Onion, thin-sliced	150g	Green bell pepper, chopped
15g	Garlic cloves, minced	0.5g	Oregano, dried, crumbled
100g	Olive oil	1g	Parsley, fresh, crumbled
15g	White wine vinegar	1g	Thyme, dried, crumbled
115g	Romano tomatoes, ripe, chopped	1g	Laurel leave dried
115g	Eggplant thin-sliced	0.5g	Coriander ground
115g	Zucchini, thin-sliced	0.5g	Fennel seeds
150g	Tomato, unripe, thin-sliced	15g	Basil leaves, fresh, shredded
150g	Red bell pepper, chopped	10g	Black pepper, fresh, ground
150g	Yellow bell pepper, chopped	10g	Salt and coarse salt

Preparation

Select fresh bell peppers with smooth skin and no blemishes for easy peeling. Wash the bell peppers and let air dry. Heat oven to 450 °F (230°C). Place the bell peppers in a single layer on the oven rack. Roast the bell peppers for 30 minutes or until the skin is blistered and blackened. Turn the peppers every few minutes until the skin charred all over. Remove the bell peppers from heat and place in a covered bowl to steam and cool. Once the peppers are cool enough to handle, put on a pair of gloves and remove skins. Cut off the stem and slice the bell pepper open. Use a knife to scrape out the seeds and membrane. Cut off strips and then in small dices. Set aside.

In a non-stick skillet pan with a removable handle, cook the onion and the garlic in 2 tablespoons of olive oil over moderately low heat, occasionally stirring, until the onion is softened. Add salt and pepper to taste and add the remaining 3 tablespoons oil and chopped Romano tomatoes and heat it over moderately high heat until it is hot but not smoking. Add the diced bake bell peppers, fennel seeds, thyme, coriander, parsley, oregano, and mix gently, cooking for 5 minutes. Put out from pan the leaves. Set aside.

Prepare a vinaigrette: In a bowl mix 3 tablespoons extra virgin olive oil (or a more neutral-flavored oil like grapeseed, canola, or vegetable), 1 tablespoon white wine vinegar (or balsamic, apple cider, rice, sherry, or other wine vinegar), 1/4 teaspoon of thyme and pinch of coarse salt. A turn of freshly ground black pepper. Set aside.

Disassemble the pan arm and put on one set of sliced Roma tomatoes, zucchini, and eggplant, forming one spiral over the pan. Scattered the vinaigrette on the spiral and cover it with aluminum foil. Bake at 300 °F (150°C) for 2 hours. After two hours, remove the aluminum foil and continue baking at 350°F (180 °C) for 30 minutes. Scatter the basil on the spiral. The ratatouille may be made 1 day in advance, kept covered and chilled, and reheated before serving.

African Peanut Stew

(https://www.budgetbytes.com/african-peanut-stew-vegan/)

Ingredients

10g	Olive oil	50g	Tomato paste
300g	Onion, finely chopped	6g	Garlic cloves, minced
300g	Sweet potato, peeled and cut into 1-inch cubes	125g	Peanut butter
6g	Jalapeno, cored and finely chopped	4g	Cumin
6g	Ginger (knob fresh), peeled and minced	1g	Cayenne
1 liter	Vegetable broth (see chapter 3 recipes)	250g	Water
1	Collard greens, bunch, stems removed and chopped	7g	Salt

Ingredients for serving side

Cilantro (fresh)
Brown Rice (cooked)
Peanut(roasted)
Lime juice

Preparation

In a large pot over medium heat, warm the olive oil. Add the onion, sprinkle with salt and cook for 3 minutes until soft. Add the garlic, jalapeño, ginger, cumin, and cayenne, stir together and cook for about 2 minutes.

Add the tomato paste, sweet potato, peanut butter, vegetable broth, and water stirring.

Stir together then bring to a boil. Reduce heat to medium-low, cover, and cook for 15 minutes. Add the chopped collard greens to the pot, stir, then cover, and continue to cook for another 15 minutes, until sweet potato is tender.

Using the back of the spoon, mash some of the sweet potatoes to help thicken the broth. Cook uncovered for 5 minutes.

Serve warm with rice and garnish with cilantro, peanuts, and lime juice.

Roasted Kumara (Sweet Potato) Salad

(https://www.food.com/recipe/roasted-kumara-sweet-potato-salad-484353)

Ingredients.

300g	Sweet Potato (Kumara), peeled and cut into 1-inch cubes
25g	Olive oil for drizzling on Kumara to roast
Several	Romaine Lettuce (leaves), chopped
8	Cherry Tomatoes, halved
4	Radishes, sliced
28g	Feta Cheese (crumbled) (Lacto-vegetarian) or 25g Soy Tofu
Dash	Olive oil (extra-virgin) for salad
Dash	Balsamic Vinegar for salad
34g	Pine Nuts
32g	Macadamia Nuts
22g	Almonds (flaked), freshly ground black pepper to taste
	Sea Salt to taste

Preparation

Place the Kumara (Sweet Potato) in a baking bowl, cover with olive oil, and sprinkle on a pinch of salt. Bake at 350 °F for 25 minutes, or until soft. Set aside to cool. Assemble lettuce, tomato, and radishes in a serving bowl. Add the sweet potato once cooled. Sprinkle on some feta cheese or soy tofu, macadamia, almonds, and pine nuts. Finally, drizzle some extra-virgin olive oil and balsamic vinegar on top. Adjust seasonings.

Aquafaba (Egg White Substitute)

[63, 64]

Ingredients.

500g	Chickpeas

Preparation

Place the chickpeas to soak overnight, in a ratio of 1:6 chickpea: water (*e.g.*, 1 glass of chickpeas and 6 glasses of water). After the soaking time, drain the chickpeas and discard the soaking water. Measure the volume of the soaked chickpeas (hydrated). Cook the hydrated chickpea using a ratio of 1:3 chickpea: water (*e.g.*, 1 glass of chickpeas and 3 glasses of water). Place the water in a bowl and bring to the boil and, when boiling, add the chickpeas. Turn the heat down to low heat, and when the mixture reaches the boil again, turn down the intensity and leave for 30-45 minutes, or until the chickpeas are soft. Remove with a foamer the soft chickpeas and allow to reduce the liquid until the liquid obtain the equivalent of a part of the chickpeas proportion used. *E.g.*, if used 1 glass of chickpeas and three glasses of water, it should remain a glass of aquafaba. Allow cooling and refrigeration. Pack in a glass jar with lid, clean, and pasteurized.

Vegan Mayonnaise

(https://minimalistbaker.com/easy-vegan-mayo-with-aquafaba/)

Ingredients

110g	Aquafaba at room temperature
7.5g	Sugar
24g	Lemon juice
12g	Vinegar
13g	Mustard
320g	Vegetal Oil
3.5g	Salt
10g	Soy Lecithin

Preparation

Whisk the aquafaba in a bowl until foaming, then add the mustard and sugar slowly and whisk together. Gradually add about half the oil, very slowly at first, whisking continuously for around 3 to 5 minutes, or until thickened. Once it adds half of the oil, whisk on the mix, a tablespoon of vinegar, this loosens the mixture slightly and gives it a paler color. Continue to add the remaining oil, whisking continuously gradually. Season with salt, a squeeze of lemon juice and the remnant vinegar, and soy lecithin if needed (by phase separation). Store in a sterilized jar in the fridge for up to one week.

Pasta and Vegan Meatballs

(Adapted from https://www.loveandlemons.com/spaghetti-and-meatballs/

Ingredients

	Ingredients of Veggie Meatballs	16g	Corn Starch
40g	Onion (white) minced	28g	Marinara or Tomato sauce
3	Garlic cloves minced	Dash	Olive oil (for sautéing)
50g	Flax Egg (see below)*	-	Salt and pepper to taste
240g	Lentil cooked	-	*Ingredients for Coating*
30g	Parmesan Cheese (vegan, see below)	36g	Breadcrumbs (vegan, see below)
5.5g	Italian seasoning	30g	Parmesan Cheese (vegan, see below)
54g	Breadcrumbs (vegan, see below)	-	-

Preparation of Veggie Meatballs

Preheat oven to 375 degrees F (190 °C) and prepare flax egg* in a small dish. In a large, deep skillet, sauté onion and garlic in 1/2 Tbsp. olive oil (adjust if altering batch size) over medium heat until soft and translucent, about 3 minutes. Set aside.

Measure out the lentils and place them in a fine-mesh strainer.

Check for discolored or broken lentils. Remove them from the batch and discard, rinse the lentils for about 1 minute under cold running water to wash them, and remove any excess dirt. Brining the lentils in a medium-sized bowl and soak in 4 cups of warm salt water (110°F/43°C) for 1 hour.

Rinse lentil for about 1 minute to discard the excess salt, and place it in a medium-sized pot. Add 3 cups of water and bring the cooking liquid to a boil, and then reduce the heat to a very gentle simmer.

Brined lentils should cook for about 10 to 15 minutes, over low heat, and with minimal agitation. Make sure to keep the lentils completely submerged, looking like porridge. Lentils should cook until tender or about 20 to 40 minutes, depending on their variety. Red and yellow lentils only need 15 to 20 minutes to cook and do not require brining, as they are more delicate in texture. Add the cooked lentils to a food processor and pulse to break down to make a dough. Then add the sautéed garlic and onion, Italian seasoning, starch, flax egg, salt, pepper, and mix, scraping down sides as needed. Make sure to form into a moldable "dough". Scoop out 1 Tbsp. of dough and roll into balls. At this time, heat the skillet to medium. Mix breadcrumbs and parmesan cheese together in a shallow dish. Add lentil balls one or two at a time and roll to coat. Add enough olive oil to form a thin layer on the bottom of your hot skillet, then add your coated lentil balls in two batches.

Do not crowd the pan. Brown for about 5 min total, shaking the pan to roll them around to brown all sides. Add browned meatballs to a baking sheet and place in the oven to bake for about 15 minutes, or longer if desired for a crispier result.

Preparation of Pasta

Prepare any pasta type (*fettuccine, conchigue, mostaccioli*) to serve with meatballs, as well as, the marinara sauce. Once meatballs are deep golden brown and fairly firm to the touch, remove them from the oven. To serve, top-cooked pasta with meatballs, marinara sauce, and a sprinkle of vegan Parmesan cheese and fresh parsley.

*Preparation of flax egg

Mix strongly one tbsp. of crushed flaxseed with two and half tbsp of water and let it for 5 minutes.

Vegan Parmesan Cheese

(Adapted from https://simpleveganblog.com/veganparmesan-cheese/)

Ingredients of Vegan Parmesan cheese

25g	Yeast (nutritional), seasoning
115g	Cashew
1.2g	Garlic powder
6g	Sea Salt

Preparation

Add, all ingredients to a food processor and mix/pulse until a fine meal is achieved. Store in the refrigerator to keep fresh. It lasts for several weeks.

Depending on how salty the vegan parmesan cheese is, it may need to add a little salt and pepper at this point.

Bread Crumbs

Ingredients

3-4 slices	bread toasted	5g	Onion powder
5.5g.	Italian seasoning	1.2g	Paprika
9.8g	Garlic powder.	-	-

Preparation

Add the ingredients to a blender or food processor. Pulse until having a crumbly mix.

Vegan Yogurt

Ingredients

125-200g	Sesame paste (*Tahini*) or coconut shredded
1liter	Water
15g	Maize Starch
6g	Agar-agar
2g)	Probiotic powder (*Lactobacillus acidophilus*)
40g	Sugar
3g	Pectin

Preparation

Mix strongly by using a blender the shredded coconut or the tahini with water and filtering to obtain the 1 liter of the grout. Mix the grout with starch and cook it until it reaches 90°C. Remove from heat and leave to rest until it reaches 35-37°C. Add the probiotic and mix well for 5 minutes. Pour into the yogurt maker and leave it following instructions from the yogurt maker manual until yogurt is done (10 hours). Place the yogurt in a fridge until to be used. Homemade yogurt keeps for about 2 weeks in the refrigerator

CONSENT FOR PUBLICATION

Not Applicable.

CONFLICT OF INTEREST

The author confirms that this chapter contents have no conflict of interest.

ACKNOWLEDGEMENT

Declared none.

REFERENCES

[1] British Nutrition Foundation (BNF). Plants: Diet and health The report of the British nutrition foundation task force. Oxford: Blackwell Publishing 2003.

[2] Beardsworth A, Keil T. The vegetarian option: varieties, conversions, motives, and careers. Sociol Rev 1992; 40(2): 253-93.
[http://dx.doi.org/10.1111/j.1467-954X.1992.tb00889.x]

[3] British Nutrition Foundation (BNF). Vegetarian nutrition: Briefing paper. Nutr Bull 2005; 30: 132-67.
[http://dx.doi.org/10.1111/j.1467-3010.2005.00467.x]

[4]   Lusk JL, Norwood FB. Some economic benefits and costs of vegetarianism. Agric Econ Res Rev 2009; 38(2): 109-24.
[http://dx.doi.org/10.1017/S1068280500003142]

[5]   Kerschke-Risch P. Vegan diet: motives, approach and duration. Initial results of a quantitative sociological study. Ernahr-Umsch 2015; 62(6): 98-103.

[6]   Phillips F. Vegetarian nutrition British Nutrition Foundation. Nutr Bull 2005; 30: 132-67.
[http://dx.doi.org/10.1111/j.1467-3010.2005.00467.x]

[7]   Goytortúa-Bores E, Civera-Cerecedo R, Rocha-Meza S, Green-Yee A. Partial replacement of red crab (*Pleuroncodes planipes*) meal for fish meal in practical diet for the white shrimp *Litopenaeus vannamei*. Effects on growth and *in vivo* digestibility. Aquacult J 2006; 256: 414-22.
[http://dx.doi.org/10.1016/j.aquaculture.2006.02.035]

[8]   Suárez López MM, Kizlansky A, López LB. Evaluación de la calidad de las proteínas en los alimentos calculando el escore de aminoácidos corregido por digestibilidad. Nutr Hosp 2006; 21(1): 47-51.
[PMID: 16562812]

[9]   Babji AS, Fatimah AS, Ghassem M, Abolhasani G. Protein quality of selected edible animal and plant protein sources using rat bio-assay. Int Food Res J 2010; 17(2): 303-8.

[10]   Hever1 J., Cronise RJ. 2017. Plant-based nutrition for healthcare professionals: implementing diet as a primary modality in the prevention and treatment of chronic disease J Geriatr Cardiol. 14(5): 355–368.

[11]   Rottka H. Health and vegetarian lifestyles.Nutritional adaption to new lifestyles. Oxford: Oxford University Press 1990; pp. 176-94.

[12]   Fraser GE. Vegetarian diets: what do we know of their effects on common chronic diseases? Am J Clin Nutr 2009; 89(5): 1607S-12S.
[http://dx.doi.org/10.3945/ajcn.2009.26736K] [PMID: 19321569]

[13]   Silva Dias J. Nutritional quality and health benefits of vegetables: A review. Food Nutr Sci 2012; 3: 1354-74.
[http://dx.doi.org/10.4236/fns.2012.310179]

[14]   Ramya V, Patel P. Health benefits of vegetables. Int J Chem Stud 2019; 7(2): 82-7.

[15]   Gagné F. Oxidative stress.Biochemical Ecotoxicology, Principles and Methods. NewYork: Academic Press/ Elsevier Inc 2014; pp. 103-15.
[http://dx.doi.org/10.1016/B978-0-12-411604-7.00006-4]

[16]   Mohora M, Greabu M, Totan A, Mitrea N, Battino M. redox-sensitive signaling factors and antioxidants. Farmacia 2009; 57(4): 399-411.

[17]   Prior RL, Cao G. Antioxidant phytochemicals in fruit and vegetables, diet and health implications. HortScience 2000; 35(4): 588-92.
[http://dx.doi.org/10.21273/HORTSCI.35.4.588]

[18]   Hyson D. The Health Benefits of Fruit and Vegetables: A Scientific Overview for Health Professionals. Wilmington, DE: Produce for Better Health Foundation 2002.

[19]   Golberg G. Plants: diet and health.The report of a British nutrition foundation task force. Oxford: Blackwell Science 2003; pp. 152-63.

[20]   The International Fruit and Vegetable Alliance (IFAVA). Fruit, vegetables, and health: A scientific overview 2006. www.5aday.co.nz

[21]   Keatinge JDH, Waliyar F, Jammadass RH, Moustafa A, Andrade M, Drechsel P, *et al.* Re-learning old lessons for the future of food: By bread alone no longer-diversifying diets with fruit and vegetables. Crop Sci 2010; 50(1): 51-62.
[http://dx.doi.org/10.2135/cropsci2009.09.0528]

[22]   Melina V, Winston CW, Levin S. Position of the American Dietetic Association: vegetarian diets. J

Acad Nutr Diet 2016; 116(12): 1970-80.
[http://dx.doi.org/10.1016/j.jand.2016.09.025] [PMID: 27886704]

[23]   Dias JS. Nutritional quality and health benefits of vegetables: A review. Food and Nutrition Sciences.A Review. Food Nutr Sci 2012; 3: 1354-74.
[http://dx.doi.org/10.4236/fns.2012.310179]

[24]   Keatinge JDH, Waliyar F, Jamnadas RH, Moustafa A, Andrade M. Relearning old lessons for the Future of Food—By Bread Alone No Longer: Diversifying Diets with Fruit and Vegetables. Crop Sci 2010; 50: 51-62.
[http://dx.doi.org/10.2135/cropsci2009.09.0528]

[25]   Hung HC, Joshipura KJ, Jiang R, *et al.* Fruit and vegetable intake and risk of major chronic disease. J Natl Cancer Inst 2004; 96(21): 1577-84.
[http://dx.doi.org/10.1093/jnci/djh296] [PMID: 15523086]

[26]   Dauchet L, Amouyel P, Hercberg S, Dallongeville J. Fruit and vegetable consumption and risk of coronary heart disease: a meta-analysis of cohort studies. J Nutr 2006; 136(10): 2588-93.
[http://dx.doi.org/10.1093/jn/136.10.2588] [PMID: 16988131]

[27]   He FJ, Nowson CA, Lucas M, MacGregor GA. Increased consumption of fruit and vegetables is related to a reduced risk of coronary heart disease: meta-analysis of cohort studies. J Hum Hypertens 2007; 21(9): 717-28.
[http://dx.doi.org/10.1038/sj.jhh.1002212] [PMID: 17443205]

[28]   Oyebode O, Gordon-Dseagu V, Walker A, Mindell JS. Fruit and vegetable consumption and all-cause, cancer and CVD mortality: analysis of Health Survey for England data. J Epidemiol Community Health 2014; 68(9): 856-62.
[http://dx.doi.org/10.1136/jech-2013-203500] [PMID: 24687909]

[29]   Amao I. Health benefits of fruits and vegetables: Review from Sub-Saharan Africa.Vegetables-Importance of Quality Vegetables to Human Health. IntechOpen 2018; p. 97.
[http://dx.doi.org/10.5772/intechopen.74472]

[30]   Office of Disease and Health Promotion Prevention (ODPHP). 2020. https://health.gov

[31]   International Food Information (IFIC). Council Foundation 2018. https://www.foodinsight.org

[32]   World Cancer Research Fund International. NDC Alliance 2017. http://www.wcrf.org

[33]   American Chemical Society (ACS). 2018. www.acs.org

[34]   American Heart Association. Vegetarian, vegan, and meals without meat 2019. http://www.heart.org

[35]   Kim H, Caulfield LE, Garcia-Larsen V, Steffen LM, Coresh J, Rebholz CM. Plant-based diets are associated with a lower risk of incident cardiovascular disease, cardiovascular disease mortality, and all-cause mortality in a general population of middle-aged adults. J. Am. Heart Assoc., 2019; 8(16):in https://www.ahajournals.org/doi/epub/10.1161/JAHA.119.012865

[36]   Gomes Silva SC, Pinho JP, Borges C, Teixeira Santos C, Santos A, Graça P, *et al.* Guidelines for a healthy vegetarian diet. Programa Nacional para a promohcao da alimentacao saudavel. Portugal. 2015

[37]   Whitten C, Haddad EH, Sabaté J. Developing a vegetarian food guide pyramid: A conceptual framework. Vegetarian Nutri. Int J 1997; 1(1): 25-9.

[38]   Haddad EH, Sabaté J, Whitten CG. Vegetarian food guide pyramid: a conceptual framework. Am J Clin Nutr 1999; 70(3) (Suppl.): 615S-9S.
[http://dx.doi.org/10.1093/ajcn/70.3.615s] [PMID: 10479240]

[39]   Baroni L. Vegetarianism in food-based dietary guidelines 2015. https://openaccesspub.org
[http://dx.doi.org/10.14302/issn.2379-7835.ijn-14-588]

[40]   Loma Linda University. School of Public 2008. http://www.vegetariannutrition.org

[41]   Amidor T. The new vegetarian and vegan diet pyramid 2014. https://health.usnews.com

http://www.veganpeace.com

[42]   European Vegetarian Union (EVU). 2015.http://www.euroveg.eu

[43]   McQuirter T. African American vegan starter guide. Simple ways to begin a plant-based lifestyle. 2016.

[44]   Simopoulos AP. The importance of the ratio of omega-6/omega-3 essential fatty acids. Biomed Pharmacother 2002; 56(8): 365-79.
[http://dx.doi.org/10.1016/S0753-3322(02)00253-6] [PMID: 12442909]

[45]   Holick MF, Chen TC. Vitamin D deficiency: a worldwide problem with health consequences. Am J Clin Nutr 2008; 87(4) (Suppl.): 1080S-6S.
[http://dx.doi.org/10.1093/ajcn/87.4.1080S] [PMID: 18400738]

[46]   Jäpelt RB, Jakobsen J. Vitamin D in plants: a review of occurrence, analysis, and biosynthesis. Front Plant Sci 2013; 4: 136.
[http://dx.doi.org/10.3389/fpls.2013.00136] [PMID: 23717318]

[47]   Heaney RP, Recker RR, Grote J, Horst RL, Armas LA. Vitamin $D_{(3)}$ is more potent than vitamin $D_{(2)}$ in humans. J Clin Endocrinol Metab 2011; 96(3): E447-52.
[http://dx.doi.org/10.1210/jc.2010-2230] [PMID: 21177785]

[48]   Watson E. Lichen-based vegan Vitamin D3 gain momentum as Nordic naturals introduce new products. 2012. Available from https://www.nutraingredients-usa.com

[49]   Lee NK, Aan B-Y. Optimization of ergosterol to vitamin D_2 synthesis in *Agaricus bisporus* powder using ultraviolet-B radiation. Food Sci Biotechnol 2016; 25(6): 1627-31.
[http://dx.doi.org/10.1007/s10068-016-0250-0] [PMID: 30263454]

[50]   Humer E, Schwarz C, Schedle K. Phytate in pig and poultry nutrition. J Anim Physiol Anim Nutr (Berl) 2015; 99(4): 605-25.
[http://dx.doi.org/10.1111/jpn.12258] [PMID: 25405653]

[51]   Messina V, Mangels AR. Considerations in planning vegan diets: children. J Am Diet Assoc 2001; 101(6): 661-9.
[http://dx.doi.org/10.1016/S0002-8223(01)00167-5] [PMID: 11424545]

[52]   Mangels AR, Messina V. Considerations in planning vegan diets: infants. J Am Diet Assoc 2001; 101(6): 670-7.
[http://dx.doi.org/10.1016/S0002-8223(01)00169-9] [PMID: 11424546]

[53]   Amit M. Vegetarian diets in children and adolescents. Paediatr Child Health 2010; 15(5): 303-14.
[PMID: 21532796]

[54]   Specker BL. Nutritional concerns of lactating women consuming vegetarian diets. Am J Clin Nutr 1994; 59(5) (Suppl.): 1182S-6S.
[http://dx.doi.org/10.1093/ajcn/59.5.1182S] [PMID: 8172121]

[55]   Sanders TAB. Essential fatty acid requirements of vegetarians in pregnancy, lactation, and infancy. Am J Clin Nutr 1999; 70(3) (Suppl.): 555S-9S.
[http://dx.doi.org/10.1093/ajcn/70.3.555s] [PMID: 10479231]

[56]   Mangels AR. Mangels AR. Vegetarian Diets in Pregnancy. In: Lammi-Keefe CJ, Couch SC, Philipson EH, eds. Handbook of Nutrition and Pregnancy. Nutrition and Health. Humana Press: XXX 2008.
[http://dx.doi.org/10.1007/978-1-59745-112-3_15]

[57]   Section on Breastfeeding. Breastfeeding and the use of human milk. Pediatrics 2012; 129(3): e827-41.
[http://dx.doi.org/10.1542/peds.2011-3552] [PMID: 22371471]

[58] Henderson A. Vitamin D and the breastfed infant. J Obstet Gynecol Neonatal Nurs 2005; 34(3): 367-72.
[http://dx.doi.org/10.1177/0884217505276157] [PMID: 15890836]

[59] Rogerson D. Vegan diets: practical advice for athletes and exercisers. J Int Soc Sports Nutr 2017; 14: 36.
[http://dx.doi.org/10.1186/s12970-017-0192-9] [PMID: 28924423]

[60] Pollan M. Food rules: An eaters Manual-Michal Pollan. 2011 Available from: https://michael pollan.com

[61] U.S. Department of Agriculture. https://it.wikipedia.org/wiki/Kerria_lacca

[62] Alencar Lopes AC, Hikichi Eda S, Pereira Andrade R, Cunha Amorim J, Ferreira Duarte W. 14 New alcoholic fermented beverages-Potentials and challenges. Fermented beverages. Sc Beverages 2019; 5: 577-603.

[63] 2020.https://www.researchgate.net/publication/339830956_produccion_de_aquafaba_a_partir_de_garbanzos_naturales

[64] Alsalman FM, Tulbek M, Ramaswamy H. Evaluation and optimization of functional and antinutritional properties of aquafaba. Corpus, ID 2020; p. 214008075.

CHAPTER 3

Foods for the Elderly

Elevina Pérez Sira[1,*]

[1] *Instituto de Ciencia y Tecnología de Alimentos, Facultad de Ciencias, Universidad Central de Venezuela, Caracas, Venezuela*

Abstract: The aging process of any population is a function of the differences in genetics, lifestyle, and health. The relationship between aging and several diseases of older adults includes loss of appetite, gustatory dysfunctions, declining basal metabolism. Moreover, the situation is aggravated by economic issues that sometimes affecting this fraction of the population. This chapter stresses the relationship between nutrition and the elderly, emphasizing some chronic conditions or clinically identifiable complications that appear during the aging process. Therefore, it is briefly discussed chronic conditions such as anorexia, presbyphagia anosmia or hyposmia, sarcopenia, hypothyroidism, osteopenia/osteoporosis, and constipation. Also, there is a brief compilation of the information on food for the elderly and some home recipes.

Keywords: Anorexia, Constipation, Foods the elderly, Health and aging, Hypothyroidism, Osteopenia/osteoporosis, Presbyphagia anosmia, Sarcopenia.

INTRODUCTION

Conventionally, "old age" has been defined as a chronological age of 65 years old or older, there is also a classification in early, middle, and late elderly [1 - 3]. The evidence on which basis is the elderly chronological definition is not clear to these authors. They believe that the definition of the elderly should be reviewed based on comprehensive evidence in all the aspects of social, cultural, and medical sciences.

Differences in genetics, lifestyle, and health play an essential role in the aging process of any population [4]. First attempt to internationally defines age was made by the World Health Organization [5], declaring that "old age" is denoted by the age of 60–65 years in the developed world.

* **Corresponding author Elevina Pérez Sira:** Instituto de Ciencia y Tecnología de Alimentos, Facultad de Ciencias, Universidad Central de Venezuela, Caracas, Venezuela; Tel: +58.212.751 4403; Fax: +58 212. 751 3871; E-mail: elevina07@gmail.com

A document published by the WHO [6] distinguishes the normal aging process from the process of aging. According to this organization, the aging process (normal aging) represents the universal biological changes that occur with age and are unaffected by disease and environmental influences. Not all these age-related changes have adverse clinical impacts. In contrast, the process of aging influenced by the effects of environmental, lifestyle, and disease is, in turn, related to or change with aging but is not due to aging itself. Often what was once thought to be a consequence of normal aging is now more appropriately attributed to factor aging-associated.

The active-aging concept, now promoted [7, 8], encourages the process of growing older without growing old by keeping an active physical, social, and spiritual life.

In 2013, the United Nations [9] stated that the elderly population would double by 2050. ONU pointed out a quick increment of the rate of growth of the elderly in the U.S. more rapidly than the rate of growth in the overall population. A phenomenon often referred to as "the graying of America" [10].

NUTRITION AND ELDERLY

Scientific research has studied the relationship between diet and several diseases of older adults, including loss of appetite, gustatory dysfunctions, declining basal metabolism, and economic issues affecting this fraction of the population [11].

In the general context, there exist recommendations to help prevent death and disability from major nutrition-related chronic diseases. This population nutrient intake and physical activity goals should contribute to the development of regional strategies and national guidelines to reduce the burden of disease related to obesity, diabetes, and cardiovascular disease, several forms of cancer, osteoporosis, and dental disease. These strategies are on the examination and analysis of the best available evidence and the collective judgment of a group of experts representing the global scope of the World Health Organization (WHO) and Food and Agriculture Organization (FAO) mandate [12].

Age is associated with a decrease in the immune response, a high rate of free radicals, accumulations of free radical damage, and decreased antioxidant activity. The decreased immune response and increased lipid peroxidation are, in turn, associated with an increase in the incidence of infections, cardiovascular disease, and cancer [13]. An optimally balanced diet with an emphasis on antioxidant contents helps an older adult to decrease the problems mentioned above. Indeed, appropriate nutrition could help many older adults with chronic conditions or clinically identifiable problems.

ANOREXIA OF AGING

The gradual tendency of older adults to eat less is known as the anorexia of aging. Anorexia of aging, or the decrease in appetite and/or food intake in old age, is a major contributing factor to under-nutrition and adverse health outcomes in the geriatric population [14, 15]. This condition of the elderly is the result of difficulties with chewing and swallowing (presbyphagia), loss of taste and smell, depression, loss of motivation to cook, impossibility to go market and find food, among others.

XEROSTOMIA, CHEW CAPACITY, AND PRESBYPHAGIA (DRY MOUTH, LOSS OF CHEW CAPACITY, AND DIFFICULTY TO SWALLOW)

Xerostomia, or dry mouth, is a common problem in the elderly population caused by decreasing in saliva secretion and composition alteration. Saliva is essential to maintain balance in the mouth. Saliva secretion is due to conditioned reflexes, the nature of the stimulus, and response according to the salivary gland. It is not a disease itself, but a symptom that occurs in various conditions, either as a side effect to head and neck radiation, the intake of some medications, or the decrease in salivary gland function. Its absence or changes in its characteristics represent a health problem.

The altered composition of the saliva makes it viscous and thick. The effects of these two problems result in poor lubrication, chewing, tasting, and ingestion difficulties. The components of saliva are of great importance since it has many functions. These functions include forming and lubricate the food bolus for deglutition, improve taste, starts digestion, prevents erosion of mucous, lubrication, improves the ability to speak, prevent dehydration of the epithelial cells and taste receptors, bacterial balance maintained, and an effect of dental remineralization. Some authors have shown that xerostomia is a significant predictor of unintentional weight loss in the elderly and nutritional deficits, which causes impairment of the function of the salivary glands, which affects the teeth with the consequence of premature edentulism and deteriorating health, creating a vicious circle [16].

Loss of chewing capacity. It has been pointed out that chewing capacity in older adults may influence their nutritional status by altering food choices [17]. Proper chewing is vital in the digestion of all foods, especially most fruits and raw vegetables, which contain indigestible cellulose membranes that must break down before the use of food by the body. Because digestive enzymes act only on the surfaces of food particles, the rate of digestion is highly dependent on the total surface area of the chewed food exposed to intestinal secretions [18].

The act of chewing has more significance than the mere preparation of food for swallowing. The food moves around the mouth, stimulate taste buds, releasing odor. Most of the satisfaction and pleasure of eating depends on these stimuli. The mastication muscles atrophied with age decrease the biting force and slowed the chewing process. The atrophy is probably caused in part by disuse because the less muscular effort is required for chewing, as a result of failing dentition or a progressively softer diet, or both. In either case, the generalized loss of muscle mass decreases the biting force and can make chewing difficult [18]. Pain in the mouth, stiffness or discomfort in the jaw muscles, or problems with the teeth can make it even tougher to chew solid foods.

Moreover, digestive functional capacity leads to changes in the gastric mucosa, decreasing the intestinal motility of the intestinal surface, which is useful for absorption, nutrient transportation capacity, and reduction of blood flow (between the mucosal cell and the vein porta). All these changes alter the overall capacity of digestion and absorption. The lower flexibility of gastric fundus in older adults results in a feeling of satiety or fullness with a lesser amount of food [19]. Health care professionals should make the appropriate suggestions to the people at risk in the elderly population to increase the intake of nutritional and nourishing dense foods [17].

Presbyphagia refers to the typical changes in the swallowing mechanism of healthy older adults that result from the normal aging process. These changes have an impact on each stage of deglutition. It can lead to impaired bolus control and transport, the slowing of the pharyngeal swallowing initiation, ineffective pharyngeal clearance, impaired cricopharyngeal opening, and the reduction of secondary esophageal peristalsis.

It is essential to differentiate presbyphagia from dysphagia. The difference between presbyphagy and dysphagia is that the normal aging of individual cause presbyphagia and the progressive and generalized reduction of muscle strength and mass can affect swallowing. In contrast, dysphagia is an alteration of swallowing, affecting both disorders to children as adults. However, it is generally more common in older individuals with some damage or neurological disorder, which includes, among others, stroke (cerebrovascular accident or CVA) and neurodegenerative diseases. Both have severe consequences for the independence and quality of life of the elderly [15, 20, 21].

To effectively identify and distinguish between presbyphagia and dysphagic symptoms in older adults and to subsequently manage their health status successfully, clinicians must have a clear understanding of how aging affects the anatomy, physiology, and functioning of the swallowing mechanism [21]. They must be more aware of the need to distinguish between dysphagia, presbyphagia (an old, yet healthy swallowing), and other related clinical diagnoses to avoid over-diagnosing and over-treating dysphagia.

Although the anatomical, physiological, psychological, and functional changes that occur in the dynamic process referred to as "aging" place older adults at risk for dysphagia, a healthy older adult's swallowing is not inherently impaired. However, age effects on the temporal evolution of isometric and swallowing pressure indicate a progression of change that, when combined with naturally diminished functional reserve (the resilient ability of the body to adapt to physiological stress) makes the old population more susceptible to dysphagia [22]. There is another important term that needs mention: sarcopenic dysphagia, which will be discussed later.

ANOSMIA OR HYPOSMIA (LOSS OF TASTE AND SMELL)

The trigeminal system-along with smell and taste forms the trigeminal somatosensory system. This system is a chemical sense and its receptors line; the nasal and oral cavities, allow the perception of chemosensory information from the environment. The trigeminal somatosensory system plays a fundamental role in chemosensation and the overall "flavor" of foods [23].

The flavor of food is one of the most significant characteristics that determine food quality and consumer acceptance. The flavor is the sensory impression of a substance (*e.g.*, a food) by the chemical and trigeminal senses. Flavor perception results from multisensory interactions and ultimate central integration, with smell and taste being the key contributors [24].

Molecular stimuli or volatile substances, such as odors or irritants, activate the trigeminal system [23, 25]. Volatile substances are perceived in the nasal cavity, while other non-volatile spices are in the oral cavity. Both the olfactory and trigeminal systems are responsible for the perception of odorants.

The senses of smell and taste are part of the somatosensory or trigeminal perception. These systems detect a variety of soluble and volatile stimulants that have different biological effects on feeding, reproduction, social interactions, mood, and territorial status [26].

The difference between the trigeminal system (TS) perceptions and the smell and taste (olfactory sensations) is that TS is in the oral cavity and the nasal cavity, while the olfactory sensations just only at the nasal cavity [27]. The trigeminal nerve is responsible for sensations in the face and mouth, such as pain, temperature, and touch, but it is not responsible for taste [28].

Based on an electrophysiological study, it has been postulated that a loss of the olfactory sensibility in humans produces a decrease in the perception of trigeminal stimuli [29].

Loss of taste and smell is affected by age. However, this loss can be affected by other factors that could be a sign of a more serious medical condition, such as nasal disease (allergies, sinuous, polyps), some medication (beta-blockers, angiotensin-converting enzyme inhibitors known as ACE), dental problems, smoking, head or facial injury, hormonal alterations, exposure to certain chemicals (insecticides and solvents), head and neck radiation for the treatment of cancers, Alzheimer's or Parkinson's diseases [27, 30 - 34]

Anosmia is the temporary or chronic loss of the sense of smell. There is a related term; hyposmia, which refers to impairment of the sense of smell olfactory ability. In the medical literature, the name "hyposmia" is to describe milder olfactory defects; which are comparatively similar in extent, with those that occur during the common head-cold [35]. Riazi [36] has described hyposmia as the diminishing sense of smell that develops over time. Carrillo *et al.* [27] define the terms of anosmia and hyperosmia as the total loss of olfactory capacity, as well as the quantitative decrease of the olfactory threshold, respectively.

A gradual loss in taste and smell perception seems to be an inevitable part of the aging process. Olfactory dysfunction in old age can cause serious problems such as; the inability to smell warning signs of imminent danger odors (fire, gas) and impair the ability to taste and enjoy food [34].

The perception of the aromas results from a combination of smell activation by odorant components released in the nasopharynx, tastes, and somatosensory sensations like texture, heat, and cold; in the elderly, this perception decreases.

In general, the loss of taste is due to the loss of olfactory retro nasal function, more than to a decrease in taste per se [27, 33]. When the elderly are suffering a loss of smell, they also lose taste. As a result, the loss of smell and taste leads to decreased appetite and poor nutrition and, sometimes, to depression [32]. Loss of smell is usually a temporary nuisance for a normal person that may persist for more extended periods, becoming a problem [37].

The causes for the loss of the taste perception in the elderly are: decrease of the turnover of taste cells, the lack of new taste buds, and a decrease of the axonal transport, due to a deficiency of the relevant nerves that innervate the taste buds [38]. Therefore, they have elevated detection thresholds for the basic tastes (sweet, sodium salt, acid, and bitter). They also experience problems discriminating between different intensities of the same taste.

These perceptions decrease can have severe consequences for the elderly, such as the inability to detect or distinguish among concentrations of sugar or salt. This inability makes it difficult for a diabetic elderly to control sugar consumption and the ability to accurately assess salt levels, which may lead hypertensive patients to stop following the prescribed low-sodium diet [38].

The deficiency of the cribriform plate causes the loss of the smell. The cribriform plate is a sieve-like structure between the anterior cranial fossa and the nasal cavity. It is a part of the ethmoid bone and supports the olfactory bulb, which lies in the olfactory fossa. The cribriform plate is crucial to the sense of smell, and any harm done to the plate can, in turn, damage the neurons that pass through it [36]. The cribriform plate is particularly vulnerable to facial trauma and is associated with CSF rhinorrhea and anosmia [39].

Functional anosmia affects up to 5% of the general population and 10% of those over 65 years [32, 40].

Although these disorders can have a substantial impact on the quality of life of older adults and may be associated with other problems, the medical community often overlooks them. Besides, older adults show a decreased appreciation for certain foods, thereby increasing the risk of a monotonous diet.

These findings highlight the need for appropriate choices in the selection of foods. It is crucial to improve and maintain the adequate quantity and quality of food intake among independently living seniors, and especially those with low sensory performance. The design of dishes for the elderly that could both compensate for these chemosensory losses and meet nutritional needs presents new challenges and opportunities for the food industry [41].

SARCOPENIA (INADEQUATE PROTEINS DIET)

In older adults, the skeletal muscle has an impaired or reduced anabolic response to amino acid ingestion [42]. The loss of skeletal muscle mass and physical function due to aging or sarcopenia is caused by a hormonal decline and decline of the numbers of neuromuscular junctions, increased inflammation, declines in activities, and inadequate nutrition [43]. Therefore, sarcopenia is the degenerative loss of skeletal muscle mass (0.5–1% loss per year after the age of 50), quality, and strength associated with aging.

Sarcopenic obesity or the prevalence of obesity in combination with sarcopenia (the age-related loss of muscle mass and strength or physical function) is increasing in the elderly population. Sarcopenic obesity is a high-risk geriatric syndrome predominantly observed in an aging population at risk of synergistic complications from both sarcopenia and obesity [44]. Excess energy intake, physical inactivity, low-grade inflammation, insulin resistance, and hormonal changes may lead to the development of sarcopenic obesity.

It was initially believed that the culprit of age-related muscle weakness was the result of a reduction in muscle mass, but it is now clear that changes in muscle composition and its quality (MQ: strength relative to its size) are a more predominant cause of muscle weakness.

The relation between obesity and muscle deficiency, either defined by low muscle mass or poor muscle strength is associated with health-related problems in older individuals.

Recent epidemiological studies suggest that this sarcopenic disorder is related to accelerated functional decline and high risk of diseases and mortality among the elderly; therefore, the identification and treatment of affected older patients should be a priority for clinicians in the geriatric field [45].

Sarcopenic dysphagia. A generalized loss of skeletal muscle mass and skeletal muscle strength also affects the muscles of the head and neck. In this way, eating and deglutition movements are also affected [46]. It is diagnosed when there is difficulty in swallowing due to sarcopenia in the chewing muscles and other groups of skeletal musculatures. It is characterized by loss of the muscle mass and strength of the swallowing muscles, including the intrinsic muscle of the tongue and mimetic, masticatory, suprahyoid, infrahyoid, palatine, pharyngeal, and esophageal muscles [47]. Consequently, sarcopenic dysphagia is the difficulty swallowing due to the sarcopenic of generalized skeletal muscles and swallowing muscles.

Sarcopenic dysphagia is also associated with age. The muscle mass losses agerelated responsible for swallowing, become evident in the geniohyoid muscle and tongue. Elderly individuals with both sarcopenia and dysphagia may have not only disease-related dysphagia but also sarcopenic dysphagia.

An assessment of the multi-factorial causes of sarcopenia, including the nutritional review is important because the rehabilitation of sarcopenic dysphagia differs depending on its etiology. The causes of adult malnutrition may also contribute to the etiology of secondary sarcopenia and sarcopenic dysphagia.

The core components of dysphagia rehabilitation are oral health care, rehabilitative techniques, and modification of the food characteristic for old people intake, for example, the food texture. Therefore, nutrition management is indispensable for sarcopenic dysphagia rehabilitation. In cases of sarcopenia with numerous complicating causes, treatment should include pharmaceutical therapies for age-related sarcopenia and comorbid chronic diseases, resistance training, early ambulation, nutrition management, protein, and amino acid supplementation, and the stressing on non-smoking [20].

The regular and adequate intake of proteins is vital in old age. The body does not have a storage system for protein; therefore, insufficient protein intake to satisfy body requirements leads to a negative protein balance (*i.e.*, protein synthesis lower than the breakdown [42].

Interventions and treatments for sarcopenia must increment, and special attention paid to analyzing the effects of exercise and nutrition on older adults [43].

The recommended dietary allowance (RDA) for protein intake in older people should be up to 1.0–1.3 g/kg/day. Furthermore, it is important to emphasize that consumption of protein in a pattern spread out through the day (approximately 30 g at each meal for a 70-kg person) to optimize the muscular anabolic response. Supplementation with essential amino acids and vitamin D (800 UI/day) that could counteract such a nutritional deficiency, has recently been shown to improve muscle mass and strength in old age [14]. In addition to the calcium requirement of 1200 mg per day, vitamin D from foods, supplements, and multivitamins is to meet this requirement.

In frail elderly individuals with malabsorption and alcoholism, there may also be a need to supplement the magnesium intake. Some elderly individuals with indications of poor nutritional status (low albumin levels) or after hip fracture might benefit from protein supplementation and a multivitamin to ensure the adequacy of other nutrients [48]. Besides rehabilitation techniques, there are other procedures for the treatment of sarcopenic dysphagia to implement, such as the modification of the texture of solid foods and the thickness of liquids.

Foods can be cut into small pieces or mashed, while liquids are thickened to slow transit through the oral and pharyngeal phases of swallowing and to avoid aspiration. Finally, sarcopenia should be treated with a combination of rehabilitation training and nutrition [47].

HYPOTHYROIDISM (LOW IODINE DIET)

Thyroid dysfunction is common in older adults [49] usually caused by iodine deficiencies that are driving them to suffer hypothyroidism [50].

Hypothyroidism is caused by an underactive thyroid gland that cannot make enough thyroid hormones (Triiodothyronine or T_3 and thyroxine or T_4) to keep the body running normally. The thyroid gland must have iodine to make thyroid hormones. The iodine comes into the body from food and travels through the blood to the thyroid. Keeping thyroid hormone production in balance requires the right amount of iodine. Taking in too much iodine can cause or worsen hypothyroidism [51].

In the elderly, thyroid dysfunctions by iodine deficiency cause the growth of clusters of autonomous thyrocytes (autonomization), resulting in the overproduction of thyroid hormones. This overproduction led to hyperthyroidism atrial fibrillation (with the risk of reduced cardiac function and embolism), osteoporosis, and lipid abnormalities with atherosclerosis in case of reduced thyroid function [52].

Correcting iodine deficiency in the elderly could help reduce this autonomization process with the normalization of thyroid-stimulating hormone (TSH) and thyroid hormones [11]. These authors confirm that milk per se is an important source of iodine if consumed in appropriate quantities.

Vitamin D and B_{12} deficiencies are associated with thyroid dysfunction. Selenium is an important component of the enzymes needed for the thyroid to function properly [52].

On the other hand, some substances can interfere with the synthesis of thyroid hormones (goitrogens) or iodine absorption (calcium, flavonoid, fiber, chromium picolinate).

The Natural Standards Database provides an extensive list of supplements that have a potential impact on thyroid functioning. Consequently, it is crucial to take the necessary precautions, and coordinating diet care with a knowledgeable practitioner is prudent [52].

OSTEOPENIA/OSTEOPOROSIS

Osteopenia and osteoporosis are among other risk factors affecting the elderly population. Osteopenia is a mild reduction of bone mass or bone mineral density (BMD), and osteoporosis is a more severe reduction of BMD. This prevalence of reduced bone density in adults varies by race and ethnicity.

The treatment of osteoporosis consists of maintaining a balanced diet and an adequate intake of calcium and vitamin D. In those cases where calcium and vitamin D are insufficient, it is recommended to prescribe them, to avoid inactivity, and perform adequate physical exercise or engage in a physical therapy program [53].

CONSTIPATION

Constipation is a decrease in defecation frequency to three or fewer per week, and Rome IV criteria for constipation is the frequent consensus definitions clinically and for research [54]. The elderly also suffer from constipation, which increases with age, particularly after the age of 65.

Marked atrophy of the muscle involved in the bowel movement and changes in mucus-secreting cells in older adults, cause structural and functional changes in the colon [19]. A poor or imbalanced diet is one of the clinical factors that impact bowel function in the elderly.

Constipation results from a combination of reduced fiber and fluid intake, decreased physical activity resulting from chronic diseases, and multiple medications [55]. Constipation is one of the most common and prevalent disorders of the pelvic floor affecting the elderly population. The normal functioning of the neuromuscular unit of the pelvic floor allows for efficient and complete elimination of stool from the rectum [56]. Treatment based on different strategies includes dietary changes, laxatives, and surgery in carefully diagnosed cases.

The most common cause of constipation is a diet low in fiber found in vegetables, fruits, and whole grains and high in fats from cheese, eggs, and meats. People who eat plenty of high-fiber foods are less likely to become constipated [57].

FOOD FOR THE ELDERLY

Specific individualized care plans should be implemented to guarantee adequate amounts of food and exercise for weight loss. Multi-stimulus programs and variations in the elaboration and presentation of food, including (food texture and flavor enhancements) and feeding assistance, may be effective in the management of older people's anorexia [14].

Seniors are becoming a significant consumer group in many countries' economies. The proportion of people over 65 years old is expected to be over 17% of the world's population by 2050 [58, 59].

As discussed before, older adults are facing severe difficulties getting proper nutrition due to their tendency to eat less. Therefore, there is a need for ready-t-eat, microwave foods, take-and-bake, and other easy-to-cook foods that can help older adults with special needs. Currently, there are not enough products available in supermarkets that can address the needs of this important group.

The elderly are a very diverse consumer group. They have different health conditions and lifestyles; so, many of them are not yet convinced of the benefits of ready meals. They believe that ready-to-eat foods do not fulfill the requirements of an excellent nutritious meal [60]. Therefore, a good marketing strategy stressing the benefits of these foods on their health, and wellbeing could be enough to convince them.

Maintaining good mental and physical health is very important to this consumer group. Some research has been done on suitable products for the elderly to address their concerns about easy-to-use and ready meals.

Older adults prefer foods that are salty and not too hard to chew [60]. They suggest that spices can be used to flavor foods to prevent the overuse of salt. They concluded that sous-vide cooking (85 °C), the use of spices to compensate for salt content, and the use of fat/oil were efficient ways to optimize the sensory characteristics of meals to meet the preferences of older adults. However, the authors emphasized that these foods must be high in energy, protein, fiber, and vitamins (especially vitamin D). They also concluded that adding selected food concentrates could be another way to enrich the nutrients content of a meal without increasing the portion size.

The packaging of products can also be modified to help the elderly. Every product designed for the elderly must be easy to handle and use. Easy-to-open, re-seal containers, easy to recognize products, attractive packaging styles, and designs, and different portion sizes for different needs are recommended.

Another research that focuses on finding solutions for anosmia and presbyphagia uses products to thicken food to make it taste better. Pregelatinized starch does not need to be heated to thicken and make it smooth so that it can use with cold food. Presenting food in a liquid form is a possible solution. Liquids, per se, are not the best way to stimulate the appetite. However, presenting food in the form of mousse is an appealing alternative.

Foods in the form of mousse are easier for older adults who have problems swallowing, to get the nutrients they need [61]. Also, ready to prepare a mix for jellies based in pre gel starch with some sources of phytochemicals (Jamaica flowers) and using natural sweeteners (stevia or lou.han.guo) can be developed.

There are numerous nutritional formulas or supplements (NS) in the markets for the elderly. NS can supply all the nutrients (by enteral or parenteral ways), to those patients who cannot handle regular food to stay healthy. Enteral nutrition (EN) is the administration of nutrients directly to the digestive system, using chemically defined formulas. The administration of EN must be prescribed and supervised by physicians. These formulas are a mixture of macro and micronutrients, used as a supplement or as a complete meal.

However, there are few food choices for older adults that do not have a medical condition or who are relatively healthy. These reasons are vast fields of prospects to be done in the area of production of ready-to-eat or cook food with all the nutritional requirements. Additionally, it needs the production of easy-to-handle packaging to senior will covers all the necessary safety requirements.

RECIPES

Breadfruit or Eggplant Purée from Pre-mix

1. Purée Pre-Mix (100g)

Ingredients

70g	Breadfruit or eggplant flour (see recipe in chapter 1)	2g	Salt
4g	Parsley leaves for ornament	1g	White Pepper
2g	Garlic powder	1g	Nutmeg
20g	Corn Starch	-	-

Preparation

Sift flour and mix with the dry ingredients to produce 100 g of the pre-mix.

2. Vegetable broth

Ingredients

200g	Carrot, peeled	50 g	Chives, roughly chopped
200g	Tomatoes, roughly chopped	50g	Leek roughly chopped
200g	Potato, chopped	4g	Garlic clove
200g	Bell Pepper, green	800ml	Water
100g	Mushrooms, roughly chopped	5 g	Salt
50g	Onion, roughly chopped	3 g	White Pepper
100g	Celery (stalks), roughly chopped	-	-
10g	Parsley, roughly chopped	-	-

Preparation

Wash the vegetables thoroughly with drinking water, and cut them into small slices. Incorporate it together with the two garlic cloves in the pot with 400 ml of preheated water, sprinkle salt and pepper to taste, and cook for 15-20 minutes. Once cooked, separate the vegetables with the foamer to obtain a base broth.

For a vegetable broth to be useful within about a week, use airtight containers and put those in the refrigerator until ready to use. For a future time (or in longer than a week) store the airtight containers with the broth in the freezer.

3. Purée

Ingredients needed for the preparation of purée at home

100g	Breadfruit or Eggplant purée premix
100g	Vegetable Broth (homemade or 8 oz. can), see recipe above
10g	Salted Butter

Preparation

Place 100 g of the vegetable broth in a large saucepan; add the purée pre-mix slowly, mixing until no lumps remain.

Cook the mixture with permanent stirring until it reaches 90°C.

Reduce heat to medium-low; to get mash consistency. Turn off the stove, add butter, and mixing inside the mash.

Cover loosely. It can be made 48 hours in advance.

Mashed Beetroot-Cocoa from Pre-mix

1. Purée Pre-Mix 100g

Ingredients

60g	Beetroot (Beta vulgaris) flour (see recipe in chapter 1)	10g	Sugar
20g	Cocoa powder	1.5g	Salt
8g	Corn Starch	0.5g	Nutmeg

Ingredients

Preparation of pre-mix

Sift flour and mix with the dry ingredients to produce 100 g of the pre-mix.

2. Sesame unhulled seed milk

Ingredients

75g	Sesame seeds, unhulled
400 ml	Water

Preparation

Mix thoroughly 75 g unhulled sesame seeds with 500ml of drinking water, by using a food processor blender. Filter the mixture through a cheesecloth into a large bowl. Sesame seed milk lasts in the fridge between 2-3 days without preservatives.

3. Purée

Ingredients needed for the preparation of purée at home

100g	Beetroot-Cocoa puree pre-mix
250g	Sesame milk from unhulled seeds

Preparation

Place 250 g of the sesame milk in the saucepan; add the purée pre-mix slowly, mixing until no lumps remain. Cook the mixture with permanent stirring until it reaches 90°C. Reduce heat to medium-low; to get mash consistency. Turn off the stove, add butter, and mixing inside the mash. Cover loosely.

Pumpkin–Coconut Crème Brùlée

Ingredients Pre-Mix 50g

20g	Pumpkin (*Cucurbita maxima*) flour (See recipe chapter 1)
25g	Sugar
4g	Corn Starch
1g	Vanillin

Ingredients needed for crème brûlée home preparation

50g	Pumpkin–Coconut *Crème Brûlée* pre-mix
20g	Coconut milk
150g	Heavy Cream (¾cups)
10g	Sugar
10g	Brown Sugar
26g	Egg yolk

Preparation

Sift flour and mix with the dry ingredients to produce 100 g of the pre-mix.

Crème Brùlée preparation

Preheat oven to 300 °F (150 °C). Beat egg yolks, and mix with the coconut milk and the pre-mix in a mixing bowl until thick and creamy. Pour heavy cream into a saucepan and stir over low heat until it almost comes to a boil. Remove the cream from heat immediately. Stir cream into the egg yolk mixture; beat until combined. Pour cream mixture into the top pan of a double boiler. Stir over simmering water until the mixture lightly coats the back of a spoon, about 3 minutes.

Remove mixture from heat immediately and pour into a shallow heat-proof dish. Bake in preheated oven for 30 minutes. Remove from oven and cool to room temperature. Refrigerate for at least 1 hour or overnight.

Preheat oven to broil. In a small bowl, combine the remaining 10g white sugar and brown sugar. Sift this mixture evenly over custard. Place dish under the broiler until sugar melts, about 2 minutes. Observe so as not to burn. Remove from heat and allow to cool. Refrigerate until the custard is set again.

Green Custard

Ingredients Pre-mix (50 grams)

23g	Spinach flour (see recipe chapter 1)
22g	Chia (*Salvia hispánica* L) seeds flour
4g	Corn Starch
0.5g	Salt
0.5g	White Pepper

Preparation

Sift flour and mix with the dry ingredients to produce 50 g of the pre-mix.

Ingredients needed for the preparation of custard at home.

50g	Green Custard pre-mix
30g	Egg yolk
250g	Sesame seed milk
0.5g	Parsley leaves as an ornament

Preparation of the custard

Heat the sesame milk in a pan over medium heat, frequently stirring, until just coming up to boiling. Set aside for 15 minutes to infuse and cool slightly. Mix the egg yolk and pre-mix in a heatproof bowl stirring to get a smooth paste.

Slowly pour the hot milk into the paste, continually stirring until thoroughly combined. Strain the mixture into a clean saucepan and, constantly stirring, cook gently over low heat until the custard thickens (at around 75°C/165°F) or coat the back of the spoon with custard and draw a line through with the finger. If the line holds, the custard is ready.

CONSENT FOR PUBLICATION

Not Applicable.

CONFLICT OF INTEREST

The author confirms that this chapter contents have no conflict of interest.

ACKNOWLEDGEMENT

Declared none.

REFERENCES

[1]   Forman DE, Berman AD, McCabe CH, Baim DS, Wei JY. PTCA in the elderly: the "young-old" *versus* the "old-old". J Am Geriatr Soc 1992; 40(1): 19-22.
[http://dx.doi.org/10.1111/j.1532-5415.1992.tb01823.x] [PMID: 1727842]

[2]   Orimo H, Ito H, Suzuki T, Araki A, Hosoi T, Sawabe M. [Reviewing the definition of elderly]. Nippon Ronen Igakkai Zasshi 2006; 43(1): 27-34.
[http://dx.doi.org/10.3143/geriatrics.43.27] [PMID: 16521795]

[3]   Zizza CA, Ellison KJ, Wernette CM. Total water intakes of community-living middle-old and oldest-old adults. Biological Sciences and Medical Sciences Series A. J Gerontol 2009; 64: 481-6.
[http://dx.doi.org/10.1093/gerona/gln045]

[4]   Singh S, Bajorek B. Defining 'elderly' in clinical practice guidelines for pharmacotherapy. Pharm Pract (Granada) 2014; 12(4): 489.
[http://dx.doi.org/10.4321/S1886-36552014000400007] [PMID: 25580172]

[5]   World Health Organization United Nations (WHO). Keep Fit for Life: Meeting the nutritional needs of older persons. Geneva: World Health Organization 2002.

[6]   World Health Organization United Nations (WHO). Men aging and health achieving health across the life span Ginebra. WHO 2008.

[7]   World Health Organization United Nations (WHO). Definition of an older or elderly person 2014.

[8]   World Health OrganizationUnited Nations (WHO). Report on Ageing and Health WHO Library Cataloguing-in-Publication Data. 2015. Available from www.who.int

[9]   United Nations (UN). Department of Economic and Social Affairs, Population Division. World population aging 2013. ST/ESA/SER.A/348. 2013.

[10]   Lohr KL. Institute of Medicine (US) Committee to design a strategy for quality review and assurance in Medicare Lohr KN, Ed. Washington (DC): National Academies Press, USA. 1990.

[11]   Watutantrige-Fernando S, Barollo S, Bertazza L, Sensi F, Cavedon E, *et al.* Iodine status in the elderly: association with milk. Intake and other dietary habits. JNHFS 2017; 5(1): 1-5.
[http://dx.doi.org/10.15226/jnhfs.2017.00189]

[12]   World Health Organization (WHO). World Health Organization (WHO). Report of the joint WHO/FAO expert consultation. Global Strategy on diet, physical activity, and health. Diet, nutrition, and the prevention of chronic diseases. WHO Technical Report Series, No. 916 (TRS 916). 2002. 2002. Available from: https://www.who.int

[13]   Fortes C, Forastiere F, Farchi S, Rapiti E, Pastori G, Perucci CA. Diet and overall survival in a cohort of very elderly people. Epidemiology 2000; 11(4): 440-5.
[http://dx.doi.org/10.1097/00001648-200007000-00013] [PMID: 10874552]

[14]   Landi F, Calvani R, Tosato M, *et al.* Anorexia of aging: risk factors, consequences, and potential treatments. Nutrients 2016; 8(2): 69.
[http://dx.doi.org/10.3390/nu8020069] [PMID: 26828516]

[15]   Cichero JAY. Age-related changes to eating and swallowing impact frailty: aspiration, choking risk, modified food texture, and autonomy of choice. Geriatrics (Basel) 2018; 3(4): 69.
[http://dx.doi.org/10.3390/geriatrics3040069] [PMID: 31011104]

[16]   DeLuca Monasterios FM, Roselló Llabrés X. Etiopathogenesis and diagnosis of dry mouth. Av Odontoestomatol 2014; 30(3): 121-8.

[17]   Mann T, Heuberger R, Wong H. The association between chewing and swallowing difficulties and nutritional status in older adults. Aust Dent J 2013; 58(2): 200-6.
[http://dx.doi.org/10.1111/adj.12064] [PMID: 23713640]

[18]   Saunders MJ, Yeh C-K. Oral health in elderly people. 2013; pp. 163-204.

[19]   Capo Pallàs M. Importancia de la nutrición en las personas de edad avanzada. Barcelona: España Novartis Consumer Health S.A. 2002.

[20]   Wakabayashi H. Presbyphagia and sarcopenic dysphagia: association between aging, sarcopenia, and deglutition disorders. J Frailty Aging 2014; 3(2): 97-103.
[PMID: 27049901]

[21]   McCoy YM, Desai RV. Presbyphagia *versus* dysphagia: Identifying age-related changes in swallow function. Perspect ASHA Spec Interest Groups 2018; 3(15): 15-21.
[http://dx.doi.org/10.1044/persp3.SIG15.15]

[22]   Humbert IA, Robbins J. Dysphagia in the elderly. Phys Med Rehabil Clin N Am 2008; 19(4): 853-866, ix-x.
[http://dx.doi.org/10.1016/j.pmr.2008.06.002] [PMID: 18940645]

[23]   Viana F. Chemosensory properties of the trigeminal system. ACS Chem Neurosci 2011; 2(1): 38-50.
[http://dx.doi.org/10.1021/cn100102c] [PMID: 22778855]

[24]   Su G, Sun-Waterhouse D, Zhao Y, He W, Zhao M. Flavor enhancement induced by taste–odor interactions Reference Module in Food Science. 2019.

[25]   Filiou R-P, Lepore F, Bryant B, Lundström JN, Frasnelli J. Perception of trigeminal mixtures. Chem Senses 2015; 40(1): 61-9.
[http://dx.doi.org/10.1093/chemse/bju064] [PMID: 25500807]

[26]   Spielman AI, Yan W, Brand JG. Chemosensory systems.Chichester. John Wiley & Sons Ltd. 2007.http://www.els.net
[http://dx.doi.org/10.1002/9780470015902.a0000038.pub2]

[27]   Carrillo B, Carrillo V, Astorga A, Hormachea D. Diagnosis in smell pathology. Rev Otorrinolaringol Cir Cabeza Cuello 2107(77): 351-60. [Review].

[28]   Scott-Thomas C. Trigeminal sensations: An emerging area for innovation. 2010. Available from: https://www.foodnavigator-usa.com

[29]   Hummel T, Barz S, Lötsch J, Roscher S, Kettenmann B, Kobal G. Loss of olfactory function leads to a decrease of trigeminal sensitivity. Chem Senses 1996; 21(1): 75-9.
[http://dx.doi.org/10.1093/chemse/21.1.75] [PMID: 8646495]

[30]   Bromley SM. Smell and taste disorders: a primary care approach. Am Fam Physician 2000; 15:61(2):427-436.

[31]   DaSilva MC, Panganiban WD. A cross-sectional study on olfactory function among young adult smokers. Philipp J Otolaryngol Head Neck Surg 2006; 21(1): 28-30.
[http://dx.doi.org/10.32412/pjohns.v21i1-2.827]

[32]   Gaines AD. Anosmia and hyposmia. Allergy Asthma Proc 2010; 31(3): 185-9.
[http://dx.doi.org/10.2500/aap.2010.31.3357] [PMID: 20615320]

[33]   Dalton P, Doty RL, Murphy C, *et al.* Olfactory assessment using the NIH Toolbox. Neurology 2013; 80(11) (Suppl. 3): S32-6.
[http://dx.doi.org/10.1212/WNL.0b013e3182872eb4] [PMID: 23479541]

[34]   Ruggiero GF, Wick JY. Olfaction: New Understandings, Diagnostic Applications. Consult Pharm 2016; 31(11): 624-32.
[http://dx.doi.org/10.4140/TCP.n.2016.624] [PMID: 28107119]

[35]   Amoore JE. Olfactory genetics and anosmia. In: Beidler LM Eds. Olfaction. Handbook of Sensory Physiology, 4/1. Berlin, Heidelberg: Springer. 1971.
[http://dx.doi.org/10.1007/978-3-642-65126-7_11]

[36]   Riazi N. To eat with your eyes.Science & Food Science & Food UCLA. Public Lecture Series 2017.

[37]   National Institute of Deafness and other Disorder (NID). Trastornos del olfato. Publicación de NIH núm. 09-3231 S. 2013.

[38]   Schiffman SS. Perception of taste and smell in elderly persons. Crit Rev Food Sci Nutr 1993; 33(1): 17-26.
[http://dx.doi.org/10.1080/10408399309527608] [PMID: 8424850]

[39] Gamble AJ, Kapinos G, Batidas N, *et al.* Depressed skull and facial fractures. In: Kusmar M, Kofke A, Levine J, Schuster J, Eds. Neurocritical Care Management of the Neurosurgical Patient. E-Book. Elsevier 2018; pp. 283-92.

[40] Neuland C, Bitter T, Marschner H, Gudziol H, Guntinas-Lichius O. Health-related and specific olfaction-related quality of life in patients with chronic functional anosmia or severe hyposmia. Laryngoscope 2011; 121(4): 867-72.
[http://dx.doi.org/10.1002/lary.21387] [PMID: 21298638]

[41] Doets EL, Kremer S. Doets EL, Kremer S. The silver sensory experience–A review of senior consumers' food perception, liking and intake Author links open overlay panel. Food Qual Prefer 2016; 48 (Part B):316-332.

[42] Thalacker-Mercer AE, Drummond MJ. The importance of dietary protein for muscle health in inactive, hospitalized older adults. Ann N Y Acad Sci 2014; 1328: 1-9.
[http://dx.doi.org/10.1111/nyas.12509] [PMID: 25118148]

[43] Santilli V, Bernetti A, Mangone M, Paoloni M. Clinical definition of sarcopenia. Clin Cases Miner Bone Metab 2014; 11(3): 177-80.
[PMID: 25568649]

[44] Batsis JA, Villareal DT. Sarcopenic obesity in older adults: aetiology, epidemiology and treatment strategies. Nat Rev Endocrinol 2018; 14(9): 513-37.
[http://dx.doi.org/10.1038/s41574-018-0062-9] [PMID: 30065268]

[45] Stenholm S, Harris TB, Rantanen T, Visser M, Kritchevsky SB, Ferrucci L. Sarcopenic obesity: definition, cause and consequences. Curr Opin Clin Nutr Metab Care 2008; 11(6): 693-700.
[http://dx.doi.org/10.1097/MCO.0b013e328312c37d] [PMID: 18827572]

[46] Dellis S, Papadopoulou S, Krikonis K, Zigras F. Sarcopenic dysphagia. A narrative review. J Frailty Sarcopenia Falls 2018; 3(1): 1-7.
[http://dx.doi.org/10.22540/JFSF-03-001] [PMID: 32300688]

[47] Patino-Hernandez D, Borda MG, Venegas Sanabria E, Chavarro-Carvajal DA, Cano-Gutiérrez CA. Sarcopenic dysphagia. Rev Col Gastroenterol 2016; 31(4): 412-7.

[48] Nieves JW. Calcium, vitamin D, and nutrition in elderly adults. Clin Geriatr Med 2003; 19(2): 321-35.
[http://dx.doi.org/10.1016/S0749-0690(02)00073-3] [PMID: 12916289]

[49] Institute of Medicine (US). 2003.https://www.ncbi.nlm.nih.gov

[50] Mayo Clinic. Patient care & health information 2019.https://www.mayoclinic.org

[51] American Thyroids Association (ATA). 2019.https://www.thyroid.org

[52] Harris C. Thyroid disease and diet nutrition play a part in maintaining thyroid health. Todays Diet 2012; 14(7): 40.

[53] Giner Ruizo V. Osteoporosis. Manejo: prevención, diagnóstico y tratamiento. 13 guías de actualización. Sociedad Española de Medicina de Familia y Comunitaria. Barcelona, España. 2014. Available from: ediciones@semfyc.es

[54] Dumic I, Nordin T, Jecmenica M, Stojkovic M, Milosavljevic T, Milovanovic T. Gastrointestinal tract disorders in older age. Can J Gastroenterol Hepato 2019; pp. 1-19.

[55] Bosshard W, Dreher R, Schnegg J-F, Büla CJ. The treatment of chronic constipation in elderly people: an update. Drugs Aging 2004; 21(14): 911-30.
[http://dx.doi.org/10.2165/00002512-200421140-00002] [PMID: 15554750]

[56] Vázquez Roque M, Bouras EP. Epidemiology and management of chronic constipation in elderly patients. Clin Interv Aging 2015; 10: 919-30.
[PMID: 26082622]

[57] University of California. 2019. https://uhs.berkeley.edu

[58] McCluskey JJ. Changing food demand and consumer preferences. Agricultural Symposium Federal Reserve Bank of Kansas City.

[59] He W, Goodkind D, Paul PUS. Census Bureau, International population reports, P95/16-1, An Aging World: 2015. Washington, DC: U.S. Government Publishing Office 2016.

[60] Heiniö RL, Pentikäinen S, Rusko E, Peura-Kapanen LP. 2014.Food for seniors https://www.vtt.fi/inf

[61] Sugimoto K. Meals for elderly people in Japan. Tokio: Innovatie Attaché 2013.www.ianetwerk.nl

CHAPTER 4

Foods for Athletes

Elevina Pérez Sira[1,*], **Frederick Schroeder**[2] and **Mily Schroeder**[3]

¹ Instituto de Ciencia y Tecnología de Alimentos, Facultad de Ciencias, Universidad Central de Venezuela, Caracas, Venezuela

² University of Arizona, Bio-medical Engineer, Tucson AZ, USA

³ St. Mary University, Education and Leadership Department, Minneapolis, MN, USA

Abstract: Concerns about athlete's alimentation begin with food availability and its versatility at the markets due that sports foods offer is reduced and low investigated. The chapter highlights foods for sports topics, food development and nutrition, and managing athlete's body composition, and their special requirements. The energy balance and availability, macro and micronutrients, and their importance in body function are also discussed. Finally, the goals of an adequate sports diet, and the use of supplements and performance enhancers, and recommendations of some recipes are mentioned.

Keywords: Athletes´ diet, Foods for athletes, Nutrition and sport.

INTRODUCTION

There are some concerns regarding the market availability of "healthy" food for athletes. Every athlete, besides the good genes, proper training, and conditioning, needs a healthy diet. The nutrient needs of the athletes not only have individual physiological and biochemical characteristics [1], but, the energy and nutrients requirements of the athletes are a function of their body structure, training load, and sporting event. Therefore, athletes need accessibility to healthy and ready-toeat food when traveling for sports events or during daily training, but it is imperative to take into consideration their body sizes and training load requirements. Unfortunately, today there are not many foods of this type in the markets. It is suitable if the athletes during training and in-season could find in the markets these types of specific healthy foods in a ready to eat or cook format. For example, fresh, gourmet, microwavable, baked, and frozen healthy meals that contain the necessary nutrients for the specific types of sports.

* **Corresponding author Elevina Pérez Sira:** Instituto de Ciencia y Tecnología de Alimentos, Facultad de Ciencias, Universidad Central de Venezuela, Caracas, Venezuela; Tel: +58.212.751 4403; Fax: +58 212. 751 3871; E-mail: elevina07@gmail.com

Therefore, it must be a commitment of the food researchers and industry to know the athlete's needs to trigger the elaboration of these types of foods.

NUTRITION AND SPORT

An active lifestyle with exercise and a balanced diet are the best system for conventional consumers to be healthy, but for athletes, the requirements are beyond those of conventional consumers. The American Dietetic Association, Dietitians of Canada, and the American College of Sports Medicine postulate that optimal nutrition enhances physical activity, athletic performance, and recovery from the exercise of the athletes. Therefore, they recommend an appropriate selection of foods and fluids, timing of intake, and supplement choices for optimal health and exercise performance [2].

A healthy diet is crucial to enhance the effects of physical activity of the athletes and varies as a function of the sport type. When feeding athletes, good alimentation and hydration improve the athletes' performance, recovery, and prevention of injury. Moreover, appropriate nutrition cover the requirements of fuel, recovery, and compositional change, which turn the athlete's body into a high-performance sports machine [3]. Athletes without enough macro and micronutrients from foods shall be tired with less performance during competition. Then, a healthy diet is not only substantial, but also rather vital for athletes, so it can help enhance their athletic performance. Carbohydrates, protein, and healthy fats, fluids, iron, vitamins, and other minerals provide the fuel needed to maintain energy.

The quantity of each macro or micronutrient that the athletes need is a function of the sport type and training time. Calories measure the energy the body gets from foods, and the energy the body spends from exercise. The number of calories necessary is different for every person and depends on inherent body factors and lifestyle, increasing as the person becomes more active and athletic [4]. However, more important than how many calories consumers take, it is where they get those calories from [4]. Other than water, the macronutrients are the sources of calories for the body as follows; Carbohydrates (4cal/g), proteins (4cal/g), and fats (9cal/g) [5].

Of all macronutrient, fats are the slowest source of energy, but it is the most efficient. If the body does not have to use the energy immediately, it is stored more easily as fat, than calories from carbohydrates and proteins [6, 7].

Since the regulator of fat storage in the adipose tissue is insulin, the reduction of insulinogenic carbohydrates (free sugars) in the diet shall reduce the body fats, even in a low-fat diet [8, 9].

MANAGING BODY COMPOSITION

According to Ackland *et al.* in 2012 [11] quantifying human body composition plays a vital in the management of the physical activity regime (particularly in gravitational, weight class, and aesthetic sports) an athlete's performance. Traditionally, the classification of the techniques for measuring body composition is according to the purpose of their application, basic and applied researches of experimental and epidemiological nature, disease diagnosis and control, or dietary and physical activity interventions in programs of body weight control. These techniques involve laboratory and clinical procedures where the target is the measure of absolute and relative body mass components [11 - 14]. In individuals the body composition and its development are crucial factors of both individuals and population health; therefore, the evaluation of the body composition is an important parameter for monitoring obesity, nutritional status, training outcomes, and general health [11].

The components of body composition are fat-free mass (FFM), fat mass (FM), and bone mineral content (BMC). FM contains two fat types; essential and storage. Essential fat is necessary for the body for important physiological body functions, contrarily FFM, which is stored around internal organs, within muscle tissue, and directly beneath the skin, provides insulation and organs protection, and ready fuel source for aerobic energy [15, 16]. The lean or FFM represents the weight of the muscles, bones, connective tissue, and internal organs. Higher lean mass is associated with higher metabolic activity and greater caloric expenditure throughout the day [17 - 19].

In this context, Siervo *et al.*, 2014 and Toomey *et al*, 2015 [14, 16] have pointed out several methods based on components numbers of body composition:

- Model of 2-component (2-C); which is the ratio of the fat-free mass (FFM) and fat mass (FM). FM and FFM are indexes used for the evaluation of nutritional requirements and energy expenditure.
- The three-component (3-C) model, where it is introduced a third component dividing FM into lean tissue mass (FFM) and bone mineral content (BMC).
- Four-component (4-C) model that divides body mass into fat, mineral, water, and protein (intracellular water, extracellular water, dry lean mass, and body fat mass).

These body composition values are used to manage dietary regimes, create optimize, and evaluate the training programs of athletes [20]. The body fat percentage [21], and the sports training effect on bone mineral content [22, 25] also have been evaluated concerning the existent concern to the effects on menstrual function in young female athletes [26].

According to Loucks [27], the objectives of the training must be optimum body size for a specific sport, body composition, and mix of energy stored for maximizing their performance. Therefore, the training program for the athletes requires the control and measure of the balances of fat, protein, and carbohydrates, separately. This procedure is feasible by monitoring biomarkers of these objectives. The skinfolds and urinary ketones may be the best biomarkers of fat stores and carbohydrate deficiency, respectively.

SPECIAL REQUIREMENTS

Every person is different in the physiological and biochemical functions that outline their nutrient needs, and the athletes; not only have these differences, but they additionally have energy and nutrient specific requirements as a function of body size and training load [28]. For example, the physiological and metabolic requirements for extreme sports varied and their nutritional need is also diverse [29]. Therefore, sports must be well-known to calculate the necessary nutrients and caloric requirements of the athletes. There is a categorization reported in the literature, which includes watersports, adventure sports, motorsports, team sports, strength sports, ball sports, mountain sports, extreme sports, and shooting sports [30, 31].

Even more, Tarnopolsky's [32] classification introduces differences in the intensity of the type of sport performed by athletes and for hence in its nutritional requirement. The author classified them as recreational (low to moderate-intensity endurance exercise), modestly trained performance, top sport, or elite endurance.

In extreme sports (alpinism, racing, ultra-endurance activities, and expedition), which demand high energy quantity, athletes must plan carefully their dietary needed. Otherwise, an inadequate diet and poor fueling strategies should impair performance and increase the risk of injury and illness during events [28, 29].

Still more, athletes also like to make different food choices based in part on cultural and lifestyle issues, but perhaps more on personal taste preferences [2]. Therefore, traveling through different countries is a challenge that athletes must undergo. Therefore, athletes need time and mental effort to establish this unknown diet. Then, it could be an excellent help, if the industry provides athletes with food with their native eating patterns at the grocery shop. Expert recommendations and athletes' preferences are useful to define in terms of sport load, in each sport the optimum requirements of the protein, carbohydrate, fat, and all the vitamins and minerals that are essential for the athletes as a function of the sports performed [2, 30 - 32]. Under these concepts, the food industry must work on the development of food for athletes accessible and easy to cook.

ENERGY BALANCE AND AVAILABILITY

Athletes are susceptible to modify their energy availability, with the consequent impairment of hormone, immune, and metabolic function, in addition to irreversible loss of bone mass, which increases the risk of fractures and injury [31]. Frequently the athletes (especially females) that participate in endurance and aesthetic sports, and sports with weight classes are chronically energy deficient. Since the energy deficiencies impair the athlete's performance growth, and health, when managing the athlete's diets, the definition of availability of energy is more valuable than the balance of energy [32].

Energy availability is the amount of dietary energy remaining after exercise training useful for all other metabolic processes [33]. And the energy balance is the relation between intake of food and output of work (as in muscular or secretory activity) that is positive when the body stores extra food as fats and negative when the body draws on stored fat to provide energy for work [34].

The energetic cost of the physical activity measure is in Metabolic Equivalents of Task (MET), or Metabolic Equivalents. One MET is defined as 1kcal /kg/hour and is roughly equivalent to the energy cost of sitting quietly. A MET also is defined as; the oxygen uptake in ml/kg/min, with one, MET equal to the oxygen cost of sitting quietly, equivalent to 3.5 ml/kg/min [35, 36].

Ainsworth *et al.*, 2011 [37], have present a well-completed coding scheme for classifying physical activity by rate of energy expenditure, *i.e.*, by intensity. The Ainsworth compendium quantify the energy cost of physical activity (PA), research studies, and, in clinical settings, to write PA recommendations and to assess energy expenditure in individuals. Table **1** shows examples of MTEs/hours of some exercises. Ainsworth *et al.*, 2011 [37] have presented a well-completed coding scheme for classifying physical activity by rate of energy expenditure, *i.e.*, by intensity.

Table 1. Examples of MTEs/hours of some exercises [38].

Activities	METs/hr.	Activities	METs/hr.
Cycling	7,5-14	Resistance/weight training	5
Jogging/brisk walking	6	Weightlifting, water aerobics, golf (not carrying clubs), leisurely canoeing or kayaking,	3.5
Running	8-16	Rowing, canoeing, kayaking vigorously, dancing (vigorous), some exercise apparatuses	6-8
Skipping	8	Slow swimming, golf (carrying clubs)	4.5
Pilates/Tai chi	3	Singles tennis, squash, racquetball	7-12
Hiking	6-7	Jogging (1 mile every 12 min), Skiing downhill or cross country, Heavy farming work	8

MACRO AND MICRONUTRIENTS

Water

Water is vital for living and depending on age and body fatness, the human body is composed of 50-75% of water. During exercise the water regulates body temperature through perspiration (heat dissipation), maintaining the physical equilibrium by the physiological homeostasis [38, 39]. Athletes must drink water before, during, and after exercise, to minimize dehydration. It is common a sensible hypohydration (>2%) in athletes who perform exercises in a warm or cold location, and in altitude by loss of sweat or diuresis [40, 41].

The recommendations for athletes must be focused on drinking the optimal water quantities needed [39]. An excessive amount of liquid can cause hyponatremia (level of blood sodium below 136 mEq/L) due to the overwhelming kidneys' ability to excrete water, and by dilution of the sodium remnant in blood after its loss by sweat [42, 43]. The normal level of sodium in the blood must be maintained by a body mechanism between 136 to 142 mEq/L [44]. Marathons, triathlons, and other endurance athletic events are associated with hyponatremia [45]. The inclusion of sodium must be when sweat losses are high, especially if exercise lasts more than about 2 h. Also during recovery from exercise, rehydration should include the replacement of both water and salts lost in sweat [40].

Other fluids different from water can be ingested during endurance exercises, and it has been pointed out that they are more effective in improving performance [46]. The drink composition to maintain fluid and electrolyte balance is a function of the intensity and duration of the exercise task, the ambient temperature and humidity, and the physiological and biochemical characteristics of the individual athlete [40, 47]. The inclusion of carbohydrates in the drink will increase the fuel but decrease the rate of water availability [48]. Adding additional beverages to daily meals should be initiated when needed at least several hours before the activity, to enable fluid absorption and allow urine output to return to normal levels [49].

In 2008 SSN has expanded some of its fragments of the requirement of nutrients of this food pyramid for adults to cover the energy and nutrient necessary for daily exercise typically performed by athletes and actives individuals [50]. For example, at the base of the pyramid (beverage), they recommend that for each additional hour of exercise, it must be drunken 400-800 ml of sports drink. As a function of the type of sports athletes must prefer water over a sports drink, the sports drik can be used shortly before, during, or after the exercise and as required, additional water can be consumed before, during, and after exercise [51].

Carbohydrates

In a fatigued muscle force production is reduced. Muscle fatigue is a main common factor that limits athletic performance and other strenuous or prolonged activity [52]. Carbohydrates, such as starch, and sugars provide energy and muscle gain to athletes. To preserve homeostasis, most of the glucose and fat absorbed must be stored to be mobilized later at rates appropriate to bring about the oxidation of a fuel mix-matching, on average, the macronutrient distribution in the diet [53].

The depletion of stored carbohydrates would be the cause of fatigue in many athletes, and it declines their performance throughout the event. Therefore, carbohydrates are the most critical fuel in extreme sports athletes, due that the glycogen utilization is during the exercise. Low glycogen levels during hard training and competition will not only decrease performance but cause muscle damage. Consequently, the damaged muscle impairs proper muscle glycogen storage capacity creating a vicious cycle and lead to overtraining [54, 55].

To have a good glycogen store within muscle and liver, it is necessary to intake carbohydrates at appropriate time and composition [56]. Good glycogen storage has a beneficial carbohydrate availability impact during exercise and subsequent exercise performance [57]. To ensure optimal muscle and liver glycogen body stores, the carbohydrates must be intake during the hours or days before the event Carbohydrates should be provided in grams relative to the athlete's body mass, rather than as a percentage of total energy intakes [54, 56, 58]. Rather than talk about high or low carbohydrate diets, it should be thought about carbohydrate availability relative to the muscle's fuel needs as is shown in Table **2**.

Table 2. Carbohydrate needs for the athlete's muscles [57, 59].

Strategy	Training Load	Carbohydrate Intake Targets (g per kg of the athlete's body mass)
Light	Low intensity or skill-based activities	3-5 g/kg
Moderate	Moderate exercise program (*i.e.* ~1 hr. per day	5-7 g/kg/d
High	Endurance program (*e.g.* 1-3 hrs. per day of mod-high intensity exercise)	*6-10 g/kg/d

*This range is depending on the gender and physical fitness level of the individual, total training load, energy expenditure, type of physical activity, and environment.

Carbohydrates are in many different foods, some of these foods include Cereals (corn tortillas, whole wheat pasta, and bread, brown rice, whole oats, or 100% whole-grain cereal), and other grains (spelt, amaranth quinoa, beans), fruits fresh, frozen or canned in its juices, starchy vegetables; like potatoes, sweet potato or other yams, milk and milk products (*e.g.*, yogurt), foods containing added sugars (*e.g.*, desserts and sodas). To elaborate diets, the athletes can consult the expanded food pyramid, of the Swiss Society of Nutrition [52]. In this pyramid, they recommend that for each hour of exercise, add 1 serving of whole grain and legumes. When exercising more than 2 hours a day, sports food /drinks can also be used instead of food from the basis pyramid. 1 serving of sports food is equal to 60-90 g of a bar, 50- 70 g carbohydrate gel, or 300- 400 ml of a regeneration drink [54].

Proteins

Proteins are biological polymers built with approximately 20 amino acids, with significant body physiological functions [60]. The amino acids building the protein can be essential (cannot are produced by the body), non-essential (the body make them in enough amounts) and conditionally essential (the body can produce them in adequate amount, but in body stressed or physiologically challenged, its production rates become inadequate) [60]. Table **3** shown that proteins require for sport type.

Unlike carbohydrates or fat, there are not protein reservoirs, however, the body has pools of amino acids. These pools are in constant go out and flow upon physiological supply and demand [61, 62].

The recommendations of protein intake for athletes from the American College of Sports [2] are: for endurance 1.2 to 1.4 g/kg per day, and for strength athletes, 1.2 to 1.7 g/kg per day, and protein intake should increase in extreme sports athletes.

Even more, San Millán [58], pointed out that protein intake with a good biological value of amino acid profile should be higher in an athlete.

Burke [59] pointed out that using the food pyramid for athletes of the Swiss Society of Nutrition, the athletes could be provided by protein intake of about 1.9 g of protein per kg body mass when eating for 3–4 hours of exercise per day. Additional servings from the meat and dairy food group of the pyramid would push the protein intake up to 3 g per kg body mass or more. Even more, the author postulated that the protein intake in sports with relatively low energy budgets, including particularly strength and sprint events, is already high with few extra servings [59].

Some protein supplements, as beta-alanine, should enhance performance in some extreme sports that involve repetitive and overcharges movements [33].

Fats

The bulk of body dietary energy is providing by the stored carbohydrates and fats. On the other hand, there is a relationship between the body's carbohydrate economy and fat intake. Fat intake and glycogen concentrations are determinants of fat oxidation, and the amount of fat has to be eaten [56].

Table 3. Protein requirement for athletes. Modified [3, 60].

Protein Requirements	
Endurance Athletes	Strength and Power Athletes
It depends upon many factors, including volume, intensity, and duration of the training, the gender of the athlete (for men are ~25% greater than those for women), energy and carbohydrate intake, and the current fitness level or training status of the athlete. It remains that recreational athletes performing low to moderate-intensity endurance activity do not have increased requirements for dietary protein, whereas modestly trained athletes may have a 25% increase in protein needs (to ~ 1.1 g/kg/day). Only elite athletes or those with exemplary fitness status and who are performing extremely high volumes of training exhibit markedly increased protein requirements, which amount to approximately 1.6 g/kg/day	Protein needs are increased when athletes are regularly performing the exercise of appropriate intensity, volume, and duration. Recent statements reveal that a protein intake of 1.2-2.0 g/kg/day could be the protein needs of exercising athletes. Other specific considerations such as energy and carbohydrate intake, gender (particularly for endurance athletes), and training status are required. Athletes do an exceptional job when consuming greater recommended amounts of protein (1.33 g/kg/day). It is evident, with which to advise athletes against protein supplementation, other factors such as optimal nutrient timing, and leucine and essential amino acid intake during acute or immediate recovery are part of these recommendations.

Vitamins and Minerals

Vitamins and minerals are micronutrients needed for the athlete's body health and to perform at best athletically. Despite this, they do not provide energy, they have important actions in the metabolism of carbohydrates and fats, contributing hence to the provision of muscle fuel during exercise and in repairing and built muscles in response to training. Vitamin and minerals act as a cofactor of enzymes that are involved in several physiological roles in the body and support growth and development, muscle contraction, hydration balance, nerve function, energy metabolism, tissue repair, bone metabolism, the transport of oxygen throughout your body, and immune function.

Regarding intake of the essential vitamins and minerals, here is a message for athletes: Eat a variety of food in an adequate amount to consuming the calories and vitamins and minerals needed, because more is not better. In case of having a dietary restriction, close the micronutrient gap by eating fortified foods or vitamins in certain circumstances (extra calcium and vitamin D for endurance exercise, and Vitamin C to avoid the risk of catching a chest cold). Intake of supplements must be in balance, including sodium, when rehydrating.

GOALS OF AN ADEQUATE SPORTS DIET

In athletic competition, the gap between triumph and defeat is small; therefore, taking care of detail could establish the difference [60]. According to Maughan [63], although athletes are supplementing their diet with protein, vitamins, minerals, and exotic compounds, several important key dietary issues are frequently neglected. It is recommended to eat a meal before the game. The preevent meal serves two purposes: To keep the athlete from feeling hungry and supply the athlete with enough energy and fluids for practice and competition.

Athlete's vital goals are to cover their need for body energy and maintaining mass and body fat at appropriate levels. Maughan [63] also has reported that during training the glycogen level is maintained with an adequate carbohydrate intake (in food type and time). During the post-exercise periods, the ingestion of protein promotes the process of adaptation in the muscle's protein synthesis.

SUPPLEMENTS AND PERFORMANCE ENHANCERS

What is a Supplement?

The DSHEA Congress [64] has defined the term "dietary supplement" in the Dietary Supplement Health and Education Act of 1994, as a product taken by mouth that contains a "dietary ingredient" intended to supplement the diet. The "dietary ingredients" in these products may include vitamins, minerals, herbs or other botanicals, amino acids, and substances such as enzymes, organ tissues, glandular, and metabolites. Dietary supplements can also be extracts or concentrates and may be found in many forms such as tablets, capsules, soft gels, gel caps, liquids, or powders. They can also be in other forms, such as a bar, but if they are, information on their label must not represent the product as a conventional food or a sole item of a meal or diet.

Dietary Supplement Health and Education Act, described also a dietary supplement as a product, other than tobacco, which is used in conjunction with a healthy diet and contains one or more of the following dietary ingredients: a vitamin, mineral, herb or other botanical, an amino acid, a dietary substance for use by man to supplement the diet by increasing the total daily intake, or a concentrate, metabolite, constituent, extract, or combinations of these ingredients [65, 66].

Maughan *et al* [67], define a dietary supplement as the following: A food, food component, nutrient, or non-food compound that is purposefully ingested in addition to the habitually consumed diet to achieve a specific health and performance benefit. While, Bishop [68] defined dietary supplements as any product taken by the mouth, in addition to foods proposed to have a performance enhancing effect.

Dietary Supplements used by Athletes are:

- D-Ribose a five-carbon sugar (D-ribose), which is synthesized by the body, but is also available in small amounts in the diet from vegetables. Researchers have postulated that the NoVo synthesis of nucleotides depends on the ribose amount in the muscle. These nucleotides shall help in turn to the restoration of the immediate muscle energy stores (ATP, ADP, and AMP), losses by the intense exercise [69]. This sugar is a well tolerate legal substance when consuming during exercise as a supplement. It has not yet checked the adverse effects [64]. The recommended dose is 3 g daily, 30 minutes before physical training. The intake of 2.5 g, 30 minutes before physical exercise, and another 2.5 g, just after finishing exercise is another possibility.

- Caffeine (1, 3, 7-trimethylxanthine) highly consumed alkaloid through coffee, tea, and cola, chocolate, and energizer drinks. It has been reported that caffeine actions are on the adenosine receptors, central nervous system, increasing $Na^+/K^+ATPase$ activity, mobilization of intracellular calcium, and increasing plasma catecholamine concentration [70]. It has been shown evidence that caffeine supports the performance-enhancing of prolonged endurance exercise. There are limited researches that have investigated the effects of caffeine on single-sprint, multiple-sprint, or team-sport performance [70]. Doses of ingestion of 3–9 mg/kg of caffeine approximately 60 min before exercise are recommended. The caffeine magnitude effect on the performance differs substantially between athletes, ranging from highly ergogenic to ergolytic. A low dose of caffeine is safe, but a high dose is associated with adverse health effects [70].

–Creatinine is a non-essential (free and phosphorylated) guanidine compound, which is stored in skeletal muscle in 95%. It can come from diet or synthesized from the amino acids glycine, arginine, and methionine [71]. Creatinine supplementation increase both total and Pcreatine (creatine), and glycogen storage in muscle. Results of the study of Kreider *et al.* [76] support that 9-56 g/d of creatine supplementation may enhance the quality of training leading to improved repetitive sprint performance and strength.

- Chromium. At conventional doses (40 to 200 µg), chromium supplementation in healthy adult athletes is safe. Chromium body store by its supplementation improves insulin efficiency, impacting the high-level athletic performance. However, there are some concerns, especially about individuals who exceed the recommended loading and maintenance chromium doses [72].

- Branched-chain amino acids (BCAAs; leucine, isoleucine, valine) are short-chain of essential amino acids. They can mitigate fatigue during exercise, acting on serotonin metabolism [73]. In addition to this potential acute effect on performance, it is also reported that BCAAs supplementation, before and after exercise, has beneficial effects for decreasing exercise-induced muscle damage and promoting muscle protein synthesis [73]. BCAAs are considered relatively safe with only mild concern that high doses may cause gastrointestinal distress or interfere with the absorption of other amino acids [74]. The supplementation strategy combined a high daily BCAAs intake (>200 mg kg-1 day-1) for a long time (>10 days); it was especially effective if taken before the damaging exercise.

ß-alanine (non-essential amino acid) is the precursor of the carnitine (ß-alanin-L-histidine). Carnitine is an important muscle buffer, which acts on the accumulation of H+ that affects muscle contraction during the exercise [75]. It also reduces the rate of anaerobic energy production, greater muscle buffering (*via* ß–alanine supplementation) may translate to improvements in multiple-sprint performance. According to Bellinger [76], the use of ß-alanine goes beyond supplementation to enhance sports performance, but also as a training aid to augment bouts of high-intensity training. The author suggests that the supplementation (4-6g/d) with β-alanine increases resistance training performance and training volume in team-sport athletes, which may allow for greater overload and superior adaptations compared with training alone.

- Alkalizing agents, (bicarbonates and citrates) are alkalizing substances that act as a buffer in an acid medium. Its effect has been demonstrated on muscle fatigue, in lactic-anaerobic exercises (short-term and intermittent efforts, with short periods of rest) due to its extracellular buffering capacity (neutralize lactic acid) and the improvement of the hydrogen ions flow of muscle blood, keeping the pH close to the normal range despite the effort physical. The ingestion of alkalinizing agents usually at 300 ppm should help to reduce the potential adverse effects of H+ accumulation on repeated-sprint and high-intensity running performance [77].

Limmer *et al.* [78], have found higher blood lactate concentrations in moderately trained participants under the alkalizing diet. It is suggesting an enhanced blood or muscle buffer capacity. Thus, an alkalizing diet may be an easy and natural way to enhance 400-m sprint performance for athletes without the necessity of taking artificial dietary supplements. It recently demonstrated that the ingestion of alkalizing agents (either sodium bicarbonate or sodium citrate) reduces the exercise-induced increase in extracellular K+ [77].

At recommended doses, alkaline supplementation is safe, but excessive doses may cause metabolic alkalosis producing heart arrhythmias. They may also cause gastrointestinal side effects (abdominal pain, nausea, cramps, and diarrhea) in some subjects [77].

–Bovine colostrum is the first milk secreted by cows. Bovine colostrum contains several proteins, immune components, and hormones that are similar to the bioactive compounds present in human colostrum. Despite the widespread use of colostrum supplementation among athletes in a dose of 10g/d, the researches on the side effects of colostrum on exercise performance are ambiguous.

It has been pointed out that supply colostrum has benefits for the immune system, intestinal barrier, and mood. It has been also reported a positive effect on endurance. Bovine colostrum effect on the anaerobic efficiency is not fully confirmed, but possible. Researchers have shown conflicting data on the impact of colostrum on the health and physical performance of athletes. Therefore, it is necessary to carry out further properly prepared clinical trials using standardized doses of colostrum and sufficiently long supplementation periods [79].

- Beta-hydroxy-beta-methyl butyrate (HMB) or Calcium-HMB-monohydrate is a natural metabolite produced endogenously in small amounts. It also comes to diet from plants (*e.g.*, citrus fruits), and animals (*e.g.*, catfish, breast milk) foods. HMB as a supplement act as an anti-catabolic agent, improve skeletal muscle mass and strength in athletes, decrease exercise-induced muscle damage, and promote the synthesis of cholesterol needed to form and stabilize cell membranes, and minimize cell breakdown and cell damages [80].

With no report of adverse effect on short-term studies (8-10 weeks) the recommended doses of HMB are 3g /d. However, there is currently no data on the long-term> 8 weeks effect of the HMB supplementation when taking more of the recommended dose [81, 82].

RECIPES

Quick Energy Bite

Ingredients

250g	Peanut butter
250g	Honey
37g	Whey Protein, vanilla (preferred brand)
500g	Oats (uncooked)
500g	Rice Krispies cereal
150g	Raisins (dried grapes)
150g	Craisins (dried cranberries)
100g	Sunflower seeds, unsalted
10g	Peanuts unsalted

Preparation

Mix peanut butter and honey in a big bowl. Add vanilla protein and mix add oat and crispy rice mixing. Add the rest of the ingredients and knead by hand. Roll the dough into balls or put the snack on a cookie sheet, freeze it for 10 minutes, then cut into bite sizes. Note: It can add, switch, or remove any ingredients.

Avocado Cocoa Smoothie

Ingredients

100g	Avocado flesh, cold (~ 1/2 Hass avocado)	60g	Greek yogurt, plain or coconut cream (vegan option)
30g	Dutch-process cocoa powder	80g	1% Low-Fat Milk, (for vegan, use non-dairy milk)
120g	Banana, cold without the peel	3g	Vanilla extract

Preparation

Blend everything in a food processor until it is very creamy. Add more milk if it is necessary to reach the desired thickness.

Protein Acai Bowl

Ingredients

	Base	-	Topping
200g	Strawberries (frozen)	20g	Strawberries (fresh)
500ml	Almond milk	20g	Banana (fresh) slides
37g	Whey Protein powder	10g	Chia seeds
30g	Acai powder	10g	Granola
60g	Banana	-	-

Preparation

Place the base ingredients in your food processor and pulse until blended. Transfer mixture to two bowls and serve with your choice of toppings.

Pumpkin Cream

Ingredients

200g	Pumpkin flour (see Chapter 2)	2g	Garlic powder
10g	Corn starch	750ml	Vegetable or Chicken Broth/stock, low sodium
37g	Soy protein powder (isolate)	250ml	Water
10g	Onion powder	-	Salt and pepper to taste

Ingredients for finished

125-185ml	Cream, half and half, or milk (for vegan, use non-dairy milk).
10g	Crouton

Preparation

Place the pumpkin flour, onion, garlic, broth, and water in a pot. Bring to a boil, continue stirring, then reduce heat and let simmer until acquire a creamy consistency, about 10 minutes. Remove from heat and add the soy protein and season to taste with salt and pepper, stir through cream (never boil the soup after adding cream, it split).

Ladle soup into bowls, drizzle over a bit of cream, and sprinkle with pepper and parsley if desired. Serve with crusty bread.

Beetroot-Chocolate Chips Cookies

(Adapted from https://veggiedesserts.com/beetroot-chocolate-chunk-cookies/)

Ingredients

100g	Beetroot flour (see chapter 1)
150g	Wheat all-purpose flour
175 g	Ghee or grass-fed butter
50g	Honey
4g	Sugar
20g	Pea protein isolate
3.5g	Baking Soda (sodium bicarbonate)
3.5g	Baking powder
3.5g	Vanilla, pure, extract
1.2g	Salt
250g	Dark Chocolate chips

Preparation

Preheat your oven to 350 °F (175 °C) and line a large cookie sheet with parchment paper. Using an electric hand mixer, cream together the ghee (or butter), honey, sugar, and vanilla until smooth on medium speed Add in the pea protein isolate and beat on low speed until combined. In a separate bowl, combine the dry ingredients, then add dry mixture to wet, beating on low speed until smooth. Stir in chocolate chips, then chill the dough for 10-15 minutes in the fridge. Using a medium cookie scoop, scoop dough onto a prepared cookie sheet about 2" apart. Bake in the preheated oven for 10 minutes or until cookies are golden brown. Allow the cookies to cool completely on the baking sheet; do not transfer them while they are cooling. Once completely cool to the touch, remove from sheet, and serve.

CONSENT FOR PUBLICATION

Not Applicable.

CONFLICT OF INTEREST

The author confirms that this chapter contents have no conflict of interest.

ACKNOWLEDGEMENT

Declared none.

REFERENCES

[1]   Wisewell A. Energy balance, body mass, and body composition. A complete nutrition guide for athletes.2013, pp 5.

[2]   Rodriguez NR, DiMarco NM, Langley LS. Dietitians of Canada; American College of Sports Medicine: Nutrition and Athletic Performance. J Am Diet Assoc 2009; 109(3): 509-27.
[http://dx.doi.org/10.1016/j.jada.2009.01.005] [PMID: 19278045]

[3]   Rodriguez NR, Di Marco NM, Langley S. American College of Sports Medicine position stand. Nutrition and athletic performance. Med Sci Sports Exerc 2009; 41(3): 709-31.
[PMID: 19225360]

[4]   Beck KL, Thomson JS, Swift RJ, von Hurst PR. Role of nutrition in performance enhancement and postexercise recovery. Open Access J Sports Med 2015; 6: 259-67.
[http://dx.doi.org/10.2147/OAJSM.S33605] [PMID: 26316828]

[5]   Dietary Guidelines for Americans. 2020. https://health.gov

[6]   Atwater WO. Methods and results of investigations on the chemistry and economy of food 1895.

[7]   Webb Kelley J. What is the difference between calories & calories from fat?
https://www.livestrong.com/article/75656-difference-between-calories-calories/

[8]   Youdim A. Carbohydrates, proteins, and fats 2018.https://www.msdmanuals.com

[9]   O'Neil CE, Keast DR, Fulgoni VL, Nicklas TA. Food sources of energy and nutrients among adults in the US: NHANES 2003–2006. Nutrients, 2012; 4(12):2097-120..

[10]   Hall KD, Bemis T, Brychta R, *et al.* Calorie for calorie, dietary fat restriction results in more body fat loss than carbohydrate restriction in people with obesity. Cell Metab 2015; 1; 22(3): 427-436..

[11]   Ackland TR, Lohman TG, Sundgot-Borgen J, *et al.* Current status of body composition assessment in sport: review and position statement on behalf of the ad hoc research working group on body composition health and performance, under the auspices of the I.O.C. Medical Commission. Sports Med 2012; 42(3): 227-49.
[http://dx.doi.org/10.2165/11597140-000000000-00000] [PMID: 22303996]

[12]   Wells JCK, Fewtrell MS. Measuring body composition. Arch Dis Child 2006; 91(7): 612-7.
[http://dx.doi.org/10.1136/adc.2005.085522] [PMID: 16790722]

[13]   Lara J, Siervo M, Bertoli S, *et al.* Accuracy of three novel predictive methods for measurements of fat mass in healthy older subjects. Aging Clin Exp Res 2014; 26(3): 319-25.
[http://dx.doi.org/10.1007/s40520-013-0169-8] [PMID: 24214485]

[14]   Siervo M, Jebb SA. Body composition assessment: theory into practice: introduction of multicompartment models. IEEE Eng Med Biol Mag 2010; 29(1): 48-59.
[http://dx.doi.org/10.1109/MEMB.2009.935471] [PMID: 20176522]

[15]   Lee SY, Gallagher D. Assessment methods in human body composition. Curr Opin Clin Nutr Metab Care 2008; 11(5): 566-72.
[http://dx.doi.org/10.1097/MCO.0b013e32830b5f23] [PMID: 18685451]

[16]   Toomey CM, Cremona A, Hughes K, Norton C. A review of body composition measurement in the assessment of health. Topics Clin Nutr 2015; 30(1): 16-32.
[http://dx.doi.org/10.1097/TIN.0000000000000017]

[17] Ellis KJ. Human body composition: *in vivo* methods. Physiol Rev 2000; 80(2): 649-80.
[http://dx.doi.org/10.1152/physrev.2000.80.2.649] [PMID: 10747204]

[18] Kuriyan R. Body composition techniques. Indian J Med Res 2018; 148(5): 648-58.
[http://dx.doi.org/10.4103/ijmr.IJMR_1777_18] [PMID: 30666990]

[19] Wilmore JH, Buskirk ER, DiGirolamo M, Lohman TG. Body Composition. Phys Sportsmed 1986; 14(3): 144-62.
[http://dx.doi.org/10.1080/00913847.1986.11709016] [PMID: 27467347]

[20] Carlson JS, Khosrozadeh H, Herndon DN. Nutritional Needs and Support for the Burned Patient. 2018.

[21] Kravitz L, Heyward V. Getting a grip on body composition. IDEA Today 1992; 10(4): 34-9.

[22] Schutz Y, Kyle UUG, Pichard C. Fat-free mass index and fat mass index percentiles in Caucasians aged 18-98 y. Int J Obes Relat Metab Disord 2002; 26(7): 953-60.
[http://dx.doi.org/10.1038/sj.ijo.0802037] [PMID: 12080449]

[23] Sinha J, Duffull SB, Al-Sallami HS. Sinha J, Duffull SB, Al-Sallami HS. (2018). A review of the methods and associated mathematical models used in the measurement of fat-free mass. 2018. Available from https://doi.org

[24] Moon JR. Body composition in athletes and sports nutrition: an examination of the bioimpedance analysis technique. Eur J Clin Nutr 2013; 67 (Suppl. 1): S54-9.
[http://dx.doi.org/10.1038/ejcn.2012.165] [PMID: 23299872]

[25] Malina RM, Geithner CA. Body composition of young athletes. Am J Lifestyle Med 2011; 5(3): 262-78.
[http://dx.doi.org/10.1177/1559827610392493]

[26] Roupas ND, Georgopoulos NA. Menstrual function in sports. Hormones (Athens) 2011; 10(2): 104-16.
[http://dx.doi.org/10.14310/horm.2002.1300] [PMID: 21724535]

[27] Loucks AB. Energy balance and body composition in sports and exercise. J Sports Sci 2004; 22(1): 1-14.
[http://dx.doi.org/10.1080/0264041031000140518] [PMID: 14974441]

[28] Burke LM. Burke LM. Energy needs for athletes. Can. J. Appl. Physiol 2011; 26 Suppl (6): S202-219

[29] Adams BB, Aliverti A, Andrianopoulos V, Bahr R, Becker J, *et al.* Extreme Sports Medicine. 2017.

[30] Mitchell JH, Gunnar Blomqvist C, Haskell WL. Classification of sports. J Am Coll Cardiol 1985; 6(6): 1198-9.
[http://dx.doi.org/10.1016/S0735-1097(85)80200-X] [PMID: 2577752]

[31] Clifford J, Maloney K. Nutrition for athletes. Colorado State University. Extension. 2018. Available from: https://extension.colostate.edu

[32] Tarnopolsky M. Protein requirements for endurance athletes. Nutrition 2004; 20(7-8): 662-8.
[http://dx.doi.org/10.1016/j.nut.2004.04.008] [PMID: 15212749]

[33] Ranchordas MK, Hudson S, Thompson SW. Nutrition for extreme sports.Extreme sports medicine. New York: Springer, Champ 2017.
[http://dx.doi.org/10.1007/978-3-319-28265-7_2]

[34] World Athletic/International Amateur Athletic Federation (IAAF). Nutrition for athletic. A practical guide for eating and drinking for health and performance in track and field. Based on an IAAF international consensus conference 2007. Updated June 2011. 2013

[35] Loucks AB, Kiens B, Wright HH. Energy availability in athletes, J Sports Sci 2011; 29(sup1): S7-S15.

[36] Loucks AB. Low energy availability in the marathon and other endurance sports. Sports Med 2007; 37(4-5): 348-52.
[http://dx.doi.org/10.2165/00007256-200737040-00019] [PMID: 17465605]

[37] Ainsworth BE, Haskell WL, Herrmann SD, *et al.* 2011 Compendium of Physical Activities: a second update of codes and MET values. Med Sci Sports Exerc 2011; 43(8): 1575-81.
[http://dx.doi.org/10.1249/MSS.0b013e31821ece12] [PMID: 21681120]

[38] TopenSports. Energy expenditure of activities 2020. https://www.topendsports.com/weight-loss/energy-met.htm

[39] Functions of Water in the Human Body. https://www.ive.edu.hk/cw/wc/html/en/cw_campus_offices_wellc_files/pdf/Function%20of%20water%20in%20the%20human%20body.pdf

[40] Ainsworth BE, Haskell WL, Herrmann SD, *et al.* The Compendium of Physical Activities Tracking Guide https://sites.google.com/site/compendiumofphysicalactivities/

[41] Helmenstine AM. How Much of Your Body Is Water? 2020. https://www.thoughtco.com/how-muc--of-your-body-is-water-609406

[42] Shirreff SM. Hydration in sport and exercise: water, sports drinks, and other drinks. FNB 2009; 34: 374-9.
[http://dx.doi.org/10.1111/j.1467-3010.2009.01790.x]

[43] Almond CS, Shin AY, Fortescue EB, *et al.* Hyponatremia among runners in the Boston Marathon. N Engl J Med 2005; 352(15): 1550-6.
[http://dx.doi.org/10.1056/NEJMoa043901] [PMID: 15829535]

[44] Sawka MN, Cheuvront SN, Kenefick RW. Hypohydration and Human Performance: Impact of Environment and Physiological Mechanisms. Sports Med 2015; 45(1) (Suppl. 1): S51-60.
[http://dx.doi.org/10.1007/s40279-015-0395-7] [PMID: 26553489]

[45] Quinn E. Proper Hydration for Athletes. 2018. Available from: https://www.verywellfit.com

[46] Mayo Clinic. https://www.mayoclinic.org/diseases-conditions/hyponatremia/symptoms-causes/s-c-20373711#:~:text=Drinking%20excessive%20amounts%20of%20water,Hormonal%20changes2007.

[47] Mitchell Rosner M, Kirven J. Exercise-associated hyponatremia. Clin. J. Am. Soc. Nephr 2007; 2(1):151-61.

[48] Vist GE, Maughan RJ. The effect of osmolality and carbohydrate content on the rate of gastric emptying of liquids in man. J Physiol 1995; 486(Pt 2): 523-31.
[http://dx.doi.org/10.1113/jphysiol.1995.sp020831] [PMID: 7473216]

[49] Verbalis JG, Goldsmith SR, Greenberg A, *et al.* Diagnosis, evaluation, and treatment of hyponatremia: expert panel recommendations. Am J Med 2013; 126(10) (Suppl. 1): S1-S42.
[http://dx.doi.org/10.1016/j.amjmed.2013.07.006] [PMID: 24074529]

[50] Garth AK, Burke LM. What do athletes drink during competitive sporting activities? Sports Med 2013; 43(7): 539-64.
[http://dx.doi.org/10.1007/s40279-013-0028-y] [PMID: 23529286]

[51] Sawka MN, Burke LM, Eichner ER, Maughan RJ, Montain SJ, Stachenfeld NS. American College of Sports Medicine position stand. Exercise and fluid replacement. Med Sci Sports Exerc 2007; 39(2): 377-90.

[52] Walter P, Infanger E, Mühlemann P. Food pyramid of the swiss society for nutrition. Ann Nutr Metab 2007; 51 (Suppl. 2): 15-20.
[http://dx.doi.org/10.1159/000103562]

[53] Samuel M. A food pyramid for Swiss athletes. Interview by Louise M. Burke. Int J Sport Nutr Exerc Metab 2008; 18(4): 430-7.
[http://dx.doi.org/10.1123/ijsnem.18.4.430] [PMID: 18708690]

[54] Murphy M. Hydration and the marathon runner 2020. http://www.mbsfitness.com/hydration- and-marathon-runner.php

[55] Wan J-J, Qin Z, Wang P-Y, Sun Y, Liu X. Muscle fatigue: general understanding and treatment. Exp Mol Med 2017; 49(10): e384-9.
[http://dx.doi.org/10.1038/emm.2017.194] [PMID: 28983090]

[56] Flatt JP. Use and storage of carbohydrate and fat. Am J Clin Nutr 1995; 61(4) (Suppl.): 952S-9S.
[http://dx.doi.org/10.1093/ajcn/61.4.952S] [PMID: 7900694]

[57] Nutrition Working Group of the International Olympic Committee; Medical and Scientific Commission of the International Olympic Committee. 2016. https://library.olympic.org

[58] SanMillán I. The importance of nutrition in extreme sports-feeding the beast 2018. Available from: https://fdocuments.in/download/the-importance-of-nutrition-in-extreme-sports-fee-ing-the-importance-of-nutrition

[59] Burke LM, Hawley JA, Wong SHS, Jeukendrup AE. Carbohydrates for training and competition. J Sports Sci 2011; 29(sup1): S17-S27.

[60] Kerksick CM, Kulovitz M. Requirements of energy, carbohydrates, proteins, and fats for athletes.Nutrition and Enhanced Sports Performance Muscle Building, Endurance, and Strength. New York: Academic PressElsevier 2013; pp. 355-66.
[http://dx.doi.org/10.1016/B978-0-12-396454-0.00036-9]

[61] Wolfe RR. Regulation of skeletal muscle protein metabolism in catabolic states. Curr Opin Clin Nutr Metab Care 2005; 8(1): 61-5.
[http://dx.doi.org/10.1097/00075197-200501000-00009] [PMID: 15586001]

[62] Wolfe RR. The underappreciated role of muscle in health and disease. Am J Clin Nutr 2006; 84(3): 475-82.
[http://dx.doi.org/10.1093/ajcn/84.3.475] [PMID: 16960159]

[63] Maughan R. The athlete's diet: nutritional goals and dietary strategies. Proc Nutr Soc 2002; 61(1): 87-96.
[http://dx.doi.org/10.1079/PNS2001132] [PMID: 12002799]

[64] Food Drug Administration (FDA). Questions and Answers on Dietary Supplements 2019.https://www.fda.gov/food/information-consumers-using-diet-ry-supplements/questions-and-answers-dietary-supplements

[65] U.S. Navy Aeromedical Reference and Waiver Guide. https://www.med.navy.mil/sites/nmotc/nami/arwg/Documents/WaiverGuide/19_Dietary_Supplements.pdf

[66] National Institute of Health. 1994.https://ods.od.nih.gov

[67] Maughan RJ, Burke LM, Dvorak J, Larson-Meyer DE, Peeling P, Phillips SM, *et al.* IOC consensus statement: dietary supplements and the high-performance athlete. Int J Sport Nutr Exerc Metab 2008; 52: 439-55.
[PMID: 29589768]

[68] Bishop D. Dietary supplements and team-sport performance. Sports Med 2010; 40(12): 995-1017.
[http://dx.doi.org/10.2165/11536870-000000000-00000] [PMID: 21058748]

[69] Seifert JG, Brumet A, St Cyr JA. The influence of D-ribose ingestion and fitness level on performance and recovery. J Int Soc Sports Nutr 2017; 14: 47.
[http://dx.doi.org/10.1186/s12970-017-0205-8] [PMID: 29296106]

[70] Pickering C, Kiely J. Are the current guidelines on caffeine use in sport optimal for everyone? Inter-individual variation in caffeine ergogenicity, and a move towards personalised sports nutrition. Sports Med 2018; 48(1): 7-16.
[http://dx.doi.org/10.1007/s40279-017-0776-1] [PMID: 28853006]

[71]   Kreider RB, Ferreira M, Wilson M, *et al.* Effects of creatine supplementation on body composition, strength, and sprint performance. Med Sci Sports Exerc 1998; 30(1): 73-82.
[http://dx.doi.org/10.1097/00005768-199801000-00011] [PMID: 9475647]

[72]   Lefavi RG, Anderson RA, Keith RE, Wilson GD, McMillan JL, Stone MH. Efficacy of chromium supplementation in athletes: emphasis on anabolism. Int J Sport Nutr 1992; 2(2): 111-22.
[http://dx.doi.org/10.1123/ijsn.2.2.111] [PMID: 1299487]

[73]   Blomstrand E. A role for branched-chain amino acids in reducing central fatigue. J Nutr 2006; 136(2): 544S-7S.
[http://dx.doi.org/10.1093/jn/136.2.544S] [PMID: 16424144]

[74]   Holeček M. Branched-chain amino acids in health and disease: metabolism, alterations in blood plasma, and as supplements. Nutr Metab (Lond) 2018; 15: 33.
[http://dx.doi.org/10.1186/s12986-018-0271-1]

[75]   Jones AM. Buffers and their role in the nutritional preparation of athletes 2014.https://www.gssiweb.org/sports-science-exchange/article/sse-124-buf-ers-and-their-role-in-the-nutritional-preparation-of-athletes

[76]   Bellinger PM. β-Alanine supplementation for athletic performance: an update. J Strength Cond Res 2014; 28(6): 1751-70.
[http://dx.doi.org/10.1519/JSC.0000000000000327] [PMID: 24276304]

[77]   Palacios Gil de Antuñano N, Manonelles Marqueta P. Suplementos nutricionales para el deportista. Ayudas ergogénicas en el deporte - 2019. Documento de consenso de la Sociedad Española de Medicina del Deporte. Arch Med Deporte 2019; 36 (Suppl. 1): 7-83.

[78]   Limmer M, Eibl AD, Platen P. Enhanced 400-m sprint performance in moderately trained participants by a 4-day alkalizing diet: a counterbalanced, randomized controlled trial. J Int Soc Sports Nutr 2018; 15(1): 25.
[http://dx.doi.org/10.1186/s12970-018-0231-1] [PMID: 29855319]

[79]   Główka N, Woźniewicz M. Potential use of Colostrum Bovinum supplementation in athletes - A review. Acta Sci Pol Technol Aliment 2019; 18(2): 115-23.
[PMID: 31256539]

[80]   Pinheiro CH, Guimarães-Ferreira L, Gerlinger-Romero F, Curi R. An Overview on Beta-hydrox--beta-methylbutyrate (HMB) Supplementation in Skeletal Muscle Function and Sports Performance Nutrition and Enhanced Sports Performance Muscle Building, Endurance, and Strength USA. Academic Press 2013; pp. 455-63.

[81]   Wilson G, Wilson JM. 2008.https://www.ncbi.nlm.nih.gov/pmc/articles/PMC2245953/

[82]   Kreider RB, Ferreira M, Wilson M, Almada AL. Int J Sports Med. Effects of calcium beta-hydrox--beta-methylbutyrate (HMB) supplementation during resistance-training on markers of catabolism, body composition and strength 1999; 20(8):503-9.

CHAPTER 5

Foods For Diabetics

Elevina Pérez Sira[1,*]

[1] *Instituto de Ciencia y Tecnología de Alimentos, Facultad de Ciencias, Universidad Central de Venezuela, Caracas, Venezuela*

Abstract: The chapter deals with diabetes overview, focuses on the relation of diet and diabetes, the conventional and non-conventional raw material for the development of foods for the diabetic. The chapter also discusses natural and synthetic sweeteners' overview. Dietary approaches to produce food for diabetic consumers also are addressed, with special emphasis on foods with insulin-secreting, insulin-sensitizing, and insulin-mimetic properties. Also, the terms: glycemic index, insulin index, and glycemic load are defined. And finally, some recipes for diabetic consumers are recommended.

Keywords: Diabetes, *Diabetes Mellitus*, Food for diabetic, Non-conventional raw material, Nutrition, Special dietary regimen, Sweeteners.

INTRODUCTION

Diabetes, often referred, as *Diabetes Mellitus* (D.M.) is a group of metabolic disorders characterized by the presence of hyperglycemia in the absence of treatment, due to defective insulin secretion, defective insulin action, or both, and disturbances of carbohydrate, fat, and protein metabolism [1 - 4]. The long-term specific effects of diabetes include retinopathy, nephropathy, and neuropathy, among other complications [5].

Diabetes prevalence, deaths attributable to diabetes, and health expenditure due to diabetes continue to rise across the globe with important social, financial, and people who have diabetes are also at increased risk of other diseases, including heart, peripheral arterial and cerebrovascular disease, obesity, cataracts, erectile dysfunction, and nonalcoholic fatty liver disease [6].

People with diabetes are also at increased risk of some infectious diseases, such as tuberculosis [4].

---

[*] **Corresponding author Elevina Pérez Sira:** Instituto de Ciencia y Tecnología de Alimentos, Facultad de Ciencias, Universidad Central de Venezuela, Caracas, Venezuela; Tel: +58.212.751 4403; Fax: +58.212.751 3871; E-mail: elevina07@gmail.com

Diabetes prevalence, deaths attributable to diabetes, and health expenditure due to diabetes continue to rise across the globe with important social, financial, and health system implications [6]. It has been reported that the diabetic prevalence has risen dramatically; therefore, diabetes contextualizes as a pandemic [7, 8].

The International Diabetes Federation (IDF) [9], has reported that the number of people with diabetes aged 20–79 years must rise to 642 million (uncertainty interval: 521–829 million) by 2040. It was postulated an expectation of 693 million by 2045 [10]. The same authors [10] estimated that in 2017, 451 million (age 18–99 years) people with diabetes worldwide, and almost half of all people (49.7%) living with diabetes are undiagnosed. Moreover, there were an estimated 374 million people with impaired glucose tolerance (IGT), and it pointed out that some form of hyperglycemia affected almost 21.3 million live births to women in pregnancy. In 2017, approximately 5 million deaths worldwide were attributable to diabetes in the 20–99 years age range [6].

The American Diabetes Association released new research in 2018 [11], estimating the total costs of diagnosed diabetes rose to $327 billion in 2017 from $245 billion in 2012. Cho *et al.* [10], concluded that the relationship between diabetes prevalence and healthcare expenditure due to diabetes presents a large social, financial, and health system burden across the world. Moreover, Elflein [12] has calculated that between 2019 and 2045, the global expenditures for diabetes treatment expect to grow from 760 billion U.S. dollars to 845 billion U.S. dollars.

Diabetes Mellitus is probably one of the oldest diseases known to man. It was first reported in the Egyptian manuscript about 3000 years ago [13]. The meaning and origin of the Diabetes Mellitus word; comes from Greek, and it means a "siphon," Thomas Willis in 1675, added the word "*Mellitus.*" Mel in Latin means "honey "associated with sweet. Consequently, diabetes mellitus means "siphoning off sweet water" [14].

Diabetes mellitus is a lifelong disorder that is markedly affected by day-to-day variations in diet, exercise, infection, and stress [15]. The chronic hyperglycemia of diabetes is associated with relatively specific long-term microvascular complications that, affecting the eyes, kidneys, and nerves, as well as an increased risk for cardiovascular disease [6, 16]. "Prediabetes" is a practical and convenient term referring to impaired fasting glucose, impaired glucose tolerance, or glycated hemoglobin of 6.0% to 6.4%, each of which places individuals at high risk of developing diabetes and its complications [3].

According to several authors, diabetes can be classified as type 1, type 2, gestational diabetes mellitus hybrid forms of diabetes, other specific types, and unclassified diabetes [3, 16, 17]. Type 1 *Diabetes mellitus* (T1DM) is an immunemediated or idiopathic disorder. The disease is manifested by progressive T-cel- mediated autoimmune destruction of insulin-producing β cells in the pancreatic islets of Langerhans, leading to insulin deficiency and a tendency to ketoacidosis [15, 18, 19]. Several authors have reported that symptomatic manifestations by the body are the production of antibodies such as glutamic acid decarboxylase (GAD65), tyrosine phosphatase-like protein ICA512 or IA-2 (secretory granule protein islet cell antigen (ICA) 512 or IA-2), -insulin, and zinc T8 transporter (ZnT8), followed the progressive loss of insulin release as the autoimmune response progresses [20].

During later stages, patients progressively develop subclinical hyperglycemia. In the final stages of development, decreased Cpeptide levels cause patients to present with overt signs of diabetes resulting from hyperglycemia [21].

Most affected people are otherwise healthy and of a healthy weight when onset occurs. Sensitivity and responsiveness to insulin are usually normal, especially in the early stages. The term "juvenile diabetes" is because it represents many of the diabetes cases in children [22].

Data on global trends in T1DM prevalence and incidence are not available, but data from many high-income countries indicate an annual increase of between 3% and 4% in the incidence of T1DM in childhood. Males and females are equally affected. Although T1DM is frequently in childhood-onset, it can occur in adults, and 84% of people who suffer from T1DM are adults [17].

As described by ADA [17], between 70% and 90% of people with T1DM at diagnosis have evidence of an immune-mediated process with β-cell autoantibodies against glutamic acid decarboxylase (GAD65), islet antigen-2 (IA2), ZnT8 transporter or insulin, and associations with genes controlling immune responses. In populations of European descent, most of the genetic associations are with HLA DQ8 and DQ2.

Type 2 *Diabetes mellitus* (DM) is a chronic metabolic disorder that occurs when the pancreas does not produce enough insulin or when insulin resistance occurs (a pathological condition in which body cells fail to respond typically to the hormone insulin) [13, 23].

Type 2 diabetes is not a single disease process but instead represents a heterogeneous constellation of disease syndromes, all leading to the final common pathway of hyperglycemia. Many factors, alone or in combination, can cause hyperglycemia; thus, the complexity of type 2 diabetes's pathogenesis reflects the heterogeneous genetic, pathologic, environmental, and metabolic abnormalities that can exist in different patients [24]. Although T1DM is frequently in childhood-onset, it can occur in adults, and 84% of people who suffer from T1DM are adults.

DM prevalence has been increasing steadily all over the world. DM is fast becoming an epidemic in some countries of the world, and the number of people affected is expecting to double in the next decade. This increment is due to an increase in the aging population, thereby adding to the already existing burden for healthcare providers, especially in poorly developed countries [25].

Several authors [13] have estimated that 439 million people would have type 2 DM by the year 2030. The authors pointed out that the incidence of this type of DM varies substantially from one geographical region to another; as a result, it has environmental and lifestyle risk factors. Type 2DM (formerly known as noninsulin dependent DM) is the most common form of DM, characterized by hyperglycemia, insulin resistance, and relative insulin deficiency [26]. DM was a component of metabolic syndrome in 1988 [27].

The metabolic syndrome is a cluster of conditions that occur together, increasing the risk of heart disease, stroke, and type 2 diabetes. The central features of metabolic syndrome are insulin resistance, visceral adiposity, atherogenic dyslipidemia, and endothelial dysfunction [28].

As it was postulated the type 2 DM results from the interaction between genetic, environmental, and behavioral risk factors, and minor lifestyle changes can significantly reduce the chances of getting type 2 diabetes [26, 29 - 31]. Therefore, Asif [31] pointed out that to prevent this condition, action should be taken regarding the modifiable factors that influence its development-lifestyle and dietary habits.

Gestational *Diabetes Mellitus* refers to glucose intolerance with onset or first recognition during pregnancy [32], and it is one of the *Diabetes Mellitus* conditions, which occur in a non-diabetic pregnant woman. This condition usually develops near the end of the 3rd trimester or the beginning of the 4th trimester of pregnancy. This condition usually returns to normal soon after delivery [15].

Hybrid forms of diabetes are as follows: slowly evolving, immune-mediated diabetes of adults, and ketosis-prone type 2 Diabetes. Other specific types include a wide variety of relatively uncommon conditions, primarily specific genetically defined forms of diabetes or diabetes associated with other diseases or drug use. Such as; Monogenic diabetes (defect of β-cell function and defect inulin action), diseases of the exocrine pancreas, endocrine disorders, infection-related diabetes, uncommon specific forms of immune-mediated diabetes, other genetic syndromes sometimes associated with diabetes

Unclassified diabetes is the usual term to describe diabetes that does not match into other categories, and there is no clear diagnostic category, especially close to the time of diagnosis.

Prevention and treatment include a healthy diet, physical exercise, not using tobacco, and a normal body weight. Blood pressure control and proper foot care are also crucial for people with the disease [33].

Differentiation among types 1, type 2, and monogenic diabetes has important implications for both therapeutic decisions and educational approaches. Diabetes's main symptoms include increased thirst and urination, blurry vision, tiredness, slow wound healing, infection frequency, weight loss, nausea and vomiting, thrush or genital itching, and increased hunger. The main risk factors are overweight, sedentary lifestyle, family history of diabetes, history of gestational diabetes, age, ethnic/racial background [33].

DIET AND DIABETES

Education regarding the effect of the available carbohydrates from diet on blood sugar is imperatively needed. Mainly in portion sizes, economic benefits of certain foods, and also highlighting vegetable consumption. Those diabetic consumers that would like to learn more about how to make healthy food choices that fit their lifestyle and taste should reach the particular eating pattern and meal plan from the American Diabetic Association [34].

The dietary patterns, according to ADA [34], are associated with loss of weight. These patterns lead to eating a daily smaller number of calories by having a balanced diet (with a high intake of grains (cereals, legumes, pseudocereal, nut among others), vegetables, fruits, fish, and mono and polyunsaturated oils. Dietary indications for diabetic consumers focus on monounsaturated fatty acids high ratio, low intake of *Trans* fatty acids, high ingestion of dietary fiber, antioxidants, and polyphenols.ADA [34] recommends controlling starch intake as a significant part of the diet. The low-starchy vegetables have less effect on insulin and blood sugar levels. The starches used as ingredients in foods are processed, and they are functional but nonnutritive. On the other hand, the fruits contain carbohydrates with low assimilation, but they give them a natural sweetness plus many vitamins, fiber, and generally few calories. Proteins do not increase insulin or blood sugar levels.

Therefore, diets characterized by a low degree of energy density overall prevents weight gain and exert a protective effect on the development of type-2 diabetes

[34]. There is no known preventive measure against type-1 diabetes. Most affected people are otherwise healthy and have a healthy weight when onset occurs. Sensitivity and responsiveness to insulin are usually normal, especially in the early stages [22]. Asif [31] agreed that a Paleolithic diet (*i.e.*, a diet consisting of lean meat, fish, shellfish, fruits and vegetables, roots, eggs and nuts, but no grains, dairy products, salt or refined fats, and sugar) was associated with marked improvement of glucose tolerance of testing subjects. Control subjects following a diet did not significantly improve their glucose tolerance despite decreases in weight and waist circumference.

The author [31] pointed out that there is no cure for diabetes but managed with diet. A balanced diet, exercise, and medicine (if prescribed) must help control weight and keep blood glucose in a healthy range. An appropriate diet can help prevent or delay complications. Many people with diabetes live long and healthy lives [35]. Conversely, people who are overweight, upper-body obesity, having a family history of diabetes, age 40 or older, and women (50% more often than men) are potentially most likely to get diabetes [16].

The nutrition therapy goals for the individual with diabetes have evolved and have become more flexible and patient-centered. The goals from the American Diabetes Association [11, 32, 36] include the following:

1. To promote and support healthful eating patterns, emphasizing a variety of nutrient-dense foods in appropriate portion sizes to improve overall health and
   ◦ Achieve and maintain body weight goals
   ◦ Attain individualized glycemic, blood pressure, and lipid goals
   ◦ Delay or prevent complications of diabetes
2. To address individual nutrition needs based on personal and cultural preferences, health literacy and numeracy, access to healthful food choices, willingness and ability to make behavioral changes, as well as barriers to change
3. To maintain the pleasure of eating by providing nonjudgmental messages about food choices
4. To provide an individual with diabetes, the practical tools for day-to-day meal planning rather than focusing on individual macronutrients, micronutrients, or single foods.

CONVENTIONAL AND NON-CONVENTIONAL RAW MATERIALS FOR DIABETIC FOOD

Many substances from the environment are useful as healthy ingredients to produce foods for diabetic consumers. But, when the sweet taste is involved in these foods, the selection must be focusing on the non-absorbable, with low calories and low glycemic index sweeteners.

The evolved taste preference of humans is still useful by helping them identify the nutrients from foods. But for those who have easy access to tasty, energy-dense foods, their sensitivities to sugary, salty, and fatty foods have also helped cause over-nutrition-related diseases, such as obesity and diabetes [37].

Diabetic consumers must balance their diet with beans, dark green leafy vegetables, citrus fruit, berries, tomatoes, fish high in omega-3 fatty acids, nuts, whole grains, milk, and yogurt. Each one of them has a load of complex carbohydrates, vitamins (A, C, E, D, folate, and K), minerals (iron, calcium, chromium, iron, magnesium, manganese, and potassium), and different phytochemicals, which can supply the nutritional needs of diabetic.

Conveniently, nature provides ingredients or foods that can supply the macro and micronutrient needs for the consumer, with additional constituents, not nutrients (phytochemicals) that have properties health benefits of consumers, especially for those with diabetes. These kinds of sources are non-conventional raw materials in food development and innovation. Therefore, in the context of industry, nonconventional sources must be developed to produce ingredients for innovation, elaborating foods that satisfy the diabetic consumer's functional and sensorial exigencies [38].

Today, the food industry focuses its efforts on developing new products with properties that provide the necessary nutrients for human food and help prevent diseases related to nutrition such as diabetes, among others [39].

Nowadays, a consensus is that the phytochemicals present in plants as secondary metabolites to protecting their cells from environmental hazards, also contribute to protecting humans against diseases due to their biological properties. According to Breslin [37] in recent years strongly support a role for phytochemicals in the prevention of several diseases, specifically polyphenols.

Oxidative stress plays a significant role in the pathogenesis and development of complications of diabetes Mellitus, such as heart disease, stroke, chronic kidney failures, foot ulcers, eye damages [40]. According to Aryaeian [41], various dietary polyphenols may prevent diabetes. Polyphenols are the most abundant antioxidants in the humans' diet and present in non-conventional sources [42].

Polyphenols are strong antioxidants that are complementary and add to the functions of antioxidant vitamins and enzymes as a defense against oxidative stress caused by excess reactive oxygen species (ROS).

Therefore, they may control and prevent diabetes complications [41]. Although most of the evidence of the antioxidant activity of polyphenols is *in vitro* studies, increasing evidence indicates they may act in ways beyond the antioxidant functions *in vivo* [43].

Polyphenols, such as flavonoids, phenolic acid, and stilbenes, are a large and heterogeneous group of phytochemicals in plant-based foods (tea, soy, coffee, cocoa, cereal grains, cinnamon, ginger, fruits, and berries) [43, 44]. Flavonoids are a class of such bioactive compounds, usually found in fruits and other plant organs [44].

Pinent *et al.* [45], have pointed out that *in vitro* and *in vivo* studies demonstrate that some flavonoids modify the insulin-secreting capacity of the cell [44], making them good candidates for the development of new functional foods with potential protective/preventive properties against diabetes mellitus [43]. Among them, there are quercetin, genistein, daidzein, pelargonidin, and resveratrol. Authors suggest that besides their antioxidant properties, they can act through other mechanisms, by interacting with protein function, modulating intracellular cascades, and modulating gene expression [44].

Studies using animals with drug-induced diabetes support the hypothesis that flavonoids can ameliorate this pathogenesis [43]. However, due to its great diversity, the structural variability of the flavonoids makes it challenging to establish their common effects in the pancreas. To date, the contribution of all these flavonoid effects to the overall improvement of experimental diabetes remains obscure [44].

Non-conventional raw material

Nuts (walnuts, almonds, hazelnuts, pecans, and Brazil nuts) do promote satiety in overweight and obese adults while maintaining stable blood glucose and insulin levels. These results suggest that mixed nuts should be studied as a potentially useful snack to prevent high glucose and insulin level [46].

Roots and tubers include those conventional crops, such as; potatoes (*Solanum tuberosum*), cassava (*Manihot esculenta*), yams (*Dioscorea* spp.), aroids (*Xanthosoma saggitifolium* and *Colocasia esculenta*), canna (*Canna edulis*), arrowroot (*Maranta arundinacea* L.), and other non-conventional such as; Peruvian carrot (*Arracacia xanthorrhiza*), ullucus (*Ullucus tuberosus*), oca (*Oxalis tuberosa*), mashua (*Tropaeolum tuberosum*), yacón (*Smallanthus sonchifolium*).

Chandrasekara and Kumar [47] pointed out that roots and tubers offer nutritional properties energy, and additionally, they provide health benefits to consumers. They have antioxidative, hypoglycemic, hypocholesterolemia, antimicrobial, and immunomodulatory properties. It is due that they contain several bioactive constituents, such as; phenolic compounds, saponins, bioactive proteins, glycoalkaloids, and phytic acids that are responsible for the observed effects.

According to the review [47], yam extracts have various bioactive components that may stimulate the hypoglycemic effect. Edible portion and extracts of sweet potato peels have shown reduced plasma glucose levels of diabetic patients and reduced insulin resistance. Extract of the white-skinned sweet potatoes reduced hyperinsulinemia in Zucker fatty rats. The ethanolic extract of *D. alata* includes hydro-Q9 chromene, γ-tocopherol, α-tocopherol, feruloyl glycerol, and dioscorin cyanidin-3-glucoside, catechin, procyanidin, cyanidin, peonidin 3-gentiobioside, and vitamins A, B, and C have shown an anti-diabetic activity in alloxan-induced diabetic rats.

Curcuma (*Curcuma longa*) plant from the *Zingiberáceas* family comes from Asia. Curcumin extracted from the curcuma root is another phytochemical proved as an ameliorator of diabetes in different mouse, rat, and hamster models studies [48, 51]. According to Seo *et al.* [52], the administration of 200 mg of curcumin/kg diet has improved insulin resistance and hyperglycemia in mice. It also has elevated insulin levels and lowered the free fatty acid, triglyceride, cholesterol, and glucose level in the blood, and reduced lipid oxidation. These data indicated that curcumin could repress inflammation and obesity and improve the chronic condition of diabetes [41].

Yacón roots (*Smallanthus sonchifolius* (Poepp. & Endl.)), is an Andean root crop related to the prevention of chronic diseases (dyslipidemia and insulin resistance), colon cancer, constipation, among other properties. Yacón has excellent potential as a functional food due to its high content of fructooligosaccharides (FOS) and inulin, promoting the development of the colonic microbiota.

Yacón leaves are used because of their phenolic compounds, which have antioxidant properties that protect cell membranes against damage caused by oxygen radicals and, consequently, cardiovascular disease and cancer.

Yacón's regular use may benefit patients with digestive and kidney diseases, as well as those with diabetes and metabolic syndrome. An alternative product from yacón may be sweet syrups and natural sweeteners for people with digestive problems and obesity, reaching a broader group of beneficiaries. Currently, several clinical studies evaluate the conditions necessary for the safe use of yacón as a dietary supplement in groups other than the populations that have traditionally used this plant in their diet [53, 54].

Ginger is another raw material of interest with evidence to prevent or control type- 2 diabetes [55]. Ginger (*Zingiber officinale*) originally from Asia, belonging to the *Zingiberaceae* family, is a plant with leafy stems (rhizomes) and yellowishgreen flowers. Ginger's rhizomes are used as a flavoring agent in food and beverage industries and from antiquity as herbal medicine to treat various diseases worldwide. The pharmacological effects of ginger come from its bioactive components [56, 57]. It has been detected in ginger more than 40 antioxidant compounds [55], and it also demonstrated that the most active ingredients in ginger are the pungent principles; gingerols, and shogaol [58, 59].

The research performed by Ajayi *et al.* [60], has shown that the rhizome contains a spectrum of biologically active compounds such as curcumin, 6-gingerol, 6shogoals, zingiberene, bisabolene, and several types of lipids that confer to it, the characteristics medicinal properties of being pungent and a stimulant [61]. Studies *in vitro*, *in vivo*, and clinical trials have shown the antihyperglycemic effect of ginger. The pharmacokinetics, bioavailability, and safety studies on ginger in regards to Diabetes Mellitus and its complications show its potential for control D.M.

Several authors have stressed that the mechanisms underlying these actions are associated with the inhibition of critical enzymes controlling both carbohydrate metabolism, and increased rate of insulin release/sensitivity, and the lipidlowering effects on insulin resistance [59, 62 - 66].

The stems or rhizomes of ginger processed for its commercial uses are available. They are marketed mostly in two forms: dried ginger and preserved (syrup) ginger. Ginger can be processed to produce flour by conventional dehydration (50 °C for 5hrs) after peeling and washing the rhizomes. Other authors have tested sun drying for three days (up to moisture content 10-12%); Oven drying at 75 °C for 20 hrs. (Up to moisture content 9-11%) and sun drying for one day at (28±2) °C, followed by oven drying at 75 °C for 10 hrs. (Up to moisture content 8-9%), microwave drying, electrohydrodynamic (EHD) drying [67 - 71].

In conclusion, the conventional drying using a cabinet dry (60 °C) produces a ginger flour with good sensorial quality and nutritional profile. As an important consideration, there are some rhizomes (*Asarum canadense*) from the *Aristolochiaceae* family or Canadian ginger (also named as wild ginger), that despite having the same sensorial properties of ginger, but it must not be used as its substitute because it contains carcinogenic concentrations of aristolochic acid [72 - 74].

Ginger usually dried and ground, to flavor sauces, curry dishes, confections, pickles, and ginger ale. The peeled root may be preserved by boiling in syrup. Sri

Lankans frequently use ginger paste or fired ginger on meat dishes. Ginger tea, prepared by cooking slices of fresh ginger for a few minutes, is a spicy and healthy drink enjoyed in Sri Lanka. It is used in chutney, pickles, preserves, and dried fruit. It is used ground in cakes and cookies [75]. Moreover, several food developments use composite flour-based ginger as a flavoring or functional ingredient. Among these researches are biscuits [76 - 78], pasta [79], cookie [80], rice noodle [81], bread and rusk [82 - 84]. Usually, it is added a pinch to a cup of hot chocolate, given to it a nice different flavor.

Fruits and vegetables are good sources of vitamins, minerals, flavonoids (antioxidants), saponins, polyphenols, carotenoids (vitamin A-like compounds), isothiocyanates (Sulphur-containing compounds), and several types of dietary fibers [85].

The fruits and vegetables prevent malnutrition and help maintain optimum health through a host of chemical components still identified, tested, and measured [31]. Therefore, whatever the arguments, there is a consensus that several fruits and vegetable sources can be a potential ingredient for food development that could have a protective or preventive effect against diabetes mellitus [86].

Ojewole and Adewunmi in 2003 [86] evaluated the effect of methanolic extract from mature and green fruits of *Musa paradisiaca* on normal (normoglycemic) and (diabetic-induced) hyperglycemic mice. As a result, the fruit induced significant, dose-related reductions in the blood glucose concentrations of both standard and diabetic mice. Today, it has been investigating the use of banana flour and starch combined with some phytochemical sources to elaborate baked goods and jellies using sweeteners to diabetic consumers.

Eggplant (*Solanum melongena* L), also known as aubergine, brinjal, berenjena, or Guinea is an important non-tuberous species of the *Solanaceae* family [87].

Eggplant fruits usually are purple, white, or striped in color. The coloration of the purple type is for the presence of anthocyanin. The purple types are more commercialized than other types [88]. Eggplant is a vegetable high valued for its content in phytochemicals, such as flavonoids (kaempferol, rutin, quercetin, apigenin, and isorhamnetin), acids (hydroxycinnamic, chlorogenic and caffeoylquinic), anthocyanins (delphinidin glucosides), acyl glycosides, carotenoids (lutein and zeaxanthin) and glycoalkaloids (α-solamargine y αsolasonine). These compounds confer to eggplants several beneficial properties for human health, such as antioxidant, anti-inflammatory, cardioprotective, anticarcinogenic, anti-obesity, and anti-diabetic properties [87, 89 - 94].

A study from the University of Massachusetts found that extracts from several eggplant varieties (purple, white, and graffiti) inhibited an enzyme that converts starch to blood sugar. The eggplant compounds restrained the glucose-releasing enzyme by as much as 60%, and the effect correlated with antioxidant activity, which also helps squelch blood sugar-generated free radicals. Other ways to help manage or even avoid diabetes [95].

Some researchers [39, 96] have demonstrated that flour elaborated from sliced eggplant dried at 45–50 °C in a drying oven is a potential ingredient for the preparation of foods with functional properties since it is rich in phenolic compounds and antioxidants.

Moreover, the results obtained by the research carried out [88] clearly showed that eggplant flour could scavenge the free radicals due to the presence of antioxidants. They conclude that eggplant flour is a functional ingredient in the processing of functional food, which is high in total dietary fiber and also high in antioxidants and nutritional value. However, the authors pointed out that the ideal drying temperature is 40°C, and that the antioxidant and inhibitory effect varies as a function of the eggplant variety.

The fruits from the passion fruit plants *(Passiflora edulis)* are another nonconventional reserve to produce foods. It is a rustic, adaptable crop, native from Brazil, used in foodstuffs and medicine at both small and industrial scales.

There is two distinct fruits form of commercial importance, the standard yellow (*Passiflora edulis* f. flavicarpa Deg.) and the purple (*Passiflora edulis* f. edulis), differing in acidity and starch content. The yellows are more acidic and less starchy, while the purples have inverse content. The hybrids of these two are available for cultivation [97]. The whole plant is a source of bioactive compounds, which could alleviate oxidative stress. The leaves contain alkaloids and several other phytoactive chemicals, such as passiflorine, a known sedative, and tranquilizer [85].

Despite its phytochemical value, the exocarp (pigmented peel) and mesocarp (pulp or white skin) are byproducts of industrial juice processing and frequently discarded. There are 3 primary groups of active chemicals in the passion fruit: alkaloids, glycosides, and flavonoids [98]. Some phenolic compounds are in *Passiflora* species, such as like C-glicosilderivatives apigenin and luteolin, as vitexin, isovitexin, orientin, schaftoside, 200-O-rhamnoside, and luteolin-7-O(2-rhamnosylglucoside) scirpusin B, piceatannol.

Passion fruit is a powerful medicinal source, but much more research needs to do to reveal its potentially potent action [99]. Dos Santos Medeiros *et al.* [100] studied the toxicological effect of the peel of passion fruits on type 2 diabetes mellitus patients. The authors have concluded well acceptance by volunteers, without adverse reactions that could jeopardize their use as food with ownership of health. Salgado *et al.* [101], evaluated the effect of the passion fruit peel flour on the blood glucose levels in diabetic rats. The results of this study showed that the passion fruit peel affects the metabolism of carbohydrates and can positively influence diabetes's metabolic control by preventing or delaying complications associated with this disease.

Moreover, flour prepared from the peels of passion fruit [102] has shown an increment of the concentration of high-density lipoproteins (HDL) in blood, reducing the concentrations of glucose, cholesterol, and LDL, as well as blood pressure and body weights in diabetic rats, and people.

Furthermore, Ramos de Queiroz *et al.*, in 2012 [103] have performed an interventional study on diabetic patients. In the study, the author has observed a statistically significant reduction in fasting plasma glucose, and a significant reduction in HbA1c values between baseline and 60 days of treatment with 30 g daily of passion fruit flour to be eaten by patients throughout the day with juices, fruits, and milk. They concluded that before the results obtained in this study, the intake of fiber-rich flour (pectin) suggests a favorable effect on insulin sensitivity during the eight weeks in the studied adults. These effects may reduce the risk of chronic complications of type 2 diabetes.

Although larger and longer trials are needed to confirm these results and elucidate the mechanisms involved, evidence-based literature is enough to encourage increased consumption of foods rich in dietary fiber. Further research [104] reported evidence that the peel of passion fruit intakes modulates in different ways the antioxidant tissue status. In this way, passion fruit peel intake could have thermogenic/ergogenic compounds in its composition. Then, further investigations about the effects of *Passiflora edulis* peel intake on health are necessary.

Some researchers [105] have prepared flour samples from passion fruit shells through a modified process to evaluate their potential use as a stabilizing agent, emulsifier, thickener, and gelling agent. They have compared these characteristics to those of low and high methoxyl pectins, xanthan gum, guar gum, and carrageenan.

The flour samples obtained have a significant stabilizing capacity, as they were able to hinder particle settling when applied to nectars. Another positive feature observed was the emulsifying potential, showing similar results to additives commonly used in mayonnaise, such as xanthan and guar gums.

The flour samples also showed good properties as a thickening and gelling agent in ice cream toppings and structured fruit. The results demonstrate that flour produced from passion fruit peel replaces the commercial hydrocolloids studied. Besides being obtained through simple procedures and associated with low cost, the flour samples showed similar technical characteristics about their stabilizing, emulsifying, thickening, and gelling power.

Recently, other researchers [106] have studied the physicochemical composition and physical properties of macerated peel flour passion fruit. The authors have proposed macerate as an ingredient for the food industry. The authors have reported that flour obtained by maceration offers greater benefits for industrial use, with 60% fewer tannins and greater thermal stability. Besides, this sample does not reabsorb moisture as easily, although the unmacerated flour also shows potential for use in dietary products, and pseudoplastic properties for its application in many industrial sectors.

Flavored leaves or seeds. Other studies have demonstrated the α-glucosidase inhibition relevant for hyperglycemia by food from *Apiaceae* (celery, parsley, fennel coriander) and *Lamiceae* (mint, sage, melissa, basil, rosemary) families. The studies suggest the high enzyme inhibitory activity, reflecting *in vitro* antihyperglycemic and antihypertensive potentials. The studies *in vitro* have indicated that consumption of these food sources would be beneficial for consumer health. Further, *in vivo* studies for type II diabetes-linked functionalities of these natural sources of antioxidants and inhibitors would confirm the human health benefits achieved through dietary intake [107].

The results of Tashakori-Sabzevar *et al.* [108] indicated that celery seed extracts effectively control hyperglycemia and hyperlipidemia in diabetic rats and demonstrate its protective effects against pancreatic toxicity resulting from STZinduction.

Godavari *et al.* [109] pointed out that the ethyl acetate and the benzene extract of fennel seeds have high enzyme inhibitory activity of two enzymes (alpha-amylase and alpha-glucosidase) that offer for the maintenance of glucose levels in diabetic patients by hydrolyzing the carbohydrates ingested in the food. Godavari *et al.* [109], also have shown the presence of phenols, saponins, terpenoids, tannins, and flavonoids in fennel extracts that can serve to maintain the glucose level in the blood and hence act as hypoglycemic agents.

Aligita *et al.* [110] concluded from their studies that the coriander leaves' ethanolic extract has the anti-diabetic activity at the dose of 400 mg/kg (mw) by improving and regenerating the pancreatic β cell and inhibiting the α-glucosidase enzyme activity. Studies have demonstrated that parsley extract has a protective effect against hepatotoxicity caused by diabetes in alloxan-treated rats [111].

The result from other investigations [112] indicated that *Menta spicata* leaf (peppermint) aqueous extract possess hypoglycemic, hypocholesterolemia, and antioxidant properties in diabetic rats. Therefore, this study suggests a promising use of it for the treatment of diabetes.

Eidi and Eidi [113] conclusions are that the traditional use of sage (*Salvia officinalis*) as an anti-diabetic agent is justified and that extracts from this plant show a dose-dependent activity that is comparable to the standard anti-diabetic drug glibenclamide. The essential oil from *M. officinalis* (melissa) is an excellent candidate as an anti-diabetic agent and worthy of further investigation [114]. The anti-diabetic properties of basil's extract may be due to its ability to suppress endogenous glucose release, inhibit glycogenolysis, and stimulate glycogenesis [115].

Mistletoe fig. Several researchers [116, 117] reported the Mistletoe fig (*Ficus deltoidea*) uses in Malaysia traditional medicine for diabetes. Other authors [118] suggested the anti-hyperglycemic actions of mistletoe fig through stimulation of insulin secretion from pancreatic β cells, enhancement of glucose uptake by adipocytes cells, and augmentation of adiponectin secretion from adipocytes cells as well. The dual pancreatic and extra-pancreatic actions of the mistletoe fig show its enormous potential as new oral anti-diabetic drugs. Moreover, the adiponectin secreting and insulin-sensitizing properties of its indicated that this plant could ameliorate systemic insulin resistance and may potentially be beneficial for type 2 diabetes mellitus related to insulin resistance.

Anti-diabetic Polysaccharides. Polysaccharides and polysaccharide complexes have shown anti-hyperglycemic and antihypercholesterolemic potential when administered *via* the oral and systemic route in various animal models with Diabetes Mellitus [119, 120]. Among them are raw polysaccharides and water extract from the several tuberous roots*Liriope spicata* (Thund, *Psacaliumde compositum*), seeds (fenugreek (*Trigonella foenum-graecum* L.), seaweed (brown seaweed; *Saccharina japonica*), and lotus plumule, endodermis of *Citrus maxima*. Moreover, certain water-soluble non-starch polysaccharides; such as oats, glucans, and guar gum, because of their ability to increase viscosity in the gastrointestinal tract, have been reported to decrease glucose absorption, gastric emptying rate and thereby reducing the postprandial rise in blood sugar as well as insulin levels in both healthy and diabetic subjects.

There are plants with related active ingredients extracted that have potential therapeutic value for diabetes treatment, for example, the active ingredient from flavonoids (*e.g.*, quercetin and kaempferol), alkaloids such as, the dieckol [121,

122].

SWEETENERS OVERVIEW

Over humans' evolution, sweetness and bitterness played a crucial role in survival. Sweetness provided the means to seek out an energy source in the form of carbohydrates; and bitterness resulted in an aversion to potentially deadly substances found in nature, *e.g.*, alkaloids and toxins [123, 124]. Therefore, the desirable taste for sugar is innate [123] and related to the human being, evolutionary survival mechanism [37]. Consequently, consumers have a selective psychological perception of the sweet taste, and it cannot be eliminated at all from the sweet food without bringing a rejecting of them. As an evolutionary mechanism, its consumption is providing quick energy and a concentrated source of calories.

There are some disadvantages when consuming too much sugar, it contributes to obesity, and it is also a significant contributor to tooth decay. The innate sweet taste preference by consumers increases the pleasure of eating; as a result, the added sugars have received considerable attention due to their association with weight gain. A higher intake of added sugars is associated with higher energy intake and lower diet quality, which can increase the risk of obesity, pre-diabetes, type 2 diabetes, and cardiovascular diseases. The main problem that a person with Diabetes faces is an increase in the threshold level of sweetness compared to nondiabetics. Therefore, a person with Diabetes needs sweeter food than a person without Diabetes to appreciate the same taste [125].

Usually, the sugar term is for tabletop sugar (sucrose); it is a type of soluble carbohydrates that provide energy in our diet. The U.S. definition for sugar in labels includes all monosaccharides and disaccharides.

Compared to other types of carbohydrates, sugars are quickly absorbed into the body, filling less. They enhance the flavor of food and drink, which makes them an attractive option for both consumers and the food and drink industry. They add sweetness, flavor, fermentable solids, and contribute other physical and chemical properties to the finished product.

Sugars and sugar substitutes are nutritional sweeteners *per se* because they are substances that sweeten. The differences among them are the number of calories they provide and their absorption on the body. Sucrose and fructose are the most representatives. However, other substances can provide fewer or no calories than sucrose.

The food industry must find uncommon sources of sweet substances (no sugar carbohydrates) to produce sweeteners with low or no calories, as well as a bulk sweetener (have a mass similar to sucrose). Some of these substances tend to have desirable sweetness but are less or not metabolized in the human body and do not provide calorie intake [126].

Therefore, sweeteners can be natural or synthetic as a function of their source, or sweet and bulk sweeteners as a function of their functional properties (sweetness and mass). Regarding the sweetness as functional properties, they have a relative sweetness lower or slightly higher than sucrose, and high-intensity sweeteners (HIS) with a relative sweetness are considerably above 1 [127].

Since some of them have received attention due to their toxicological acceptance and commercial development, the two types of sweeteners usually handled are natural from plant origin and artificial or synthetic sweeteners.

Natural sweeteners are saccharide (sugars) and non-saccharides.

Saccharides

From a chemical point of view, the saccharides are organic compounds polyhydroxy aldehydes, ketones, or polymers. Biologically, saccharides are the unit structure of carbohydrates, such as monosaccharides, disaccharides, oligosaccharides, and polysaccharides. Then, sucrose, fructose, glucose, starch hydrolysates (glucose syrup, high-fructose syrup), and other isolated sugar preparations used as such or added during food preparation and manufacturing are saccharides [128].

Sucrose, glucose, and fructose are the most common nutritional sweeteners in nature.

Glucose is always less sweet than sucrose, whereas fructose sweetener is highly dependent on temperature; for example, fructose is sweeter than sucrose at low temperatures, whereas the sweetening effect decreases as the temperature rises [129]

Sucrose (table sugar) is present naturally in several foods and is one of the most common natural sweeteners added to the human diet [129]. Commercially sucrose comes from two plants, cane, and beetroot. Both plants are useful to extract and prepare refined tabletop sugar.

Adverse health effects associated with sucrose intake include the facilitation of excess caloric intake, excess weight gain, dilutional effects of essential nutrients, and increased risk for dental caries, type 2 diabetes, and cardiovascular diseases [130 - 137].

Consequently, by consensus, sucrose was excluded entirely from the diet or meal diabetics plan and substituted by alternative sweeteners. However, recently it has been pointed out that the total caloric value (VCT) depends on the patient's nutritional status and the level of activity physics patients perform.

Therefore, foods containing sucrose can be useful if they are considered in the final carbohydrate count and covered with the appropriate insulin dose. However, it should be moderate its consumption to avoid caloric excess [138]. On the other hand, technologically sucrose cannot merely be replaced by these types of intense sweeteners, due to the question of bulk, quality, the intensity of sweetness, and physical characteristics [139].

Fructose, named fruit sugar (levulose) is a monosaccharide component of sucrose, which delivers a similar amount of energy as sucrose. Fructose is in fruit, honey, and table sugar. Sources of dietary fructose include agave, the richest natural source of fructose, with 85% of carbohydrate in this form; honey with approximately 50%; and fruit juices.

High-fructose corn syrup (HFCS) is made from acid- or amylase-treated corn starch and contains 42–55% fructose [140].

Fructose term 'slow sugar, is because it metabolizes slower than sucrose. The metabolic pathway of fructose in a well-controlled diabetic has a positive flux towards the formation of glycogen (glycogenesis), and glycogenolysis (the breakdown of glycogen to glucose) occurs as and when required at a slow and steady pace. While in uncontrolled diabetes, glycogenesis occurs at the same pace, but glycogenolysis occurs rapidly. Glycogenesis causes a swift rise in the blood glucose levels in these patients. In either case, the metabolism of fructose is slower than that of sucrose [138].

Fructose is metabolized even in the absence of insulin, which is vital in a person with Diabetes. Hence, fructose causes an overall slower rise in blood glucose levels than glucose. An increased intake of fructose may cause hypertriglyceridemia, especially in patients with uncontrolled Diabetes.

Consumption of fructose up to 50–60 g per day has no adverse effect on blood glucose, glycosylated hemoglobin, and serum lipids. The recommendation of 2 to 3 servings of fruit per day holds well in a well-controlled diabetic [129, 138, 141]. Glucose usually used as syrup is from starch sources, mainly maize. Sirop offers alternative functional properties, as well as economic benefits. Glucose syrups are extremely versatile sweeteners and are widely used in food manufacturing and other industries [142].

Glucose has a Relative Sweetness Factor of 74, and as a function of its Dextrose Equivalent (DE) value, the Relative Sweetness Factor of the syrup can vary from 23-48 as compared to a value of the glucose of 100. They are a crucial ingredient in confectionery products, beer, soft drinks, sports drinks, jams, sauces, ice creams, and pharmaceuticals, and industrial fermentations [143].

Non-saccharides

The non-saccharides comprise sweet glycosides (stevioside and rebaudioside), aldehyde (perillaldehyde), saponins (glycyrrhizin, osladin). They also encompass dihydrochalcone (Neohesperidin dihydrochalcone), sweet proteins (thaumatins, mabinlin, pentadin, brazzein, curculin, monellin, miraculin), terpenoid (hernandulcin), and luo-han-guo).

Glycosides: (steviosides and rebaudioside). Stevia leaves (*Stevia rebaudiana* Bertoni), and its products have the potential for commercial uses as sweetener or therapeutic. The stevia plant is native to Paraguay and has been consumed by Paraguayan a long time ago [144, 145]. The stevia plant produces around 30 steviol glycosides that have a sweetener role, but its best-known molecules are the stevioside and rebaudioside A [146].

According to Pérez *et al.* [147], the questioned role of other sweeteners by consumers leads to stevia and its derivatives being a solution. The authors conclude that other patients can use glycosides from stevia because they offer other important therapeutic benefits. There exists production of stevia worldwide, with established procedures for isolation and purification of its glycosides, and one of them approved for food use. Consequently, a solid market for processed products must emerge to meet these consumers' requirements for reducing or controlling the disease. The acceptable daily intake or ADI is 4 mg/kg bw/day to steviol glycosides [148].

Aldehydes (perillaldehyde). The perilla (*Perilla frutescens* L.) is grown in many world regions, and it is a flavoring ingredient that adds spiciness and citrus taste to foods [149]. Perillartin (or perilla sugars) is a highly sweet semisynthetic analog prepared from a natural monoterpenoid perillaldehyde from perilla herb.

According to Surana *et al.* [150], the perilla sugar with a mint-cinnamon-like flavor is 2000 times sweeter than sucrose but with low water solubility and potential allergenicity.

Regarding the concerns about perillaldehyde toxicity, the studies of Hobbs *et al.* [151] do not indicate any potential genotoxic effect for perillaldehyde.

Saponins (Glycyrrhizin). Glycyrrhizin is the principal active constituent of licorice root (*Glycyrrhiza glabra*) and has been used in traditional medicine to alleviate bronchitis, gastritis, and jaundice [152]. Besides being a potent inhibitor of replication of viruses [153], it is 50–100 times sweeter than sucrose and has a slow onset of sweetness followed by a lingering licorice-like aftertaste [154, 155]. According to Gloria (2003) [155], it exhibits a sweet woody flavor, which limits its use as a pure sweetener.

Glycyrrhizin enhances food flavors, masks bitter flavors, and increases the perceived sweetness level of sucrose. It has the potential for providing functional characteristics, including foaming, viscosity control, gel formation, and possibly antioxidant characteristics. Its uses are as a coating for candies and chewing tobacco. Ingestion of large amounts of these foods may cause headache, lethargy, sodium and water retention, and excessive excretion of potassium, high blood pressure, and sometimes heart failure. Hence it behaves like a mineralocorticoid [138].

Dihydrochalcones. Such as the Neohesperidin dihydrochalcone. (NHDC) which is an artificial sweetener derived from citrus, prepared by alkaline hydrogenation of the biflavanoid neohesperidin present in Seville (bitter) oranges (*Citrus aurantium*) [155]. NHDC is non-cariogenic, with a caloric value of 2 kcal/g. Due, little of the compound is absorbed unchanged from the small intestine. After cleavage of the glycosidic side chain by the intestinal mucosal or bacterial glycosidases, the residual primary metabolites are partly excreted unchanged in the bile and partly metabolized further [155]. Owing to its intense and long-lasting sweetness, NHDC generally used at concentrations of less than 100 mg/kg [155].

Due to its ability to reduce bitterness and its flavor-enhancing properties is particularly effective in masking the bitter tastes of other compounds found in citrus, including limonin and naringin [155].

The European Union approved NHDC's use as a sweetener in 1994 but not approved as a sweetener in the United States. It is listed as a Generally Recognized as Safe flavor enhancer by the Flavour and Extract Manufacturers' Association but does not have FDA GRAS status as of 2019 [155].

Sweet Proteins. Miraculin, although not sweet, has the property of modifying sour food's taste into a delightfully sweet taste. It is a glycoprotein consisting of amino acids and carbohydrate chains. Chemically it occurs as a tetramer, a combination of four monomers grouped into dimers. It is 400,000 times sweeter than sucrose on a molar basis. Interestingly, a mixture of miraculin with citrate did not elicit sweetness. FDA denied Miraculin approbation for sweetener purposes. Miraculin also has no legal status in the European Union [138, 156].

Terpenoids (hernadulcin). Hernandulcin is a sesquiterpene, and it is the main sweet component isolated from*Lippia dulcis* Trev, obtained as a colorless oil. It was a judge for a test of panelists to be more than three orders of magnitude sweeter than sucrose. However, it was detected aftertaste as well as some bitterness [157, 158].

Siraitia grosvenori or luo-han-guo is an herbaceous perennial plant of the *Cucurbitaceae* family, native to southern China and northern Thailand. Its fruit extract used in Chinese traditional medicine contains potent sweet glycosides of triterpenes with sweetness several hundred times higher than table sugar [159]. In 1995 Procter and Gamble Company developed and patented a non-caloric sweetener from luo-han-guo extract [160]. As is described in the patent, the fruit itself, though sweet, has too many additional flavors that would make it unsuitable for widespread use as a sweetener, so P&G developed a method for processing it to eliminate the undesired flavors. The Suzuki *et al.,* studies [159] indicate that luo-han-guo extract supplementation may prevent complications, attenuate pathological conditions for type 2 diabetes, and its sweetness characteristic.

Fructooligosaccharides (FOS). Fructooligosaccharides (FOSs) are non-digestible carbohydrates with functional and physiological attributes like low sweetness, non-carcinogenicity, low caloric value, prebiotic, hypolipidemic, and hypocholesterolemic properties [161]. They are composed of linear chains of fructose units linked by beta (2-1) bonds. Small intestinal glycosidases do not hydrolyze dietary fructooligosaccharides, reach the cecum structurally unchanged. They are metabolized by the intestinal microflora to form short-chain carboxylic acids, L-lactate, CO_2, hydrogen, and other metabolites [162].

Fructans or fructooligosaccharides (FOS), also referred to as fructofibers, exhibit sweetness levels between 30 and 50 percent of sugar. They come from natural sources, such as blue Agave, bananas, onions, wheat, chicory root, garlic, asparagus, artichoke, jícama, yacón tomato, honey, and leeks. FOS contains inulin and oligofructose, both of which are inert polysaccharides that go through unabsorbed in the body.

Fructofibres provide added benefit as it gives the bulk to the diet and helps prevent constipation. It lowers blood glucose levels and serum lipids. The effects of fructofibres may be insignificant as used in minimal quantities in sweeteners [53, 138, 163 - 165].

Although FOSs are present in trace amounts in natural foods, commercial production uses microbial transferase such as fructosyl transferase or βfructofuranosidase [166, 167].

In the food industry, inulin is widely in foodstuff as a prebiotic, fat replacer, sugar replacer, texture modifier, and for the development of functional foods to improve health due to its beneficial role in gastric health [163]. When using to replace fat, inulin increases the texture and softness of foodstuff, increasing sweet taste and mouthfeel.

Artificial sweeteners

Most of the currently available sweeteners in the world market are synthetic compounds, but their use depends on the granting of legislative approval, for which individual countries have their regulatory requirements [168].

The artificial sweeteners currently in use are polyol, aspartame, neotame, acesulfame K, sucralose, cyclamate, saccharin, tagatose, and alitame [169, 170].

Besides the previously artificial sweeteners mentioned, United approve for uses the luo-han-guo fruit extract, and stevia [133]. It is important to mention that both last sweeteners were previously discussed as natural, although they have an industrial patent for their extraction and crystallization.

Despite the considerable market value of synthetic sweeteners, problems are perceived with some of these compounds in terms of their safety, stability, cost, and quality of taste [150]. The sugar substitutes are up to several hundred times sweeter than sucrose and provide negligible calories. Sugar substitutes named low-calorie sweeteners (LCSs) added to many foods and beverages impact beverages as they can reduce the energy content to zero while maintaining palatability [171].

Polyols are polymers from dextrose (glucose), which provides fewer calories than sucrose. They are thermostable (up to 160°C) and absorbed by passive diffusion and metabolized slowly by the body, producing a low glycemic response. Its disadvantage is a laxative effect causing abdominal cramps and diarrhea when consuming large amounts [172], but they do not produce dental caries, and they are also bulk agents improving taste, mouthfeel, and texture when using in food.

Erythritol is the most used because it has the best tolerance level among all polyols [138].

Aspartame is a combination of methyl ester of the amino acid, aspartic acid, and phenylalanine (aspartyl-phenylalanine methyl ester) that is about 200 times sweeter than table sugar. Aspartame approved in 1981, is not heat stable and not recommended for phenylketonuric consumers. It is an all-purpose sweetener used in beverages, breath mints, chewing gum, cocoa mixes, frozen desserts, gelatins, puddings, powdered soft drinks, and as a tabletop sweetener in Equal. The FDA has confirmed it is safe to consume, except for anyone with phenylketonuria, a genetic disorder of metabolism [173].

Neotame is a blend of two amino acids: aspartic acid and phenylalanine. The derivative of aspartame, more stable than aspartame, and approved 2002. It is 7,000 to 13,000 times sweeter than sucrose. Neotame is stable at high temperatures. It is a general all-purpose sweetener that has both cooking and baking applications. Neotame used in baked goods, beverages, candies, chewing gum, dairy products, frozen desserts, puddings, yogurt-type products, is a tabletop sweetener [139, 174].

Acesulfame-K used blended with other sweeteners (usually sucralose or aspartame) is a high-intensity sweetener heat-stable. Acesulfame-K is 200 times most sweet than sucrose and has a grittier texture than direct sugar, but it has a slightly bitter aftertaste [138, 139].

Caution is required in individuals on a restricted potassium diet or having a sulpha antibiotic-based allergy. It is in dairy products, Chiclet, frozen dessert, baked goods, and effervescent drinks [138, 175, 176].

Sucralose is an extremely versatile high-intensity sweetener with about 600 times the sweetness of sucrose. It is merely a modification of the sucrose molecule (a chlorinated version known as trichlorogalacto-sucrose). It does not cause any rise in blood glucose levels because it is not absorbed and gets excreted unchanged in the body [138].

Sucralose retains its sweetness over a wide range of temperatures and is used in place of or in combination with sucrose in baked goods. However, the caramelization, cooking time, flavor, moisture retention, texture, and volume may vary. Complete substitution of sucralose for sugar is possible in some beverages, cheesecakes, fruit pie fillings, glazes, and sweet sauces [174].

Cyclamate is a sweetener substance derived from N-cyclo-hexyl-sulfamic acid utilized as a non-caloric artificial sweetener in foods and beverages as well as in the pharmaceutical industry [177]. Cyclamate is 30 times sweeter than sucrose. It has a bitter off-taste but has good sweetness synergy with saccharin. It is soluble in water, and its solubility increased by preparing the sodium or calcium salt [178]. Expert committees, such as FDA, FAO-WHO, and the Scientific Committee for Foods (SCF) of the European Union, evaluated the cyclamate carcinogenicity. These evaluations had concluded that cyclamate is not a carcinogen. Cyclamate has continued to be approved in many countries worldwide, and its acceptable daily intake (ADI) is yet 0-11 mg/kg/day. The SCF is currently evaluating new data on the safety of cyclamate [179].

Saccharine (benzoic sulfimide), a petroleum derivative, is a white crystalline artificial sweetener about 200 to 700 times sweeter than sucrose. It is one of the most studied food ingredients and the foundation of many low-calorie and sugarfree products worldwide. It is one of the oldest non-nutritive sweeteners, whose use is allowed in the US, but banned in other countries. The International Agency for Research on Cancer (IARC) initially classified saccharin in Group 2B ("possibly carcinogenic to humans") based on rat studies. However, it downgraded it to Group 3 ("not classifiable as to the carcinogenicity to humans") upon review of the subsequent research. In the United States, saccharin is in restaurants in pink packets; the most popular brand is "Sweet 'N Low". Saccharine is heat stable and is used to sweeten products such as drinks, candies, medicines, and toothpaste, canned fruit, jams, salad dressing, chewing gum, tabletop sweeteners, baked goods, jams, and dessert toppings [139, 180].

Tagatose is similar in sweetness and physical bulk to sucrose but metabolized like other high-intensity sweeteners [174, 181]. Its production is by purification and crystallization of the galactose isomerized under alkaline conditions. Chewing gum, dairy products, diet soft drinks, frostings, frozen yogurt, hard, and soft confectioneries, health bars, non-fat ice cream, and ready-to-eat cereals use tagatose. Due to its bulk, tagatose is in small amounts in baking and products subjected to high temperatures [174].

Alitame is an intense sweetener with sweetness potency 200 times greater than that of sucrose. It is a dipeptide of L-aspartic acid and D-alanine with a terminal N-substituted tetra methylthietanyl-amine moiety [139]. Alitame is readily absorbed in the GI tract and then rapidly metabolized and excreted. It has two main components, aspartic acid, and alanine amide. The aspartic acid component is metabolically normal, and the alanine amide passes through the body with minimal metabolic changes. In humans, the glucuronic derivative of D-alanine tetramethyl thietane amide is the major urinary metabolite. JEFCA reviewed safety data on alitame in 2002. The committee concluded that there was no evidence that alitame is carcinogenic. An ADI of 0–1 mg/kg body weight was allocated based on the NOAEL of 100mg/kg body weight/day to an 18-month study in dogs. Mexico, Colombia, China, Australia, and New Zealand approve Alitame [139]

The sweeteners have different functional properties that may affect the perceived taste or use in different food applications [182]. All sweeteners approved for use in the United States are determined to be "GRAS" (Generally Recognized As Safe) [130, 183]. Even after decades of scientific research demonstrating the safety of artificial sweeteners, some consumers remain unconvincing. The main reason for searching for a natural sweetener that can pass all tests of toxicity [136, 184] and many of them not challenged, because they are unnatural or because they are less sweet, laxative [172] do not caramelize, expensive or leave an aftertaste [144, 145].

It is the position of the Academy of Nutrition and Dietetics [130] that consumers can safely enjoy a range of sweeteners when consumed within an eating plan that is guided by current federal nutrition recommendations, such as the Dietary Guidelines for Americans and the Dietary Reference Intakes, as well as, individual health goals and personal preference.

DIETARY APPROACHES TO PRODUCE FOOD FOR DIABETIC CONSUMERS

The philosophical principles *"La vie est une fonction chimique,"* wielded by Antoine-Laurent Lavoisier in the 18th century and the aphorisms and sentences of Hippocrates 337 BC, "Let your food be your medicine and your medicine be your food," confirm the tight relationship between health and food [185]. Today, the food industry develops several foods with changes in their composition and with decrease, elimination, or addition of nutrients to avoid the nutritional deficiencies of the consumers and prevent excesses harmful to health. Indeed, there exist the terms Food for Special Regimes [186], and functional ingredients.

The foods prepared with these sources are foods for special dietary use (FSDU), Food for Medical Purpose (FMP), or Functional Food (FF) as a function of their nutritional or medical supervision [187, 188]. However, these foods should be included in the usual diet, because their effects go beyond being simple contributors of nutrients. They can prevent or control diseases, including Diabetes.

Today numerous consumers have a vast scientific knowledge of the food's constituents and its relationship with disease control or prevention. Consequently, there is a wide demand from the consumer of food with these constituents. Since ancient times, humans look for defeating diseases and therefore prolonging their life. Thus, all foods related to disease prevention, anti-aging, energy, and immunity have all the consumer's attention.

The marketing of food products for the prevention of diseases and treatments has a commonplace, which is why the concepts of foods for special diets and functional foods arise. The offer must be for consumers suffering from Diabetes, obesity, stress, heart disease, osteoporosis, high cholesterol, and cancer. The vision of food as preventive medicine continues to grow. The presence of phytochemicals and nutrients in plant products and grains continues to induce the consumer to get closer to healthy states through food. At the same time, the market for "nutraceutical" or functional products and special regimes mature, offering food and drinks, not only to improve lifestyle and sports but for those consumers with risk factors and in chronic conditions of significant diseases. The diet pattern for a person with Diabetes can prevent and reverse the disease. As more knowledge about Diabetes, dietary patterns for diabetics have been changing.

The traditional approach to Diabetes focuses on limiting refined sugars and foods that release sugars during digestion-starches, bread, fruits. However, with carbohydrates reduced, the diet may contain an unhealthful amount of fat and protein [189]. Consequently, it has been taken care of to limit fats, especially saturated fats that can raise cholesterol levels and limit protein for people with impaired renal function [190].

Fat is a concern in a diabetic diet because the more fat there is in the diet, the harder time insulin has in getting glucose into the cells. Conversely, minimizing fat intake and reducing body fat help insulin do its job much better [31]. The new diet pattern reduces meats, high-fat dairy products, and oils, and recommends diabetic consumers to eat grains, legumes, fruits, and vegetables.

SOURCES OF FOODS WITH INSULIN SECRETING, INSULIN MIMETIC, AND INSULIN SENSITIZING PROPERTIES

As was previously discussed, *Diabetes Mellitus* (DM) is a group of metabolic disorders characterized by the presence of hyperglycemia due to defective insulin secretion, defective insulin action, or both [1].

Pancreatic β-cell dysfunction plays a vital role in the pathogenesis of both types 1 and 2 diabetes [191]. Insulin, a key metabolic hormone produced in β-cells [191], is a vital hormone required to maintain glucose homeostasis [192, 193].

Insulin causes cells in the liver, skeletal muscles, and fat tissue to absorb glucose from the blood [194]. In the liver and skeletal muscles, glucose is store as glycogen, and in fat cells (adipocytes), glucose is store as triglycerides [195]. Insulin acts on specific receptors located on the cell membrane of practically every cell, but their density depends on the cell type: liver and fat cells are very rich. The insulin receptor is a receptor tyrosine kinase (RTK), a glycoprotein consisting of α and β subunits [194]. The α-subunits carry insulin-binding sites, while the β subunits have tyrosine kinase activity. Insulin stimulates glucose transport across the cell membrane by ATP-dependent translocation of glucose transporter GLUT4 to the plasma membrane [194].

Over a period, insulin also promotes the expression of the genes directing the synthesis of GLUT4. Genes for many enzymes and carriers are regulated by insulin through Ras/Raf and MAP-Kinase pathway, as well as through the phosphorylation cascade system [194].

Insulin is synthesized as pre-proinsulin and processed to proinsulin. Proinsulin is then converted to insulin and C-peptide and stored in secretory granules awaiting release on demand [192]. In healthy subjects, insulin release is strictly exact to meet the metabolic demand, specifically, β-cells sense changes in plasma glucose concentration and response by releasing corresponding amounts of insulin. The βcells respond to many nutrients in the blood circulation, including glucose, other monosaccharides, amino acids, and fatty acids [191, 192].

Glucose is evolutionarily the primary stimuli for insulin release in some animal species. Although multiple factors control insulin biosynthesis, glucose metabolism is the most critical physiological event that stimulates insulin gene transcription and mRNA translation [195].

According to Fu *et al.* [192], β-cells do not appear to contain membrane-bound glucose receptors but are equipped with several sensing devices that measure circulating glucose as follows

1. Glucose equilibration in β-cells *via* glucose transporter 2-mediated facilitated diffusion and the glucokinase enzyme, that function as a glucose sensor in β-cell.
2. Products derived from the metabolism of pyruvate β-cells. They can act as insulin secretion signals, which include NADPH, malonyl-CoA, and glutamate. Two ways metabolize pyruvate
   a. After being metabolized to acetyl-CoA, it enters glucose oxidation.
   b. Anaplerosis is the act of replenishing TCA cycle intermediates extracted for biosynthesis. Pyruvate oxidation through the tricarboxylic acid cycle (TCA) by mitochondria is the major signaling pathway coupled to "ATP-sensitive potassium (KATP) channel-dependent insulin release".

This signaling pathway runs to increase the intracellular ATP/ADP ratio, sequentially leading to the closure of KATP channels, depolarization of the plasma membrane, the opening of voltage-dependent Ca^{2+} channels, the influx of Ca^{2+}, and eventual activation of exocytosis of insulin-containing granules.

3 . Formation of glycerol-3-phosphate (Gly3P) coming from the metabolism of pyruvate to dihydroxyacetone phosphate. Gly3P can also replenish NAD+ to promote β-cell glycolysis *via* the mitochondrial Gly3P NADH shuttle process,

which then activates mitochondrial energy metabolism and triggers insulin secretion.

Insulin secretion is extremely sensitive to changes in blood glucose. The stimulus for insulin secretion by glucose takes place with an increase in the intracellular ATP levels. In the intracellular medium, the increase of ATP levels leads to the closure of ATP-sensitive K+ channels (KATP), resulting in the membrane depolarization capable of opening the voltage-dependent Ca^{2+} channels, which promote the influx of extracellular Ca^{2+}, inducing insulin secretion [196].

According to Kazeen and Davies [197], several sources of foods have the potential to modulate insulin. They can control insulin secretion or action due to the presence of different phytochemicals in their composition, as was previously discussed.

-Sources of foods with insulin-secreting properties.

Phytochemicals are natural antioxidants and effective medicines for humans. The phytochemicals are chemical compounds produced by plants, generally to help them thrive or thwart competitors, predators, or pathogens [198], which are useful for humans' health, mainly its anti-diabetic effect. These phytochemicals showed activities that stimulate or potentiate insulin secretion in the pancreatic islets, acting on insulin secretagogues.

They improve the performance of pancreatic tissues by increasing insulin secretion or decreasing the intestinal absorption of glucose [199].

Several of them are for use individually, for example, flavonoids, phenolic, triterpenes and derivatives, phytosterols, stilbene, and iridoid glycoside, among others. They also have been studied and used as plant extracts [199 - 201].

Plants extracts come from conventional and non-conventional plants such as *Acacia arabica, Achyranthes aspera, Acosmium panamense, Aegle marmelose, Allium sativum* (garlic), Aloe barbadensis Miller, Andrographis paniculata, Annona squamosa, Argyreia nervosa, Artemisia herba, Averrhova bilimbí, Azadirachta indica, Barleria prionitis, Biophytum sensitivum, Brassica nigra, Bryonia alba, Caesalpinia bonducella, Cajanus cajan, Carum carvi, Casearia esculenta, Chamaemelum nobile, Cichorium intybus, Citrulus colocynthis, Coriandrum sativum, Dorema aucheri, Eclipta alba, Fraxinus excersior, Helicteres isora, Hypoxis hemerocallidea, Lepidium sativum, Mangifera indica, Myrcia bella, Nigella sativa, Ocimum sanctum, Origanium vulgare, Phyllanthus amarus, Prangos ferulacea (L.) lindl, Rhus coriaria (sumac), Salacia reticulate Securinegra virosa, and Ocimum sanctum.

The concentration of blood glucose triggers the mechanism of insulin secretion because insulin secretion is quite sensitive to changes in blood glucose. Glucose stimulates insulin secretion due to the increment of intracellular ATP levels. The increment of the ATP levels leads to the closure of ATP-sensitive K+ channels with consequent membrane depolarization and opening of the Ca^{2+} channels (voltage-dependents). This membrane opening promotes the influx of extracellular Ca^{2+}, inducing insulin secretion.

Even though glucose is the most potent stimulator of insulin secretion; other nutrients are also capable of triggering insulin release or amplifying glucosestimulated insulin secretions (GSISs) [193, 202]. Indeed, the same authors have postulated that flavonoids from some foods can act on insulin secretagogues because they are capable of triggering insulin release or amplify glucosestimulated insulin secretions. The authors explain that flavonoids can modulate insulin secretion through alterations in Ca^{2+} fluxes by L-type Ca^{2+} channels. They also pointed out that flavonoids can act by other mechanisms, such as intracellular cAMP accumulation, activation by protein-kinase-A, activation of Ca^{2+}/calmodulin-dependent protein kinase, or by the transcription factors or its products (genes). They conclude that flavonol and isoflavones have shown better activities of modulation.

According to several researchers [203, 204], the triterpenes have several ant diabetic mechanisms. They can inhibit enzymes involved in glucose metabolism, prevent the development of insulin resistance and normalize plasma glucose and insulin levels [203]. The use of triterpenes as advanced glycation end products (AGEs) inhibitors may be a potentially effective strategy to prevent diabetic complications [204]. Many triterpenoid compounds are present in fruits and vegetables, most of them found in the peel of the fruit, especially within the cuticle.

The Iridoid lyonofolin B potentiates glucose-induced insulin secretion and thus can serve as a new insulin secretagogue for the treatment of diabetes [205].

Iridoids are a large group of cyclopenta[c]pyran monoterpenoids that occur widely in nature, mainly in dicotyledonous plant families like *Apocynaceae, Scrophulariaceae, Diervillaceae, Lamiaceae, Loganiaceae, and Rubiaceae* [206].

The resveratrol, and its derivatives, particularly the 3(OH) ST, inhibited adipocyte differentiation and enhanced glucose uptake in the myotubes, resulting in an improvement in glucose tolerance *in vivo* [207]. Plants containing resveratrol have been used in traditional medicine for a long time [208]. Resveratrol is in some plants, fruits, and derivatives, such as red wine.

In recent times some studies identified phytosterols as one of the key modulators of glucose metabolism, which could lead through the AMP-activated kinase (AMPK) activation or peroxisome proliferator-activated receptors (PPARs) to transcriptional regulation pathways [209].

-Sources with insulin-mimetic properties.

Other of the examples is the elaboration of foods for special dietary is by using insulin-mimetic compounds. The application of insulin-mimetic compounds, *i.e.*, substances that induce GLUT4 translocation in the absence of insulin, represents a promising strategy for the prevention and treatment of type 2 diabetes mellitus [210].

The translocation of glucose transporter 4 (GLUT4) to the plasma membrane from intracellular storage compartments, results in an increased uptake of glucose in muscle and adipose tissue in the absence of insulin, known as insulin-mimetic properties [211]. The insulin-mimetic triggers insulin signaling, which is characterized by rapid activation of insulin receptor substrate-1, Akt, and glycogen synthase kinase-3 independent of insulin receptor phosphorylation [212, 213].

Various phytochemicals induce the translocation of GLUT4 *in vitro* such; as, such as gallic acid, tannic acid, abscisic acid, caffeic acid, and quercetin [210].

- Sources with insulin-sensitizer properties

The reduced response of the body's tissues to the hormone insulin is the most prominent feature common in Diabetes, the insulin sensitizer work mainly by reducing insulin resistance. An insulin-sensitizer is a compound that allows insulin to work more effectively on cells, decreasing the blood glucose concentration without augments in the concentration of insulin. Moreover, evidence shows that insulin sensitizers have not only beneficial effects on glycemic control but also have multiple effects on lipid metabolism and atherosclerotic vascular processes that could prove to be beneficial [214].

Recent studies suggest that insulin-sensitizer changes mitochondrial metabolism and metabolic signals that coordinate downstream cell function. As it was postulated [215], the insulin-sensitizer binds directly to a protein complex in the inner membrane of the mitochondria, the small organelles in each cell that carry out oxidative metabolism. This complex in the mitochondria contains proteins that comprise a route through which pyruvate, an intermediate at the crossroads of metabolism, enters the mitochondria.

The effect of the insulin-sensitizer is to modify the entry of pyruvate at this site, and this adjustment affects the metabolism of other nutrients. These modifications, in turn, result in signals that coordinate cell function changes to match the perceived availability of nutrients. These changes include regulation of the expression of gene networks specific for that cell. Thus, fitting with all available data, over-nutrition predisposes to insulin resistance and favors the progression of the diseases associated with insulin resistance. Insulin sensitizers can counter this metabolic dysfunction [212].

Robertson *et al.* [216], pointed out that resistant starch might modulate insulin sensitivity, although the precise mechanism of this action is unknown. Also, the role of vitamin D in restraining adipose tissue inflammation and fibrosis as well as hepatic insulin resistance and suggests that normalizing 25(OH)D levels could have metabolic benefits in targeted individuals [217, 218]. Moreover, the conclusion of Belenchia *et al.* [219] highlights that the correction of poor vitamin D status through dietary supplementation may be an effective addition to the standard treatment of obesity and its associated insulin resistance. Later, Bhattacharya [218] suggests that vitamin D deficiency contributes to further insulin resistance and poorer long-term diabetic control in type 2 diabetes mellitus subjects.

On the other hand, data reported by Lin *et al.* [220] have indicated that low Pi (phosphorus) in diet regulates glucose homeostasis, partly *via* enhancing insulin sensitivity through upregulating insulin signals and insulin-induced glucose uptake in skeletal muscles.

Oleanolic acid (OA), a natural component of many plant food and medicinal herbs is endowed with a wide range of pharmacological properties whose therapeutic potential has only partly been exploited. Although it directly modulates enzymes connected to carbohydrate metabolism and insulin signaling, the main OA contributions appear derived from its interaction with critical transduction pathways [221].

GLYCEMIC AND, INSULINIC INDEX AND GLYCEMIC LOAD

Glycemic Index (GI)

The glycemic index (GI) is a measure of the blood glucose-raising ability of the available carbohydrate in foods [222]. The glycemic index (GI) defined by Jenkins *et al.* [223], as the incremental blood glucose area (0-2 h), following the ingestion of 50 g of available carbohydrates as a percentage of the corresponding area following an equivalent amount of carbohydrate from a standard reference product.

The glycemic response to a food, which affects the insulin response, depends on the rate of gastric emptying, as well as on the rate of digestion and absorption of carbohydrates from the small intestine [224].

It agreed that the size of the carbohydrate affects the GI. However, Björck *et al.* [225] pointed out other food factors that are different from the carbohydrate component's molecular size, which is the determinant of glycemic response. Therefore, different food products or meals with the same amount of carbohydrates show differences in glycemic and insulinemic responses. The author highlights the food structure, starch, gel-forming types of dietary fiber, organic acids, amylase inhibitors, fructose/glucose-ratio among these foods factor. In such cases as ground, ripened, fermented food, the GI could be high.

Both the quantity and quality (*i.e.*, nature or source) of carbohydrates influence the glycemic response. The GI compares equal quantities of carbohydrates and provides a measure of carbohydrate quality, but not quantity [226].

Glycemic Load (GL)

The concepts of glycemic load (GL) allow comparisons of the likely glycemic effect of realistic portions of different foods, calculated as the amount of carbohydrate in one serving times the GI of the food [224]. The glycemic load (GL) is an equation that considers the planned portion size of food as well as the glycemic index of that food.

Glycemic Load = [Glycemic Index/100] x net of planned carbohydrate*

*Net carbohydrate (g) = Carbohydrate Total (g) - Dietary Fiber (g).

In theory, a large amount of low GI food may increase your blood sugar as much as a small amount of a high GI food.

Insulin Index (FII)

The insulin index (FII) of food represents how much food elevates insulin concentration during the two hours after its ingestion. Its range varies from 0-100. FII can help to identify foods that minimize lifetime insulin secretion. It is of great information for metabolic flexibility and overall health and longevity.

FII measures the postprandial increase of insulin secretion of whole food. It depends on carbohydrates, the quantity, and quality of protein and fat, and its interactions [227, 228].

Holt *et al.*, in 1997 [229] have suggested that consideration of insulin scores may be relevant to the dietary management and pathogenesis of non-insulin-dependent diabetes mellitus and hyperlipidemia and may help increase the accuracy of estimating pre-prandial insulin requirements.

Due to the inconsistencies in the results of GI *versus* GL of foods, data must be completed by glycated hemoglobin (A1C) assays before adopting as useful antidiabetic foods.

To be explicit and to understand the concerns, the measurement of glycated proteins, primarily glycated hemoglobin, is effective in monitoring long-term glucose control in people with Diabetes. Glycosylated or glycated hemoglobin is the hemoglobin subfractions formed by the glycation of the alpha or beta chains of the hemoglobin A1 (HbA). During the normal 120-day life span of the red blood cell (RBC), glucose molecules react with hemoglobin, forming glycated hemoglobin. Once glycated, it remains in this form.

In people without diabetes, about 4% to 6% have hemoglobin glycosylated. Red blood cells (RBCs) contain the hemoglobin circulating in the bloodstream for three to four months before being broken down and replaced. During that time, the RBC can bond, irreversibly, to glucose in the bloodstream. A build-up of glycated hemoglobin within the red blood cell reflects the average level of glucose to which the cell is exposed during its life cycle. Thus, A1C readings higher than about 6% indicate higher than normal amounts of glucose roaming the bloodstream in the past 120 days [230].

RECIPES

Eggplant Dip and Chips

Ingredients

1.5kg	Eggplants
2	Garlic (cloves)
10g	Sesame seeds (ground)
5g	Olive oil
1g	Cumin (ground)
45g	Lemon juice
1g	Salt

Preparation

Eggplant Dip

Preheat the oven to 180°C/350°F. Cut the eggplants in half and place face down on a greased baking tray, and pinhole the skin with a fork. Put the garlic cloves on the eggplant Place the tray in the oven and bake it for 45min or until the eggplant is soft inside. Remove the tray from the oven and once the eggplant is let to cool, scoop out the eggplant flesh with a spoon and place it in a bowl, discard the skins. Add to the eggplant flesh the baked garlic cloves, ground sesame seed, lemon juice, cumin, and salt in a food processor to blend. Drizzle the dip with olive oil over the top and side. Serve with eggplant chips.

Eggplant Chips

Preheat the oven to 131 °F (55 °C). Use a mandolin to cut the eggplant thinly as possible. Tossing it in a little sesame oil, and salt. Dehydrate at 130 °F (55 °C) for 24 hours, cool for 30 minutes. Fully dehydrated eggplant store for at least 6 months at room temperature. If eggplant chips are yet moist, turn off the oven and let them sit and dry out.

Grilled Eggplant

Ingredients

300g	Eggplant	Pinch	Black Pepper
0.5g	Coriander seed (ground)	Pinch	Cayenne pepper
0.5g	Cumin seed (ground)	26g	Olive oil

Preparation

Preheat the grill to medium-hot 350 °F (180 °C). Sliced the eggplant using a mandolin or knife into 1/2-inch rounds. In a bowl, mix olive oil with coriander, cumin, salt, cayenne, and pepper (condiment mix). Drizzle the sliced eggplant with the olive oil-condiment mix. Let sit for 5 to 10 minutes. Grill it at a mediumhot temperature, about 4 minutes per side.

Eggplant, Tomato and Passion Fruit Chutney

Ingredients

350g	Eggplants (chopped)		
450g	Tomatoes (peeled, diced, and pitted)		
225g	Passion Fruit (chopped mesocarp)		
175g	Onion (chopped)		
1	Garlic clove		
100g	Raisin (pitted and roughly chopped)		
12g	Stevia granulated leaf extract		
10ml	Passion fruit juice		
300ml	Apple cider vinegar		
1	Lime (zest and juice)		
5g	Ginger powder		
10g	Spice mix (5g cumin, 2g black pepper)	5g	Salt

Preparation

Combine tomatoes, garlic clove, onions, apple cider vinegar, salt, the zest and juice lime, powdered ginger, spice mix, raisins in a heavy-bottomed 4-6 quart pot. Bring to a boil, then reduce to a simmer and let cook up to 2 hours, or until slightly thickened (often stirring to prevent scorching). Add stevia powder and season to taste. If canning, transfer the chutney into canning jars, leaving ¼ space at the top. Bring the canning water bath to a boil and submerge at a medium boil for 10 minutes. Remove jars and cool for 24 hours before storing in a cool, dark place.

Passion Fruit Jam

Ingredients

3.5kg	Passion Fruit (about 12 large)
1.5 l	Water (6 cups)
80ml	Lemon juice (1/3 cup)
20g	Stevia (granulate leaf extract)

Preparation

Remove pulp from passion fruit and reserve it for later. Place skins in a large saucepan, add water and lemon juice, cover, bring to boil, reduce heat, simmer, covered, 20 to 30 minutes, or until pulpy (mesocarp) remains inside skins puff up and become soft enough to remove from the outer layer. The inside pulpy part (cooked mesocarp) should be a burgundy color and should scrape away easily with a teaspoon. Drain and reserve this cooking liquid. Scrape all skins until they are free from the pulp, discard outer skins (exocarp). Measure pulp; allow 12g sweeteners to each cup of pulp. Place pulp and sweetener in a large saucepan with reserved liquid; mixture should not be more than 5cm deep at this stage. Stir constantly, without boiling, until sweetener is dissolved, bring to boil rapidly, without stirring, until mixture sets when tested on a cold saucer; this takes about 40 minutes. Add reserved passion fruit pulp, stand 10 minutes before pouring into hot sterilized jars, and seal it when cold, storing it in a cool dark place.

Passion Fruit-Yogurt Ice Cream

Ingredients and equipment

1.7kg	Passion fruit (about 6 large)	450g	Greek plain Yogurt (skimmed)
80g	Lemon juice	240g	Passion-Fruit pulp (thawed frozen)
10g	Sweetener (sucralose o stevia leaf extract)	-	Ice cream maker

Preparation

Ice cream bowl: Cut by half the passion fruits. Remove pulp from it. Freeze the pulp and reserve; to add to ice cream later. Place skins in a large saucepan, add water and lemon juice, cover, bring to boil, reduce heat, simmer, covered, 20 to 30 minutes or until pulpy remains inside skins puff up and become soft enough to remove the outer layer. The inside pulpy part (cooked mesocarp) should be a burgundy color, and soft. Drain the liquid. Carefully with a knife cut all outer pigmented skin (exocarp) and discard it. Leave to cold.

Ice cream: Whisk together sweetener and skimmed Greek plain yogurt. Stir in the passion-fruit pulp, cover, and chill, until cold. Freeze mix in ice cream maker. Serve in each bowl a serving of the ice cream. Transfer to an airtight container and put it in the freezer to harden.

Plantain-Ginger Men Cookies

Ingredients

350g	Plantain (2/12oz green plantain cooked; green)
30g	Plantain flour for rolling out; see chapter 1 recipes
5g	Bicarbonate of soda
3g	Ginger (ground)
2.7g	Cinnamon (ground)
125g	Butter
12g	Stevia (leaf extract granulated)
55g	Egg

Preparation

Clean the whole green plantains carefully with plenty of potable water and cook in boiling water for 20 minutes. Leave to cold and peeling, discard peel.

Mix cooked edible portion of green plantain, ginger, cinnamon, baking soda, nutmeg, and salt in a food processor. Set aside. Beat butter and stevia in a large bowl with an electric mixer on medium speed until light and fluffy. Add egg and vanilla; mix well. Gradually beat in plantain mixture on low speed until well mixed. Press dough into a thick flat disk and cover with plastic wrap. Refrigerate 4 hours or overnight. Preheat the oven at 350 °F. Roll out the dough to 1/4-inch thickness on a lightly floured work surface. Cut into gingerbread men shapes with a 5-inch cookie cutter. Place 1 inch apart on ungreased baking sheets. Bake 8 to 10 minutes or until edges of cookies setting and begin to brown. Cool on baking sheets for 1 to 2 minutes. Remove to wire racks; cool completely and store cookies in an airtight container for up to 5 days.

Ginger/Mistletoe/Almond Biscuit

Ingredients

38g	Mistletoe Fig (mashed pulp)	15g	Butter, melted
100g	Almond meal	15g	Water
100g	Oat or plain whole meal flour	2g	Cloves spice (ground)
55g	Egg whole	2.5g	Cinnamon spice (ground)
Pinch	Salt	5g	Ginger finely (fresh and grated)
9g	Stevia leaf extract granulated	-	-

Preparation

Preheat oven at 350°F (180°C). Add the ingredients into the food processor, and mix thoroughly until forming a dough. Over an ungreased baking tray, mold the dough into a roll. Roll the dough into balls, pressing gently on top of each one to flatten out molding sized as a cookie. Bake it at 180 °C/350 °F for 15 minutes.

Once they have cooled, store them in an airtight container at room temperature.

CONSENT FOR PUBLICATION

Not Applicable.

CONFLICT OF INTEREST

The author confirms that this chapter contents have no conflict of interest.

ACKNOWLEDGEMENT

Declared none.

REFERENCES

[1]　Craig ME, Hattersley A, Donaghue KC. Definition, epidemiology and classification of diabetes in children and adolescents. Pediatr Diabetes 2009; 10 (Suppl. 12): 3-12.
[http://dx.doi.org/10.1111/j.1399-5448.2009.00568.x] [PMID: 19754613]

[2]　Brink S, Lee W, Pillay K. Diabetes in children and adolescents: basic training for healthcare professionals in developing countries.Practical Pediatric Endocrinology in a Limited Resource Setting. 1st ed. New York: Academic Press 2013; pp. 243-84.
[http://dx.doi.org/10.1016/B978-0-12-407822-2.00012-8]

[3]　Goldenberg R, Punthakee Z. Classification and diagnosis of diabetes, pre-diabetes, and metabolic syndrome. 2013; 37(Suppl 1): S8-11.
[http://dx.doi.org/10.1016/j.jcjd.2013.01.011]

[4]　WHO. Organización Mundial de la Salud (OMS). Classification of Diabetes Mellitus. Geneva: World Health Organization; 2019. Licence: CC BY-NC-SA 3.0 IGO. 2019.. 2019.

[5]　Leontis LM, Hess-Fischl A. Type 2 Diabetes Complications How to Prevent Short- and Long-term Complications. 2020 from https://www.endocrineweb.com/conditions/type-2-diabetes/type-2-diabtes-complications

[6]　Cho NH, Shaw JE, Karuranga S, *et al.* IDF Diabetes Atlas: Global estimates of diabetes prevalence for 2017 and projections for 2045. Diabetes Res Clin Pract 2018; 138: 271-81.
[http://dx.doi.org/10.1016/j.diabres.2018.02.023] [PMID: 29496507]

[7]　WHO. Organización Mundial de la Salud (OMS). Diabetes. Día Mundial de la Diabetes. Available from: . http://who.int/diabetes/es/index.html2013.

[8]　Johnston CA, Stevens B, Foreyt JP. The role of the low-calories sweeteners in Diabetes. US Endocrinol 2013; 13-21.
[http://dx.doi.org/10.17925/USE.2013.09.01.13]

[9] Ogurtsova K, da Rocha Fernandes JD, Huang Y, *et al.* IDF Diabetes Atlas: Global estimates for the prevalence of diabetes for 2015 and 2040. Diabetes Res Clin Pract 2017; 128: 40-50.
[http://dx.doi.org/10.1016/j.diabres.2017.03.024] [PMID: 28437734]

[10] Cho NH, Shaw JE, Karuranga S, *et al.* IDF Diabetes Atlas: Global estimates of diabetes prevalence for 2017 and projections for 2045. Diabetes Res Clin Pract 2018; 138: 271-81.
[http://dx.doi.org/10.1016/j.diabres.2018.02.023] [PMID: 29496507]

[11] American Diabetes ADA. Association®. Economic Costs of Diabetes in the U.S. in 2017. Diabetes Care 2018; 43(7): 1-12.care.diabetesjournals.org [Cited: 25th June 2020].

[12] Elflein J. 2019.Elflein J. Estimated global healthcare expenditure to treat Diabetes in 2019 and 2045 (in billion U.S. dollars). Health & Pharm 2019. Available from: https://www.statista.com

[13] Olokoba AB, Obateru OA, Olokoba LB. Type 2 diabetes mellitus: a review of current trends. Oman Med J 2012; 27(4): 269-73.
[http://dx.doi.org/10.5001/omj.2012.68] [PMID: 23071876]

[14] Suresh Lal B. Chapter-5. Diabetes: Causes, symptoms, and treatments.Public Health Environment and Social Issues in India: Publisher. Serials Publications 2016.

[15] Shivashankar M, Mani T. A brief overview of diabetes. Int J Pharma Sci 2011; 3 (Suppl. 4): 22-7.

[16] American Diabetes ADA. American Diabetes Association. Diagnosis and classification of diabetes mellitus. Diabetes Care 2014; 37 (Suppl. 1): S81-90.
[http://dx.doi.org/10.2337/dc14-S081] [PMID: 24357215]

[17] American Diabetes ADA. ADA.American Diabetes Association®. Classification of Diabetes mellitus. Geneva: World Health Organization; License: CC BY-NC-SA 3.0 IGO. 2019a.

[18] Dell AJ, Lernmark A. Autoimmune (type 1) Diabetes.The Autoimmune diseases. 5th ed. New York: Academic Press 2014; pp. 575-86.
[http://dx.doi.org/10.1016/B978-0-12-384929-8.00041-1]

[19] Burrack AL, Martinov T, Fife BT. T Cell-Mediated Beta Cell Destruction: Autoimmunity and Alloimmunity in the Context of Type 1 Diabetes. Front Endocrinol (Lausanne) 2017; 8: 343.
[http://dx.doi.org/10.3389/fendo.2017.00343] [PMID: 29259578]

[20] Michels AW, Eisenbarth GS. Immunologic endocrine disorders. J Allergy Clin Immunol 2010; 125(2) (Suppl. 2): S226-37.
[http://dx.doi.org/10.1016/j.jaci.2009.09.053] [PMID: 20176260]

[21] Piya A, Michels AW. Understanding the immunology of type 1 diabetes. An overview of current knowledge and perspectives for the future. US Endocrinol 2012; 8(1): 70-4.
[http://dx.doi.org/10.17925/USE.2012.08.01.12]

[22] Shouip HA. Diabetes Mellitus. Faculty of Pharmacy & Pharmacology Industries: Sinai University 2014.

[23] American Diabetes Association. Diagnosis and classification of *diabetes mellitus.* Diabetes Care 2009; 32 (Suppl. 1): S62-7.
[http://dx.doi.org/10.2337/dc09-S062] [PMID: 19118289]

[24] Hupfeld CJ, Courtney CH, Olefsky JM. Chapter 41. In: Type 2 Diabetes Mellitus: Etiology, Pathogenesis, and Natural History; 2016 pp., 765-787.

[25] Ginter E, Simko V. Type 2 diabetes mellitus, pandemic in 21st century. Adv Exp Med Biol 2012; 771: 42-50.
[http://dx.doi.org/10.1007/978-1-4614-5441-0_6] [PMID: 23393670]

[26] Maitra A, Abbas AK. The endocrine system. Pathologic Basis of Disease. Philadelphia: Elsevier Saunders 2005; pp. 1155-226.

[27] Shin J-A, Lee J-H, Lim S-Y, *et al.* Metabolic syndrome as a predictor of type 2 diabetes, and its clinical interpretations and usefulness. J Diabetes Investig 2013; 4(4): 334-43.
[http://dx.doi.org/10.1111/jdi.12075] [PMID: 24843675]

[28] Huang PL. A comprehensive definition for metabolic syndrome. Dis Model Mech 2009; 2(5-6): 231-7.
[http://dx.doi.org/10.1242/dmm.001180] [PMID: 19407331]

[29] Chen L, Magliano DJ, Zimmet PZ. The worldwide epidemiology of type 2 diabetes mellitus--present and future perspectives. Nat Rev Endocrinol 2011; 8(4): 228-36.
[http://dx.doi.org/10.1038/nrendo.2011.183] [PMID: 22064493]

[30] Murea M, Ma L, Freedman BI. Genetic and environmental factors associated with type 2 diabetes and diabetic vascular complications. Rev Diabet Stud 2012; 9(1): 6-22.
[http://dx.doi.org/10.1900/RDS.2012.9.6] [PMID: 22972441]

[31] Asif M. The prevention and control of type-2 diabetes by changing lifestyle and dietary pattern. J Educ Health Promot 2014; 3:1.26ADA. American Diabetes Association®. Eating patterns and meal planning. 2017. Available from: www.diabetes.org

[32] American Diabetes Association. Gestational diabetes mellitus. Diabetes Care 2003; 26 (Suppl. 1): S103-5.
[http://dx.doi.org/10.2337/diacare.26.2007.S103] [PMID: 12502631]

[33] Godswill Awuchi C, Kate Echeta Chinelo K, Igwe SV. Diabetes and the Nutrition and Diets for its prevention and treatment: A systematic review and dietetic perspective. Health Sciences Research 2020; 6(1): 5-19.

[34] ADA. 2020.American Diabetes Association https://www.diabetes.org/nutrition/meal-planning

[35] American Diabetes ADA. American Diabetes Association. Association®. Lifestyle management: Standard of medical care in Diabetes -2019. Diabetes Care 2019; 42 (Suppl. 1): S46-60. b
[http://dx.doi.org/10.2337/dc19-S005] [PMID: 30559231]

[36] Gray A, Threlkeld RJ. Nutritional Recommendations for Individuals with Diabetes. [Updated 2019 Oct 13]. In: Feingold KR, Anawalt B, Boyce A, *et al.*, editors. Endotext [Internet]. South Dartmouth (MA): MDText.com, Inc. Available from https://www.ncbi.nlm.nih.gov

[37] Breslin PAS. An evolutionary perspective on food and human taste. Curr Biol 2013; 23(9): R409-18.
[http://dx.doi.org/10.1016/j.cub.2013.04.010] [PMID: 23660364]

[38] Sampaio Cutrim C, Sloboda Cortez MA. A review on polyphenols: Classification, beneficial effects and their application in dairy products. Int J Dairy Technol 2018; 71(3): 564-78.
[http://dx.doi.org/10.1111/1471-0307.12515]

[39] Rodriguez-Jimenez JR, Amaya-Guerra CA, Baez-Gonzalez JG, Aguilera-Gonzalez C, Urias-Orona V, Nino-Medina G. Physicochemical, functional, and nutraceutical properties of eggplant flours obtained by different drying methods. Molecules 2018; 23(12): 3210.
[http://dx.doi.org/10.3390/molecules23123210] [PMID: 30563127]

[40] Sruthi G, Pillai HH, Ullas N, Jiju V, Abraham E. Role of antioxidants in the management Diabetes Mellitus. Int J Pharm Sci Nanotechnol 2017; 10(4): 3763-7.

[41] Aryaeian N, Sedehi SK, Arablou T. Polyphenols and their effects on diabetes management: A review. Med J Islam Repub Iran 2017; 31: 134.
[http://dx.doi.org/10.14196/mjiri.31.134] [PMID: 29951434]

[42] Han X, Shen T, Lou H. Dietary polyphenols and their biological significance. Int J Mol Sci 2007; 8(9): 950-88.
[http://dx.doi.org/10.3390/i8090950]

[43] Tsao R. Chemistry and biochemistry of dietary polyphenols. Nutrients 2010; 2(12): 1231-46.
[http://dx.doi.org/10.3390/nu2121231] [PMID: 22254006]

[44]   Pandey KB, Rizvi SI. Plant polyphenols as dietary antioxidants in human health and disease. Oxid Med Cell Longev 2009; 2(5): 270-8.
[http://dx.doi.org/10.4161/oxim.2.5.9498] [PMID: 20716914]

[45]   Pinent M, Castell A, Baiges I, Montagut G, Arola L, Ardévol A. Bioactivity of flavonoids on insulin-secreting cells. Compr Rev Food Sci Food Saf 2008; 7(4): 299-308.
[http://dx.doi.org/10.1111/j.1541-4337.2008.00048.x] [PMID: 33467792]

[46]   Godwin N, Roberts T, Hooshmand S, Kern M, Hong MY. Mixed nuts may promote satiety while maintaining stable blood glucose and insulin in healthy, obese, and overweight adults in a two-arm randomized controlled trial. J Med Food 2019; 22(4): 427-32.
[http://dx.doi.org/10.1089/jmf.2018.0127] [PMID: 30897012]

[47]   Chandrasekara A, Josheph Kumar T. Roots and tuber crop as functional foods: a review on phytochemical constituents and their potential Health Benefits. Int J Food Sci 2016; 2016: 3631647.
[http://dx.doi.org/10.1155/2016/3631647] [PMID: 27127779]

[48]   Mesa MD, Ramírez-Tortosa MC, Aguilera CM, Ramírez-Boscá A, Gil A. Pharmacological and nutritional effects of *Curcuma longa* L. extracts and curcuminoids. Ars Pharm 2000; 41(3): 307-21.

[49]   Asai A, Miyazawa T. Dietary curcuminoids prevent high-fat diet-induced lipid accumulation in rat liver and epididymal adipose tissue. J Nutr 2001; 131(11): 2932-5.
[http://dx.doi.org/10.1093/jn/131.11.2932] [PMID: 11694621]

[50]   Pari L, Murugan P. Antihyperlipidemic effect of curcumin and tetrahydrocurcumin in experimental type 2 diabetic rats. Ren Fail 2007; 29(7): 881-9.
[http://dx.doi.org/10.1080/08860220701540326] [PMID: 17994458]

[51]   Jang EM, Choi MS, Jung UJ, *et al.* Beneficial effects of curcumin on hyperlipidemia and insulin resistance in high-fat-fed hamsters. Metabolism 2008; 57(11): 1576-83.
[http://dx.doi.org/10.1016/j.metabol.2008.06.014] [PMID: 18940397]

[52]   Seo KI, Choi MS, Jung UJ, *et al.* Effect of curcumin supplementation on blood glucose, plasma insulin, and glucose homeostasis related enzyme activities in diabetic db/db mice. Mol Nutr Food Res 2008; 52(9): 995-1004.
[http://dx.doi.org/10.1002/mnfr.200700184] [PMID: 18398869]

[53]   Pérez Sira EE. Capítulo 9. Raíces y Tubérculos.De tales harinas, tales panes Granos harinas y productos de panificación en Iberoamérica Programa Iberoamericano de Ciencia y Tecnología para el Desarrollo. Córdoba, Argentina: CYTED 2007; pp. 363-401.

[54]   Choque-Delgado GT, Marostica Jr M, da Silva Tamashiro WM, Pastore GM. Choque-Delgado GT, Marostica Jr, M, da Silva Tamashiro WM, Pastore GM. Yacón (Smallanthus sonchifolius): A functional food. Plant Foods Hum Nutr 201; 68(3):222-228.

[55]   Shirdel Z, Mirbadalzadeh R, Madani H. Anti-diabetic and antilipidemic effect of ginger in alloxan monohydrate diabetic rats in comparison with glibenclamide. Iran J Diabetes Lipid Disord 2009; 9: 7-15.

[56]   Rahmani AH, Shabrmi FM, Aly SM. Active ingredients of ginger as potential candidates in the prevention and treatment of diseases *via* modulation of biological activities. Int J Physiol Pathophysiol Pharmacol 2014; 6(2): 125-36.
[PMID: 25057339]

[57]   57 Zadeh JB, Kor NM. Physiological and pharmaceutical effects of Ginger (*Zingiber officinale* Roscoe) as a valuable medicinal plant. Eur J Exp Biol 2014; 4(1): 87-90.

[58]   de Lima RMT, Dos Reis AC, de Menezes APM, *et al.* Protective and therapeutic potential of ginger (*Zingiber officinale*) extract and [6]-gingerol in cancer: A comprehensive review. Phytother Res 2018; 32(10): 1885-907.
[http://dx.doi.org/10.1002/ptr.6134] [PMID: 30009484]

[59]   Li L-L, Cui Y, Guo X-H, Ma K, Tian P, Feng J, *et al.* Pharmacokinetics and tissue distribution of gingerols and shogaols from ginger (*Zingiber officinale* Rosc.) in rats by UPLC–Q-Exactive–HRMS. Molecules 2019; 24(3): 512-24.
        [http://dx.doi.org/10.3390/molecules24030512]

[60]   Ajayi OB, Akomolafe SF, Akinyemi FT. Food value of two varieties of ginger (*Zingiber officinale*) commonly consumed in Nigeria. ISRN Nutr 2013; 2013: 359727.
        [http://dx.doi.org/10.5402/2013/359727] [PMID: 24967255]

[61]   Oluwatoyin A. Physicochemical characterisation, and antioxidant properties of the seeds and oils of ginger (*Zingiber officinale*) and garlic (*Allium sativum*). Sci J Chem 2014; 2(6): 44-50.
        [http://dx.doi.org/10.11648/j.sjc.20140206.11]

[62]   Li Y, Tran VH, Duke CC, Roufogalis BD. Preventive and protective properties of Zingiber officinale (Ginger) in Diabetes Mellitus, diabetic complications, and associated lipid and other metabolic disorders: A Brief Review. Evid-Based Complementary Altern Med 2012; pp. 1-10.

[63]   Mozaffari-Khosravi H, Talaei B, Jalali B-A, Najarzadeh A, Mozayan MR. The effect of ginger powder supplementation on insulin resistance and glycemic indices in patients with type 2 diabetes: a randomized, double-blind, placebo-controlled trial. Complement Ther Med 2014; 22(1): 9-16.
        [http://dx.doi.org/10.1016/j.ctim.2013.12.017] [PMID: 24559810]

[64]   Arablou T, Aryaeian N, Valizadeh M, Sharifi F, Hosseini A, Djalali M. The effect of ginger consumption on glycemic status, lipid profile and some inflammatory markers in patients with type 2 diabetes mellitus. Int J Food Sci Nutr 2014; 65(4): 515-20.
        [http://dx.doi.org/10.3109/09637486.2014.880671] [PMID: 24490949]

[65]   Fensker WA, Brill A, Nall R, Pabitch S, Punt M, Daniels M, *et al.* Prostaglandin E2 (PGE2) levels as a predictor of type 2 diabetes control in humans subjects: a cross-sectional view of initial cohort study data. FASEB J 2017; 31(1): Supplement.

[66]   Lindstedt I. Ginger and Diabetes: A mini-review. Arch Gen Intern. Med 2018; 2(2): 29-33.

[67]   Adebayo-Oyetoro AO, Olatidoye OP, Ogundipe OO, Akande EA, Isaiah CG. Production and quality evaluation of complementary food formulated from fermented sorghum, walnut, and ginger. J Appl Biosci 2012; 54: 3901-10.

[68]   Shirshir RI, Hossain M, Hossain M. Processing of ginger powder. Bangladesh Res Pub J 2012; 7(3): 277-82.

[69]   Norhidayah A, Noriham A, Rusop M. The effect of drying methods on physicochemical properties of nanostructured *Zingiber officinale* Rosc. (ginger) rhizome. Adv Mat Res 2013; 667: 458-63.
        [http://dx.doi.org/10.4028/www.scientific.net/AMR.667.458]

[70]   Sangwan A, Kawatra A, Sehgal S. Nutritional composition of ginger powder prepared using various drying methods. J Food Sci Technol 2014; 51(9): 2260-2.
        [http://dx.doi.org/10.1007/s13197-012-0703-2] [PMID: 25190894]

[71]   Sumariyah J, Khuriati A, Fachriya E. Electrohydrodynamic (EDH) drying of ginger slices (*Zingiber officinale*). J Phys 2018; 1025: 1.

[72]   Schaneberg BT, Applequist WL, Khan IA. Determination of aristolochic acid I and II in North American species of Asarum and Aristolochia. Pharmazie 2002; 57(10): 686-9.
        [PMID: 12426949]

[73]   Bogusz MJ, Al-Tufail M. Aristolochic acid Forensic Science. Handbook of Analytical Separations. 2nd ed. Elsevier 2008; 6: pp. 357-82.

[74]   Debelle FD, Vanherweghem J-L, Nortier JL. Aristolochic acid nephropathy: a worldwide problem. Kidney Int 2008; 74(2): 158-69.
        [http://dx.doi.org/10.1038/ki.2008.129] [PMID: 18418355]

[75]   Takeda J, De Silva S, Muthuraman P, Rahman SM, Kawet L. Spices in Sri Lanka, India, and Bangladesh with special reference to the usages and consumptions. Bull. Fac. Agr. Saga Univ 2008; 9: 1-25.

[76]   Akinwande BA, Ade-Omowaye BIO, Olaniyan SA, Akintarom OO. Quality evaluation of ginger-flavoured soy-cassava biscuit. Nutr Food Sci 2008; 38(5): 473-81.
[http://dx.doi.org/10.1108/00346650810906994]

[77]   Filipčev B, Šimurina O, Sakač IM, Sedej I, Jovanov P, Pestorić M, *et al.* Feasibility of use of buckwheat flour as an ingredient in ginger nut biscuit formulation. Food Chem 2011; 125(1): 164-70.
[http://dx.doi.org/10.1016/j.foodchem.2010.08.055]

[78]   Gbenga-Fabusiwa FJ, Oladele EP, Oboh G, Adefegha SA, Oshodi AA. Polyphenol contents and antioxidants activities of biscuits produced from ginger-enriched pigeon pea–wheat composite flour blends. J Food Biochem 2018; 42(4): e12526.
[http://dx.doi.org/10.1111/jfbc.12526]

[79]   Mishra P, Kumar Bhatt D. A Study on development of fortified pasta with ginger powder. IOSR-JESTFT 2016; 8(10): 14-8.
[http://dx.doi.org/10.9790/2402-1008011418]

[80]   Adebayo-Oyetoro AO, Ogundipe OO, Azoro CG, Adeyeye SAO. Production and evaluation of ginger spiced cookies from wheat-plantain composite flour. Pac J Sci Technol 2016; 17(1): 280-7.

[81]   Quaisie J, Liao L, Wu W. Effect of blending ginger starch (*Zingiber officinale*) on the dynamic rheological, pasting, and textural properties of rice flour. Afr J Food Sci 2017; 11(8): 263-72.
[http://dx.doi.org/10.5897/AJFS2017.1596]

[82]   Martinez-Villaluenga C, Horszwald A, Frias J, Piscula M, Vidal-Valverde C, Zielinsky H. Effect of flour extraction rate and baking process on vitamin B1 and B2 contents and antioxidant activity of ginger-based products. Eur Food Res Technol 2009; 230: 119.
[http://dx.doi.org/10.1007/s00217-009-1146-5]

[83]   Balestra F, Cocci E, Pinnavaia GG, Romani S. Evaluation of antioxidant, rheological and sensorial properties of wheat flour dough and bread containing ginger powder. LWT-Food Sci Techno 2011; 44(3): 700-5.
[http://dx.doi.org/10.1016/j.lwt.2010.10.017]

[84]   Soluman Almasodi AG. Production and evaluation of some bakery products containing ginger powder. J Food Nutr Res 2018; 6(4): 205-15.
[http://dx.doi.org/10.12691/jfnr-6-4-2]

[85]   Silva Dias J. Nutritional Quality and Effect on Disease Prevention of Vegetables 2019.https://cwww.intechopen.com/books/nutrition-in-health-and-disease-our-chal-enges-now-and-forthcoming-time/nutritional-quality-and-effect-on-disease-prevention-of-vegetables
[http://dx.doi.org/10.5772/intechopen.85038]

[86]   Ojewole JA, Adewunmi CO. Hypoglycemic effect of methanolic extract of *Musa paradisiaca* (Musaceae) green fruits in normal and diabetic mice. Methods Find Exp Clin Pharmacol 2003; 25(6): 453-6.
[http://dx.doi.org/10.1358/mf.2003.25.6.769651] [PMID: 12949631]

[87]   Bohs L, Weese TL. Eggplant origins: Out of Africa, into the Orient. Taxon 2010; 59(1): 1.

[88]   Uthumporn U, Fazilah A, Tajul AY, Maizura M, Ruri AS. Physico-chemical and antioxidant properties of eggplant flour as a functional ingredient. Adv J Food Sci Techn 2016; 12(5): 235-43.
[http://dx.doi.org/10.19026/ajfst.12.2905]

[89]   Kwon YI, Apostolidis E, Shetty K. *In vitro* studies of eggplant (*Solanum melongena*) phenolics as inhibitors of key enzymes relevant for type 2 diabetes and hypertension. Bioresour Technol 2008; 99(8): 2981-8.
[http://dx.doi.org/10.1016/j.biortech.2007.06.035] [PMID: 17706416]

[90]   Ma C, Whitaker BD, Kennelly EJ. New 5-O-caffeoylquinic acid derivatives in fruit of the wild eggplant relative Solanum viarum. J Agric Food Chem 2010; 58(20): 11036-42.
[http://dx.doi.org/10.1021/jf102963f] [PMID: 20886887]

[91]   Qonita NR, Zulhaida M, Sudiarto T, Tjahjone HA. The effect of eggplant (*Solanum melongena* L.) extract peroal against blood glucose level of white rat (*Ratus novergicus*) wistar strain diabetic model. Int J Pediatr Endocrinol 2013; (Suppl. 1)O33.
[http://dx.doi.org/10.1186/1687-9856-2013-S1-O33]

[92]   Plazas M, Andújar I, Vilanova S, Hurtado M, Gramazio P, Herraiz FJ, *et al.* Breeding for chlorogenic acid content in eggplant: interest and prospects. Not Bot Horti Agrobot Cluj-Napoca 2013; 41(1): 26-35.
[http://dx.doi.org/10.15835/nbha4119036]

[93]   Gürbüz N, Uluişik S, Frary A, Frary A, Doğanlar S. Health benefits and bioactive compounds of eggplant. Food Chem 2018; 268: 602-10.
[http://dx.doi.org/10.1016/j.foodchem.2018.06.093] [PMID: 30064803]

[94]   Potter BJ. Understanding type II Diabetes: The chemistry of Diabetes. 1st ed., New York 2018.

[95]   Dole. Eggplant *vs.* blood sugar. 2019. Available from: http://www.dole.com

[96]   Rodriguez-Jiménez J, Amaya-Guerra C, Núñez-González A, Báez-González JG, Aguilera-Gonzalez C. Caracterización bromatológica y tecnofuncional de la harina de berenjena (*Solanum melongena*) y quínoa (*Chenopodium quinoa*). Invest Desarro Cien y Tecnol Alimentos 2017; 2: 417-42.

[97]   Tripathi PC. Passion fruit. In: Perter KV (ed). Horticultural crops of high nutraceutical value, Brillion Pub. New Delhi. Pp. 245-270.

[98]   Akanbi B, Bodunrin O, Según O. Phytochemical screening and antibacterial activity of Passiflora edulis. 2011 @inproceedings {Akanbi2011PhytochemicalSA

[99]   Joy PP. Passion fruit Production Technology (Ad hoc). Pineapple Research Station (Kerala Agricultural University). 2010. District, Kerala, India. Available from: https://www.researchgate.net

[100]   Dos Santos Medeiros J, Melo Diniz MF, Oliveira Sabaa Srur AU, Barbosa Pessoa M, Alves Cardoso MA, Franklin de Carvalho D. Ensaios toxicológicos clínicos da casca do maracujá-amarelo (*Passiflora edulis*, f. flavicarpa), como alimento com propriedade de saúde. RevBras Pharmacog 2009; 19(2A): 394-9.

[101]   Salgado M, Dias Bombarde ITA, Niero Mansi ID, de Stefano Piedade SM, Molina Meletti LM. Effects of different concentrations of passion fruit peel (*Passiflora edulis*) on the glicemic control in diabetic rat. Food Sci Technol (Campinas) 2010; 30(3): 784-9.
[http://dx.doi.org/10.1590/S0101-20612010000300034]

[102]   Smith RE, da Silva Menezes EM, Sabaa-Srur A, Wycoff WG. Potential Health Benefits of Passion Fruit Peel Flour. Nat Prod J 2012; 2(2): 104-7.
[http://dx.doi.org/10.2174/2210315511202020104]

[103]   de Queiroz MdoS, Janebro DI, da Cunha MA, *et al.* Effect of the yellow passion fruit peel flour (*Passiflora edulis* f. flavicarpa deg.) in insulin sensitivity in type 2 diabetes mellitus patients. Nutr J 2012; 11: 89.
[http://dx.doi.org/10.1186/1475-2891-11-89] [PMID: 23088514]

[104]   DaSilva JK, Betim Cazarin CB, Batista AG. Marostica Jr.M. Effects of passion fruit (*Passiflora edulis*) byproduct intake in antioxidant status of Wistar rats tissues. LWT-Food Sci Techn 2014; 59: 1213-9.
[http://dx.doi.org/10.1016/j.lwt.2014.06.060]

[105] Monteiro Coelho E, Guttierres Gomes R, Souza Machad BA, Santos Oliveira R, Dos Santos Lima M. Passion fruit peel flour–Technological properties and application in food products. Food Hydrocoll 2016; 62: 158-64.
[http://dx.doi.org/10.1016/j.foodhyd.2016.07.027]

[106] Coelho EM, de Azevêdo LC, Viana AC, *et al.* Physico-chemical properties, rheology and degree of esterification of passion fruit (Passiflora edulis f. flavicarpa) peel flour. J Sci Food Agric 2018; 98(1): 166-73.
[http://dx.doi.org/10.1002/jsfa.8451] [PMID: 28556245]

[107] Saleem F. Anti-Diabetic Potentials of Phenolic Enriched Chilean Potato and Select Herbs of Apiaceae and Lamiaceae Families Masters Theses 1911 Amherst ScholarWorks@UMass Amherst. University of Massachusetts 2010.

[108] Tashakori-Sabzevar F, Ramezani M, Hosseinzadeh H, *et al.* Protective and hypoglycemic effects of celery seed on streptozotocin-induced diabetic rats: experimental and histopathological evaluation. Acta Diabetol 2016; 53(4): 609-19.
[http://dx.doi.org/10.1007/s00592-016-0842-4] [PMID: 26940333]

[109] Godavari A, Amutha K, Manicka Moorthi N. *In-vitro* hypoglycemic effect of Foeniculum vulgare Mill, seeds on the carbohydrate hydrolyzing enzymes, α-amylase and α-glucosidase. Int J Pharm Sci Res 2018; 9(10): 4441-4.

[110] Aligita W, Susilawati E, Septiani H, Atsil R. Anti-diabetic activity of coriander (*Coriandrum Sativum* L) leaves' ethanolic extract. Int J Pharm Phytopharm Res 2018; 8(2): 59-63.

[111] Mahmoud KA. Anti-diabetic and antioxidant effects of parsley extract (*Petroselinum crispum*) on diabetic rats. Isotope Radiation Res 2011; 43(2): 341-57.

[112] Bayani M, Ahmadi-Hamedani M, Jebelli Javan A. Study of hypoglycemic, hypocholesterolemic and antioxidant activities of Iranian Mentha spicata leaves aqueous extract in diabetic rats. Iran J Pharm Res 2017; 16 (Suppl.): 75-82.
[PMID: 29844778]

[113] Eidi A, Eidi M. Anti-diabetic effects of sage (*Salvia officinalis* L.) leaves in normal and streptozotocin-induced diabetic rats. Diabetes Metab Syndr 2009; 3(1): 40-4.
[http://dx.doi.org/10.1016/j.dsx.2008.10.007]

[114] Yen H-F, Hsieh C-T, Hsieh T-J, Chang F-R, Wang C-K. *In vitro* anti-diabetic effect and chemical component analysis of 29 essential oils products. Yao Wu Shi Pin Fen Xi 2015; 23(1): 124-9.
[http://dx.doi.org/10.1016/j.jfda.2014.02.004] [PMID: 28911435]

[115] Ezeani C, Ezenyi I, Okoye T, Okoli C. *Ocimum basilicum* extract exhibits antidiabetic effects *via*inhibition of hepatic glucose mobilization and carbohydrate metabolizing enzymes. J Intercult Ethnopharmacol 2017; 6(1): 22-8.
[http://dx.doi.org/10.5455/jice.20161229054825] [PMID: 28163956]

[116] Hassan WE. Healing Herbs of Malaysia. Kuala Lumpur: Federal Land Development Agency 2006.

[117] Bunawan H, Amin NM, Bunawan SN, Baharum SN, Mohd Noor N. *Ficus deltoidea* Jack: A review on its phytochemical and pharmacological importance. Evid Based Complement Alternat Med 2014; 2014: 902734.https://www.hindawi.com [Cited: 25th June 2020].
[http://dx.doi.org/10.1155/2014/902734] [PMID: 24772185]

[118] Adam Z, Khamis S, Ismail A, Hamid M. *Ficus deltoidea*: A potential alternative medicine for Diabetes Mellitus. Evid Based Complement Alternat Med 2012; 2012: 632763.
[http://dx.doi.org/10.1155/2012/632763] [PMID: 22701507]

[119] Wang P-C, Zhao S, Yang B-Y, Wang Q-H, Kuang H-X. Anti-diabetic polysaccharides from natural sources: A review. Carbohydr Polym 2016; 148(5): 86-97.
[http://dx.doi.org/10.1016/j.carbpol.2016.02.060] [PMID: 27185119]

[120] Dave DT, Shah GB. Pharmacological potential of naturally occurring non-starch polysaccharides (NSP). J Phytopharm 2015; 4(6): 307-10.

[121] Yang N, Zhao M, Zhu B, Yang B, Chen C, Chun Cui C, *et al.* Anti-diabetic effects of polysaccharides from *Opuntia monacantha* cladode in normal and streptozotocin-induced diabetic rats. Innov Food Sci Emerg Technol 2008; 9: 570-4.
[http://dx.doi.org/10.1016/j.ifset.2007.12.003]

[122] Mao XQ, Yu F, Wang N, *et al.* Hypoglycemic effect of polysaccharide enriched extract of Astragalus membranaceus in diet induced insulin resistant C57BL/6J mice and its potential mechanism. Phytomedicine 2009; 16(5): 416-25.
[http://dx.doi.org/10.1016/j.phymed.2008.12.011] [PMID: 19201177]

[123] Abou-Arab AE, Abou-Araband AA, Abu-Salem MF. Physico-chemical assessment of natural sweeteners steviosides produced from *Stevia rebaudiana* Bertoni plant. Afr J Food Sci 2010; 4: 269-81.

[124] Kokotou MG, Asimakopoulos AG, Thomaidis NS. 13a Sweeteners.Food Analysis by HPLC, Chapter: Sweeteners, Publisher. CRC Press 2012; pp. 493-514.

[125] Shah J, Dion C. Sweet taste perception is impaired in NIDDM but not in IDDM patients.Chandalia HB, Shah J. The Research Society Grant Medical College 1996; pp. 178-9.

[126] Chattopadhyay S, Raychaudhuri U, Chakraborty R. Artificial sweeteners - a review. J Food Sci Technol 2014; 51(4): 611-21.
[http://dx.doi.org/10.1007/s13197-011-0571-1] [PMID: 24741154]

[127] Stone h, Oliver SM. Measurement of the Relative Sweetness of Selected Sweeteners and Sweetener Mixtures. J Food Sci 2006; 34(2): 215-22.

[128] Yeung CA, Goodfellow A, Flanagan L. The truth about sugar. Dent Update 2015; 42(6): 507-510, 512.
[http://dx.doi.org/10.12968/denu.2015.42.6.507] [PMID: 26506805]

[129] Mohan Rao L, Ramalakshmi K. Ingredients of soft drinks 2011.
https://www.sciencedirect.com/topics/food-science/sweetener
[http://dx.doi.org/10.1533/9780857093653.3.189]

[130] American Diabetes ADA. Association®. Position of the academy of nutrition and dietetics: Use of nutritive and non-nutritive sweeteners. J Am Diet Assoc 2012; 1112: 739-58.

[131] Coulston AM, Hollenbeck CB, Donner CC, Williams R, Chiou YA, Reaven GM. Metabolic effects of added dietary sucrose in individuals with noninsulin-dependent diabetes mellitus (NIDDM). Metabolism 1985; 34(10): 962-6.
[http://dx.doi.org/10.1016/0026-0495(85)90146-5] [PMID: 3900632]

[132] Coulston AM, Hollenbeck CB, Swislocki ALM, Chen YDI, Reaven GM. Deleterious metabolic effects of high-carbohydrate, sucrose-containing diets in patients with non-insulin-dependent diabetes mellitus. Am J Med 1987; 82(2): 213-20.
[http://dx.doi.org/10.1016/0002-9343(87)90058-1] [PMID: 3544839]

[133] Fitch C, Keim KS. Academy of Nutrition and Dietetics. Position of the Academy of Nutrition and Dietetics: use of nutritive and nonnutritive sweeteners. J Acad Nutr Diet 2012; 112(5): 739-58.
[http://dx.doi.org/10.1016/j.jand.2012.03.009] [PMID: 22709780]

[134] Caballero B. Sucrose: Dietary sucrose and disease Encyclopedia of human nutrition. 3rd ed., Amsterdam: Elsevier 2013.

[135] Shankar P, Ahuja S, Sriram K. Non-nutritive sweeteners: review and update. Nutrition 2013; 29(11-12): 1293-9.
[http://dx.doi.org/10.1016/j.nut.2013.03.024] [PMID: 23845273]

[136] Kendig MD, Lin CS, Beilharz JE, Rooney KB, Boakes RA, Boake R. Maltodextrin can produce similar metabolic and cognitive effects to those of sucrose in the rat. Appetite 2014; 77: 1-12.
[http://dx.doi.org/10.1016/j.appet.2014.02.011] [PMID: 24582585]

[137] Mohamed GA, Ibrahim SRM, Elkhayat ES, El Dine RS. Natural anti-obesity agents. Bull Fac Pharm Cairo Univ 2014; 53: 269-84.
[http://dx.doi.org/10.1016/j.bfopcu.2014.05.001]

[138] Modi SV, Borges VJ. Artificial sweeteners: boon or bane? Int J Diabetes Dev Ctries 2005; 25: 1-8. [Review].
[http://dx.doi.org/10.4103/0973-3930.26753]

[139] Chattopadhyay S, Raychaudhuri U, Chakraborty R. Artificial sweeteners - a review. J Food Sci Technol 2014; 51(4): 611-21.
[http://dx.doi.org/10.1007/s13197-011-0571-1] [PMID: 24741154]

[140] Bloomgarden ZT. Nonnutritive sweeteners, fructose, and other aspects of diet. Diabetes Care 2011; 34(5): e46-51.
[http://dx.doi.org/10.2337/dc11-0448] [PMID: 21525491]

[141] Berg JM, Tymoczko JL, Stryer L. Biochemistry, 5th edition. New York: W H Freeman Ed., 2002; 277(35):31646–31655.

[142] Hull P. Syrup applications: An overview. In: Glucose Syrups: Technology and Applications 2010. Wiley-Blackwell.

[143] Hull P. Glucose syrups: Technology and applications. Wiley-Blackwell 2010; pp. 61-75.
[http://dx.doi.org/10.1002/9781444314748.ch5]

[144] González C, Tapia MS, Pérez E, Dornier M, Morel G. Caracterización de cultivares de *Stevia rebaudiana* Bertoni de diferentes procedencias. Bioagro- 2014; 26: 79-88.

[145] González C, Tapia M, Pérez E, Pallet D, Dornier M. Main properties of steviol glycosides and their potential in the food industry: A review. Fruits 2014; 69: 127-41.
[http://dx.doi.org/10.1051/fruits/2014003]

[146] Martinez Cruz M. Stevia rebaudiana (Bert.) Bertoni. Una revision. Cultrop 2015; 36 (Suppl. 1): 5-15. [Stevia rebaudiana (Bert.) Bertoni. A review].

[147] Pérez E, González C, Vaillant F, Lares M. Stevia derivative and its potential uses in diabetic directed foods. J Nutr 2016; 3(1): 1-20. [Review].

[148] Jorge K. Soft drinks chemical composition. In: Encycl food Sci Nutr, 2nd edn. Elsevier Ltd, London, 2003, pp 5346–5352.

[149] Lee Y-J, Yang C-M. Growth behavior and perillaldehyde concentration of primary leaves of *Perilla frutescens* (L.) Britton growing in different seasons. Crop Envirom Bioinform 2006; 3: 135-48.

[150] Surana SJ, Gokhale SB, Rajmane RA, Jadhav B. Non-saccharide natural intense sweeteners. An overview of current status. Nat Prod Radiance 2002; 5(4): 270-9.

[151] Hobbs CA, Taylor SV, Beevers C, *et al.* Genotoxicity assessment of the flavouring agent, perillaldehyde. Food Chem Toxicol 2016; 97: 232-42.
[http://dx.doi.org/10.1016/j.fct.2016.08.029] [PMID: 27593899]

[152] Ramos-Tovar E, Muriel P. Phytotherapy for the Liver.Dietary Interventions in Liver Disease Foods, Nutrients, and Dietary Supplements. New York: Academic Press, Elsevier 2019; pp. 101-21.
[http://dx.doi.org/10.1016/B978-0-12-814466-4.00009-4]

[153] Cinatl J, Morgenstern B, Bauer G, Chandra P, Rabenau H, Doerr HW. Glycyrrhizin, an active component of liquorice roots, and replication of SARS-associated coronavirus. Lancet 2003; 361(9374): 2045-6.
[http://dx.doi.org/10.1016/S0140-6736(03)13615-X] [PMID: 12814717]

[154] Glória MBA. Intense sweeteners and synthetic colorants. Food analysis by HPLC. New York: Marcer Dekker, Inc 1997; pp. 523-74.

[155] Glória MBA. Sweeteners. Encyclopedia of Food Sciences and Nutrition. 2nd ed. New York: Academic Press 2003; pp. 42-7.
[http://dx.doi.org/10.1016/B0-12-227055-X/01404-8]

[156] Izawa K, Amino Y, Kohmura M, Ueda Y, Kuroda M. 2010.Human-Environment Interactions-Taste.
[http://dx.doi.org/10.1016/B978-008045382-8.00108-8]

[157] Compadre CM, Pezzuto JM, Kinghorn AD, Kamath SK. Hernandulcin: an intensely sweet compound discovered by review of ancient literature. Science 1985; 227(4685): 417-9.
[http://dx.doi.org/10.1126/science.3880922] [PMID: 3880922]

[158] Sauerwein M, Yamazaki T, Shimomura K. Hernandulcin in hairy root cultures of *Lippia dulcis.* Plant Cell Rep 1991; 9(10): 579-81.
[http://dx.doi.org/10.1007/BF00232336] [PMID: 24220716]

[159] Suzuki YA, Tomoda M, Murata Y, Inui H, Sugiura M, Nakano Y. Antidiabetic effect of long-term supplementation with *Siraitia grosvenori* on the spontaneously diabetic Goto-Kakizaki rat. Br J Nutr 2007; 97(4): 770-5.
[http://dx.doi.org/10.1017/S0007114507381300] [PMID: 17349091]

[160] Dawson GE, Maxwell MW, Harper HJ, Mohlenkamp MJ, Rizzi GP Jr, Romer K, *et al.* Process and composition for sweet juice from Cucurbitaceae fruit, U.S. patent 5,411,755, 1995.

[161] Khanvilkar S, Arya S. Fructooligosaccharides: Applications and health benefits- A review. Agro Food Ind Hi-Tech 2015; 26(6): 8-12.

[162] Sabater-Molina M, Larqué E, Torrella F, Zamora S. Dietary fructooligosaccharides and potential benefits on health. J Physiol Biochem 2009; 65(3): 315-28.
[http://dx.doi.org/10.1007/BF03180584] [PMID: 20119826]

[163] Manrique I, Gonzales R, Valladolid V, Blas R, Lizárraga L. Yacon (Smallanthus sonchifolius (Poepp. & Endl.)) seeds production through controlled pollination techniques. Ecol Apl 2014; 13(2): 135-8.
[http://dx.doi.org/10.21704/rea.v13i1-2.464]

[164] Shoaib M, Shehzad A, Omar M, *et al.* Inulin: Properties, health benefits and food applications. Carbohydr Polym 2016; 147(147): 444-54.
[http://dx.doi.org/10.1016/j.carbpol.2016.04.020] [PMID: 27178951]

[165] Fasura CB, da Cruz AG, Ferreira M. Inulin: Technological Applications and Health Benefits.Inulin: Chemical Properties, Uses and Health Benefits. Series Biochemistry Res Trends. Food Sci Tech. Nova Science Publisher 2017.

[166] Sangeetha PT, Ramesh MN, Siddalingaiya P. Fructooligosaccharide production using fructosyl transferase obtained from recycling culture of *Aspergillus oryzae* CFR 202. Process Biochem 2005; 40(3-4): 1085-8.
[http://dx.doi.org/10.1016/j.procbio.2004.03.009]

[167] Lara-Fiallo M, Lara-Gordillo P, Julian-Ricardo MC, *et al.* Advance on the inulin production. RTQ 2017; 37(2): 252-266.

[168] Carniel Beltrami M, Döring T, Dea J. Sweeteners and sweet taste enhancers in the food industry. Food Sci Technol (Campinas) 2018; 38(2): 181-7.
[http://dx.doi.org/10.1590/fst.31117]

[169] Sardesai VM, Waldshan TH. Natural and synthetic intense sweeteners. J Nutr Biochem 1991; 2: 236-44.
[http://dx.doi.org/10.1016/0955-2863(91)90081-F]

[170] Godshall MA. The expanding world of nutritive and non-nutritive sweeteners. Sugar J 2007; 69: 12-20.

[171] Cook D, Haslam D, Weir C. The role of low-calorie sweeteners in weight management: Evidence and practicalities. Supplement to Diabetes Digest 2013; 12: 1-4.

[172] Oku T, Okazaki M. Laxative threshold of sugar alcohol erythritol in human subjects. Nutr Res 1996; 16: 577-89.
[http://dx.doi.org/10.1016/0271-5317(96)00036-X]

[173] Aldarete-Velasco J, López-García R, Zúñiga-Guajardo S, Riobó-Serván P, Serra-Majem L, Suverza-Fernández A, *et al.* Análisis de la evidencia disponible para el consumo de edulcorantes no calóricos. Documento de expertos. Med Int Méx 2017; 33(1): 61-83.

[174] Marcus JB. Culinary Nutrition. Carbohydrate basics: Sugars, starches, and fibers in foods and health.The Science and Practice of Healthy Cooking. New York: Academic Press 2013; pp. 149-87.

[175] Nabors LO. Sweet choices: sugar replacements for foods and beverages. Food Technol 2002; 56: 28-32.

[176] Horne J, Lawless HT, Speirs W, Sposato D. Bitter taste of saccharin and acesulfame-K. Chem Senses 2002; 27(1): 31-8.
[http://dx.doi.org/10.1093/chemse/27.1.31] [PMID: 11751465]

[177] Martins AT, Azoubel R, Lopes RA, Sala di Matteo MA, Ferraz de Arruda JG. Effect of sodium cyclamate on the rat fetal liver: a karyometric and stereological study. Int J Morphol 2005; 23(3): 221-6.
[http://dx.doi.org/10.4067/S0717-95022005000300005]

[178] Bopp BA, Sonders RC, Kesterson JW. Toxicological aspects of cyclamate and cyclohexylamine. Crit Rev Toxicol 1986; 16(3): 213-306.
[http://dx.doi.org/10.3109/10408448609037465] [PMID: 2420530]

[179] Takayama S, Renwick AG, Johansson SL, *et al.* Long-term toxicity and carcinogenicity study of cyclamate in nonhuman primates. Toxicol Sci 2000; 53(1): 33-9.
[http://dx.doi.org/10.1093/toxsci/53.1.33] [PMID: 10653518]

[180] Okoduwa SIR, Ebiloma GU, Baba J, Ajide S. The metabolism and toxicology of saccharin. Infohealth Awareness 2013; 1(1): 14-9.

[181] Van Nostrand's Scientific Encyclopedia. 2005.

[182] Sjöström LB, Cairncross SE. Role of sweeteners in food flavor. Use of sugars and other carbohydrates in the food industry. Cambridge, Mass: Arthur D. Little, Inc. 1955; p. 108.
[http://dx.doi.org/10.1021/ba-1955-0012.ch015]

[183] O'Mullane M, Fields B, Stanley G. Food Additives: Sweeteners. Encyclopedia of Food Safety 2014; (2): 477-484.

[184] Rosenman K. Benefits of saccharin: a review. Environ Res 1978; 15(1): 70-81.
[http://dx.doi.org/10.1016/0013-9351(78)90080-4] [PMID: 340218]

[185] Grammaticos PC, Diamantis A. Useful known and unknown views of the father of modern medicine, Hippocrates and his teacher Democritus. Hell J Nucl Med 2008; 11(1): 2-4.
[PMID: 18392218]

[186] FDA (Food and Drugs Administration). 2018.https://www.accessdata.fda.gov

[187] Ross S. Functional foods: the Food and Drug Administration perspective. Am J Clin Nutr 2000; 71(6) (Suppl.): 1735S-8S.
[http://dx.doi.org/10.1093/ajcn/71.6.1735S] [PMID: 10837331]

[188] Doyon M. Functional foods: A conceptual definition. Br Food J 2008; 110(11): 1133-49.
[http://dx.doi.org/10.1108/00070700810918036]

[189] Lim A. Heart Healthy Diet for Diabetic Patients 2020.https://foryoursweetheart.ph/article/heart-healthy-diet-for-diabetic-patients/

[190] Cholesterol and Chronic Kidney Disease. DaVita Kidney Care 2020. https://www.davita.com/education/kidney-disease/risk-factors /cholesterol-and-chronic-kidney-disease

[191] Kahn SE. Clinical review 135: The importance of β-cell failure in the development and progression of type 2 diabetes. J Clin Endocrinol Metab 2001; 86(9): 4047-58. [PMID: 11549624]

[192] Fu Z, Gilbert ER, Liu D. Regulation of Insulin Synthesis and Secretion and Pancreatic Beta-Cell Dysfunction in Diabetes 2013. [http://dx.doi.org/10.2174/157339913804143225]

[193] Soares JMD, Pereira Leal AEB, Silva JC, Almeida JRGS, de Oliveira HP. Influence of flavonoids on mechanism of modulation of insulin secretion. Pharmacogn Mag 2017; 13(52): 639-46. [http://dx.doi.org/10.4103/pm.pm_87_17] [PMID: 29200726]

[194] Pathophysiology V. Physiologic Effects of Insulin 2020. http://www.vivo.colostate.edu/hbooks/ pathphys/endocrine/pancreas/insulin_phys.html

[195] Anatomy and Physiology. Metabolic States of the Body. 2020. Available in: https://opentextbc.ca/anatomyandphysiologyopenstax/chapter/metabolic-states-of-the-body

[196] Ashcroft FM. ATP-sensitive potassium channelopathies: focus on insulin secretion. J Clin Invest 2005; 115(8): 2047-58. [http://dx.doi.org/10.1172/JCI25495] [PMID: 16075046]

[197] Kazeen MI, Davies TC. Anti-diabetic functional foods as sources of insulin secreting, insulin sensitizing, and insulin mimetic agents. J Funct Foods 2016; 20: 122-38. [http://dx.doi.org/10.1016/j.jff.2015.10.013]

[198] Molyneux RJ, Lee ST, Gardner DR, Panter KE, James LF. Phytochemicals: the good, the bad and the ugly? Phytochemistry 2007; 68(22-24): 2973-85. [http://dx.doi.org/10.1016/j.phytochem.2007.09.004] [PMID: 17950388]

[199] Kooti W, Farokhipour M, Asadzadeh Z, Ashtary-Larky D, Asadi-Samani M. The role of medicinal plants in the treatment of diabetes: a systematic review. Electron Physician 2016; 8(1): 1832-42. [http://dx.doi.org/10.19082/1832] [PMID: 26955456]

[200] Hannan JM, Marenah L, Ali L, Rokeya B, Flatt PR, Abdel-Wahab YH. Ocimum sanctum leaf extracts stimulate insulin secretion from perfused pancreas, isolated islets and clonal pancreatic beta-cells. J Endocrinol 2006; 189(1): 127-36. [http://dx.doi.org/10.1677/joe.1.06615] [PMID: 16614387]

[201] Chan C-H, Ngoh G-C, Yusoff R. A brief review on anti diabetic plants: Global distribution, active ingredients, extraction techniques and acting mechanisms. Pharmacogn Rev 2012; 6(11): 22-8. [http://dx.doi.org/10.4103/0973-7847.95854] [PMID: 22654401]

[202] Rauf A, Uddin G, Siddiqui BS, *et al.* Antinociceptive and anti-inflammatory activities of flavonoids isolated from *Pistacia integerrima* galls. Complement Ther Med 2016; 25: 132-8. [http://dx.doi.org/10.1016/j.ctim.2016.02.002] [PMID: 27062961]

[203] Nazaruk J, Borzym-Kluczyk M. The role of triterpenes in the management of *diabetes mellitus* and its complications. Phytochem Rev 2015; 14(4): 675-90. [http://dx.doi.org/10.1007/s11101-014-9369-x] [PMID: 26213526]

[204] Xu F, Huang X, Wu H, Wang X. Beneficial health effects of lupenone triterpene: A review. Biomed Pharmacother 2018; 103: 198-203. [http://dx.doi.org/10.1016/j.biopha.2018.04.019] [PMID: 29653365]

[205] Hussain N, Hameed A, Ahmad MS, *et al.* New iridoids from *Lyonia ovalifolia* and their anti-hyperglycemic effects in mice pancreatic islets. Fitoterapia 2018; 131: 168-73. [http://dx.doi.org/10.1016/j.fitote.2018.08.016] [PMID: 30149098]

[206] Tundis R, Loizzo MR, Menichini F, Statti GA, Menichini F. Biological and pharmacological activities of iridoids: recent developments. Mini Rev Med Chem 2008; 8(4): 399-420.
[http://dx.doi.org/10.2174/138955708783955926] [PMID: 18473930]

[207] Ito-Nagahata T, Kurihara C, Hasebe M, *et al.* Stilbene analogs of resveratrol improve insulin resistance through activation of AMPK. Biosci Biotechnol Biochem 2013; 77(6): 1229-35.
[http://dx.doi.org/10.1271/bbb.121000] [PMID: 23748787]

[208] Burns J, Yokota T, Ashihara H, Lean MEJ, Crozier A. Plant foods and herbal sources of resveratrol. J Agric Food Chem 2002; 50(11): 3337-40.
[http://dx.doi.org/10.1021/jf0112973] [PMID: 12010007]

[209] Zakłos-Szyda M. 5. Phytosterols in type 2 diabetes and obesity. Molecular mechanisms of action.Plant Lipids Science, Technology, Nutritional Value and Benefits to Human Health. Kerala, India: Research Signpost 2015; pp. 201-19.

[210] Haselgrübler R, Stadlbauer V, Stübl F, *et al.* Insulin Mimetic Properties of Extracts Prepared from *Bellis perennis.* Molecules 2018; 23(10): 2605.
[http://dx.doi.org/10.3390/molecules23102605] [PMID: 30314325]

[211] Martel J, Ojcius DM, Chang CJ, *et al.* Anti-obesogenic and antidiabetic effects of plants and mushrooms. Nat Rev Endocrinol 2017; 13(3): 149-60.
[http://dx.doi.org/10.1038/nrendo.2016.142] [PMID: 27636731]

[212] Saltiel AR, Kahn CR. Insulin signalling and the regulation of glucose and lipid metabolism. Nature 2001; 414(6865): 799-806.
[http://dx.doi.org/10.1038/414799a] [PMID: 11742412]

[213] García-Vicente S, Yraola F, Marti L, *et al.* Oral insulin-mimetic compounds that act independently of insulin. Diabetes 2007; 56(2): 486-93.
[http://dx.doi.org/10.2337/db06-0269] [PMID: 17259395]

[214] Zangeneh F, Kudva YC, Basu A. Insulin sensitizers. Mayo Clin Proc 2003; 78(4): 471-9.
[http://dx.doi.org/10.4065/78.4.471] [PMID: 12683699]

[215] Colca JR. The TZD insulin sensitizer clue provides a new route into diabetes drug discovery. Expert Opin Drug Discov 2015; 10(12): 1259-70.
[http://dx.doi.org/10.1517/17460441.2015.1100164] [PMID: 26479699]

[216] Robertson MD, Bickerton AS, Dennis AL, Vidal H, Frayn KN. Insulin-sensitizing effects of dietary resistant starch and effects on skeletal muscle and adipose tissue metabolism. Am J Clin Nutr 2005; 82(3): 559-67.
[http://dx.doi.org/10.1093/ajcn/82.3.559] [PMID: 16155268]

[217] Lontchi-Yimagou E, Kang S, Zhang K, Goyal A, You JP, Kishore P, *et al.* Insulin sensitising effects of vitamin D mediated through reduced adipose tissue inflammation and fibrosis 2018.

[218] Bhattacharya J. Assessment of vitamin D status and its association with insulin resistance among type 2 diabetic subjects. IJRMS 2018; 6(12): 3825-31.
[http://dx.doi.org/10.18203/2320-6012.ijrms20184877]

[219] Belenchia AM, Tosh AK, Hillman LS, Peterson CA. Correcting vitamin D insufficiency improves insulin sensitivity in obese adolescents: a randomized controlled trial. Am J Clin Nutr 2013; 97(4): 774-81.
[http://dx.doi.org/10.3945/ajcn.112.050013] [PMID: 23407306]

[220] Lin Y, Berger L, Sun Z. Regulation of insulin sensitivity by phosphorus 2018.
[http://dx.doi.org/10.2337/db18-1772-P]

[221] Castellano JM, Guinda A, Delgado T, Rada M, Cayuela JA. Biochemical basis of the antidiabetic activity of oleanolic acid and related pentacyclic triterpenes. Diabetes 2013; 62(6): 1791-9.
[http://dx.doi.org/10.2337/db12-1215] [PMID: 23704520]

[222]   Henry CJK, Thondre PS. The glycaemic index: concept, recent developments and its impact on diabetes and obesity. London, UK: Smith Gordon Pub 2013; pp. 154-75.

[223]   Jenkins DJ, Wolever TM, Taylor RH, *et al.* Glycemic index of foods: a physiological basis for carbohydrate exchange. Am J Clin Nutr 1981; 34(3): 362-6.
[http://dx.doi.org/10.1093/ajcn/34.3.362] [PMID: 6259925]

[224]   Arvidsson-Lenner R, Asp NG, Axelsen M, Bryngelsson S, Haapa E, Järvi A, *et al.* Glycaemic index. Relevance for health, dietary recommendations, and food labelling. Scand J Nutr 2003; 48(2): 84-94.
[http://dx.doi.org/10.1080/11026480410033999]

[225]   Björck I, Liljeberg H, Östman E. Low glycaemic-index foods. Br J Nutr 2000; 83 (Suppl. 1): S149-55.
[http://dx.doi.org/10.1017/S0007114500001094] [PMID: 10889806]

[226]   Foster-Powell K, Holt SH, Brand-Miller JC. International table of glycemic index and glycemic load values: 2002. Am J Clin Nutr 2002; 76(1): 5-56.
[http://dx.doi.org/10.1093/ajcn/76.1.5] [PMID: 12081815]

[227]   Bao J, de Jong V, Atkinson F, Petocz P, Brand-Miller JC. Food insulin index: physiologic basis for predicting insulin demand evoked by composite meals. Am J Clin Nutr 2009; 90(4): 986-92.
[http://dx.doi.org/10.3945/ajcn.2009.27720] [PMID: 19710196]

[228]   Sampson KL, Franz M, Brand Miller J, Willett W. Beyond glycemic index: new food insulin index 2019.https://www.nutrientdataconf.org

[229]   Holt SHA, Miller JC, Petocz P. An insulin index of foods: the insulin demand generated by 1000-kJ portions of common foods. Am J Clin Nutr 1997; 66(5): 1264-76.
[http://dx.doi.org/10.1093/ajcn/66.5.1264] [PMID: 9356547]

[230]   Balatbat J. . Glycated (Glycosylated) Hemoglobin: HbA1c New directions to diagnose Diabetes. Contin Educ Topics Issues 2010; 112-115. Available from: http://americanmedtech.org

CHAPTER 6

Food For Phenylketonuric Consumers

Elevina Pérez Sira[1,*] and **Antonieta Mahfoud**[2]

[1] *Instituto de Ciencia y Tecnología de Alimentos, Facultad de Ciencias, Universidad Central de Venezuela, Caracas, Venezuela*

[2] *Instituto de Estudios Avanzados IDEA. Unidad de Errores Innatos del Metabolismo, Venezuela*

Abstract: Phenylketonuria (PKU) is an inborn error of amino acid metabolism, characterized by persistent hyperphenylalaninemia. There is no cure for PKU, however, early diagnosis and treatment during the first month of life, make it possible to prevent all the mentioned consequences. The treatment of classic and moderate PKU is nutritional, based on a diet restricted in *Phe*, and supplemented with special formulas free of *Phe*. The chapter is handling phenylketonuria (PKU) overview, highflying the treatment strategies, incidence, nutrition, and PKU Diet, and development and innovation of food for PKU including some home recipes.

Keywords: Foods for phenylketonuric, Hyperphenylalaninemia diet, Nutrition and PKU, PKU food development.

INTRODUCTION

Phenylketonuria (PKU) is an inborn error of amino acid metabolism, characterized by persistent hyperphenylalaninemia. PKU is an autosomal recessive metabolic, genetic disorder caused by mutations in the phenylalanine hydroxylase enzyme (PAH) gene [1 - 4].

Mutations in the PAH gene result in a decreased catalytic activity affecting the catabolic pathway of phenylalanine (*Phe*) by the absence of PAH [5]. It is autosomal recessive, meaning that both copies of the gene must be mutated for the condition to develop.

Those with one copy of a mutated gene typically do not have symptoms. It is one of the several ways to pass down through families a trait, disorder, or disease [6].

[*] **Corresponding author Elevina Pérez Sira:** Instituto de Ciencia y Tecnología de Alimentos, Facultad de Ciencias, Universidad Central de Venezuela, Caracas, Venezuela; Tel: +58.212.751 4403; Fax: +58.212.751 3871; E-mail: elevina07@gmail.com

The PAH gene provides instructions for producing the enzyme PHA. PAH is a hepatic enzyme responsible for the first step in processing phenylalanine, which is an essential amino acid that, the building block of proteins obtained through the diet.

All proteins and some artificial sweeteners contain Phe. Also, for the efficient enzymatic activity of PAH, the system needs as a cofactor the tetrahydrobiopterin (BH4) [7, 8], molecular oxygen, and iron [9]. Deficiency in PAH or its cofactor BH4 results in the accumulation of excess phenylalanine, whose toxic effects can cause severe and irreversible intellectual disability if remains untreated.

Other clinical features associated with untreated PKU may include autistic behaviors, motor deficits, eczematous rash, and seizures. Behavioral impairment, as well as psychiatric disturbances, can become apparent with age [10, 11].

In turn, to explain the functional mechanism of the PAH system, Kure and Shintaku [8] reported that in the L-*Phe* metabolism of mammals it acts mainly as the enzyme PAH or phenylalanine 4-monooxygenase, classified as EC 1.14.16.1; L-phenylalanine, tetrahydropteridine: oxygen oxidoreductase [12]. Therefore, PAH is necessary for the hepatic hydroxylation of phenylalanine to tyrosine. The para-hydroxylation of L-*Phe* produces L-*Tyr* in the presence of (6R)-L-erythro-5, 6, 7, 8-BH4 as a cofactor, O_2, and iron as an additional substrate [9, 13]. After the catalytic reaction of L-Phe by PAH, the pterin-4a-carbinolamine (4-OH-BH4) is regenerated to its functional tetrahydro-form (BH4) by two enzymes, the pterincarbinolamine dehydratase (PCD) and the dihydropteridine reductase (DHPR).

PCD catalyzes the dehydration of 4-OH-BH4, which produces the quinonoid 7,8dihydrobiopterin (q-BH2). The NAD-(P)-H-dependent DHPR reduces q-BH2 back to BH4. The authors highlight that the PAH system to optimal mechanism needs to include these two BH4-regenerating enzymes, PCD and DHPR, in addition to the PAH. The rate-limiting in the PAH system is the enzymatic activity of PAH.

Approximately 75% of the L-*Phe*, which contains the diet and proteins, is catabolized by the PAH system under a regular diet with the remainder 25%, used for protein synthesis [14, 15].

In healthy conditions, phenylalanine (*Phe*) does not require the process of protein synthesis to convert in the liver to tyrosine (Tyr) [16]. If PKU disorder remains untreated, the levels of L-*Phe* in the blood increase, and consequently, the L-*Phe* forms phenylpyruvic acid and its derivatives (phenylactic and phenylacetic acids) [2, 17] causing intellectual disability and other serious health problems.

Alternatively, Tyr is a nonessential amino acid formed by the hydroxylation of phenylalanine in the liver [18]. Since tyrosine is necessary to produce neurotransmitters like epinephrine, norepinephrine, and dopamine [19], it becomes an essential amino acid in PKU patients because, without PAH, the body through the breakdown of phenylalanine not produced Tyr.

The treatment guidelines of the American College of Medical Genetics and Genomics state that the clinical treatment goal for individuals with PKU is to maintain blood L-*Phe* within the range of (120–360μmol/L) for individuals of all ages and that treatment should be lifelong. Treatment of PKU eventually is individualized with multiple medications, and medical foods available to tailor the therapy. The primary goal of therapy should be to lower blood L-*Phe*, and any interventions, including medications, or combinations of therapies that help to achieve that goal in an individual, without other negative consequences [20].

A PKU unaffected individual contains in blood 1mg/dl (60 μmol/L) of Phe. On this basis different categories of PKU were determined as follows: 1. based on the diagnostic Phe level; 2. mutation testing (if performed), and the amount of *Phe* that an individual can tolerate [21].

• Classical PKU is the most common form of PKU. It results when there are two severe mutations of the PAH gene, and as a result, there is little or no PAH enzyme activity to convert phenylalanine to tyrosine. These are the most severely affected patients. *Phe* level in blood: Above 20 mg/dl (>1200 μmol/L).

• Moderate/Mild PKU is associated with elevated *Phe* levels that require treatment but are lower than those observed in Classical PKU. *Phe* level in blood: Above 6 mg/dl but less than 20 mg/dl (360- 1200μmol/L).

• Hyperphenylalanemia (HyperPhe) is used to describe those people whose blood *Phe* level is above normal but still low enough that they may not require dietary treatment. *Phe* level in blood: less than 6 mg/dl (<360 μmol/L).

González Muñoz [22] reports a comparative Table **1** of the classification of the PKU and PAH for various authors. Later, Vockley *et al.* [20] highlight that PAH deficiency presents a spectrum of severity, and several different classification schemes are proposed to assist in clinical management. Most severe are individuals with complete PAH deficiency whose untreated blood L-*Phe* levels are typical>1,200 μmol/l (mean normal level: 60 μmol/l); this phenotype is consistently termed "classical PKU." Infants diagnosed and treated earlier in life might have a peak L-*Phe* level <1,200 μmol/l and still have complete PAH deficiency.

Table 1. Comparative classification of PKU and HPA [22].

Classification	Beltmont *et al.*, 2012		Feillet *et al.*, 2010		Ramirez *et al.*, 2010	
	mg/dl	µM	mg/dl	µM	mg/dl	µM
Benign HPA	2-6	120-360	2-10	120-600	2-4	120-240
Clinically significant PKU	>6-10	>360-600	-	-	>4-10	>240-600
Moderate/Mild PKU	>10-6.6	>600-1000	>10-20	600-1200	>10-16.6	>600-1000
Classical PKU	>16.6	>1000	>20	>1200	>16.6	>1000

HPA= Hyperphenylalanemia.

For the Therapeutic Committee of the American College of Medical Genetics and Genomics in 2014, PKU can be classified based on blood L-*Phe* levels at diagnosis and dietary *Phe* tolerance [23].

González Muñoz *et al.* [22] also have reported that after the *Phe* level, the serum level of tyrosine (*Tyr*) and its quotient are the most frequent criterion used to classify the disease. Differences are in the typical values of the *Phe/Tyr* ratio since some authors consider a quotient of 1.5 and others up to 3.0 to be pathological. Several researchers also include dietary tolerance to *Phe* as a criterion, quantified by a specific challenge test.

The diagnosis must be through a neonatal screening program done between 48 and 72 hours after the birth of the children. The diagnosis is through the determination of phenylalanine on a blood sample [24] (from the baby's heel. The concentrations accepted as normal up to 2-2.5 mg/dL (120-150 mol/l).

The diagnostic criteria are constant values of phenylalanine higher than 16 to 20 mg/100ml, tyrosine values lower than 3mg/100ml, presence of phenylpyruvic, hydroxyphenylpyruvic acids in urine, and inability to tolerate oral provocation of phenylalanine. Infants with higher levels of phenylalanine than 8-12 mg/100ml should receive treatment [25]

The commercial formulas for an innate error of metabolism were regulated as drugs, later as Foods for Special Dietary Use, and recently they have been named as medical foods. From a point of view, like food security, there are no obligations for the food industry to produce food for PKU consumers. Today, the gap still exists, and there are no commitments for the food industry to produce foods in a wide gastronomic variety for PKU consumers. Not only formulas for new-born and babies, but also consumers of all ages.

TREATMENT STRATEGIES

Mahfoud *et al.* [10] have indicated that early diagnosis and treatment during the first month of life make it possible to prevent all the consequences. The authors point out that the treatment of classic and moderate PKU is nutritional, based on a diet restricted in *Phe*, and supplemented with special formulas free of *Phe*.

The main goal of treatment for PKU is to keep plasma phenylalanine levels within safe limits of 120-360 umol/L (2-6 mg/dL) (for pregnant women of 120-240 umol/L) to prevent mental retardation, to ensure normal growth and normal life with good health through adulthood [26 - 28]. This goal is, as previously reported, reached through a prudently planned and monitored diet.

Consequently, people with PKU need to follow a diet that limits foods with phenylalanine [29]. Indeed, there is not a standard meal plan for PKU patients. However, there is a list of allowed, restricted, allowed/monitored, and sometimes free food, with a full complement of nutrients except for the offending nutrient (phenylalanine-free). Until recently, lifelong dietary phenylalanine restriction was the only therapy available [22] requiring the administration of special phenylalanine-free protein supplements. Even though the consumer can find at the market some special medical formula that supplies vitamins, minerals, and all essential fatty acid and amino acids except *Phe*, there are not a wide range of offers for PKU consumers.

On the other hand, industries have developed and commercialize innovative biopharmaceuticals. Among them, the U.S. Food and Drug Administration (FDA) in 2007 [30] has approved the drug sapropterin dihydrochloride for the treatment of PKU [30 - 32]. It is a form of BH4, which is a substance in the body that helps break down phenylalanine. Though, having too little BH4 is only one reason a person may not break down phenylalanine. Therefore, the drug only helps some people reduce phenylalanine in their blood. Even if the medication helps, it not decreases the phenylalanine to the desired amount and must be used together with the PKU diet.

Besides, there are new and more palatable foods based on glycomacropeptide GMP that contains a minimal amount of aromatic amino acids, the administration of large neutral amino acids to prevent phenylalanine entry into the brain or tetrahydropterina cofactor capable of increasing residual activity of phenylalanine hydroxylase.

Providing high concentrations of the other Large Neutral Amino-acids (LNAAs) different of *Phe,* such as; histidine, isoleucine, leucine, lysine, methionine, threonine, tryptophan, tyrosine, valine might block the entry of *Phe* as well as enhancing brain levels of these critical precursors [33].

Needs for improved treatment options have led to the development of new therapeutic strategies. Therefore, human trials were performed with subcutaneous administration of phenylalanine ammonia-lyase.

Further efforts are underway to develop an oral therapy containing phenylalanine ammonia-lyase. Gene therapies also seem to be a promising approach [2]. To date, this approach has not been studied in humans but has shown encouraging results in the PAH emu2/emu2 mice involving the use of the adeno-associated virus, causing prolonged lowering of blood *Phe* [33].

Another therapy could be liver cell transplantation/repopulation. It is a technique where the liver is repopulated with phenylalanine hydroxylase (PAH)-expressing cells. And follow by a hepatocyte or hematopoietic stem cell transplantation as a possible novel treatment approach for PKU.

Successful therapeutic liver repopulation requires both a stimulus for liver regeneration at the time of cell transplantation and a selective growth advantage for the PAH+ donor cells [34]. Normal functioning liver cells are introduced to the PKU-liver and if the cells provide 10-20% of the liver activity, the disease cure. A Clinical Trial is now ongoing in Pittsburgh, USA [33].

INCIDENCE OF PKU

In spite, there is no difference in frequency of occurrence between males and females; the incidence of PKU varies among ethnic groups and geographic regions worldwide.

Prevalence rates of PKU in white Europeans and Chinese are similar (~ 1/10,000) with Taiwan 1 in 55,057. It is rare in Finland (1:100.000 birth) and Japan (1:108,000). A high rate was found in some countries such as Ireland (1 in 4,500) and Turkey (1 in 3,627). The Czech Republic's prevalence is around 1:5295, in the Islamic Republic of Iran is 1:3,627, and South African showed 1/20,000. In the United States, PKU occurs in 1 in 10,000 to 15,000 newborns.

Analysis based on available information from several Latin American new-borns screening programs shows incidence values of 1:23,518 in PKU and 1:20,759 in hyperPKU. However, individual analysis of incidence by country indicates that phenylketonuria ranges from 1:12,473 to 1:161,748 live newborns. It has been reported 1 in 50,000 in the African American population. The findings of Scriver *et al.*, 1995 support the hypothesis that the PKU phenotype is rare in African populations and arose after the out-of-Africa migration of H. sapiens [4, 35 - 44].

Some developed countries have research programs where most PKU cases are detected shortly after birth by new-borns screening, and treatment must start promptly. As a result, the severe signs and symptoms of classic PKU are rarely seen. In Latin America, there are 3 pioneering countries in terms of implementation of organized NBS programs for PKU at a national level -Cuba in 1986, Costa Rica in 1990, and Chile in 1992. Today, only 6 other countries in Latin America have implemented national or regional NBS programs -Argentina (1995, 1999, and 2000 regional; 2006 national), Brazil (2001), and more recently Uruguay (2007), Paraguay (2007), Panama (2008), and Ecuador (2011). Other countries like Mexico, Venezuela, Peru, and Guatemala have implemented NBS activities with varying degrees of success and coverage. In Venezuela, the newborns screening program started in 1985, and the prevalence is around 1:35000 [45].

Whereas countries like Colombia, Bolivia, Nicaragua, and the Dominican Republic only offer screening testing for PKU in the private sector by request and without a formal program structure. The most critical situation observed in El Salvador, Honduras, and Haiti, where NBS for PKU is virtually non-existent [46]. However, Borrajo [46] highlighted that a detailed analysis by country showed that the incidence of PKU and HPA in countries located above the equatorial line was significantly lower than in South American countries, a fact probably linked to ethnic composition.

NUTRITION AND PKU DIET

Phenylketonuria (PKU) was the first inherited metabolic disease in which dietary treatment prevents the disease's clinical features. The dietary treatment has been effective in the prevention of impaired cognitive development, but it still has its shortcomings [2].

According to MacLeod and Ney [47], elevated *Phe* concentrations may occur due to illness, excessive or inadequate *Phe* intake, or inadequate intake of essential amino acid (AA) formula. Therefore, an individualized dietary prescription is needed to meet nutrient requirements with intake monitored through assessment of blood *Phe* levels.

Long-term dietary requirements, physical activity, growth, and intellectual skills need monitoring in patients with PKU. Consequently, an experienced team of healthcare professionals, including a physician, psychologist, metabolic dietician, nurse, and genetic counselor, should accomplish the nutritional management of PKU.

Diet consists of restriction, long life, of natural proteins through the elimination of all sources of animal protein, legumes, and nuts, as well as limited intake of bread, pasta, rice, and some vegetables in the diet. Patients with PKU must avoid protein-rich foods like meat and meat products, seafood, eggs, milk, and dairy products, nuts, and bread [48] and also foods and drinks that have aspartame, as well as soya, flour, beer, or cream liqueurs in the food formulations [28].

The only products that contain no phenylalanine are sugar, oil, and pure starch. Low-protein products made from starch provide needed energy and increase variety.

Nevertheless, the expected growth of PKU people needs limited amounts of phenylalanine [49]. This amount was provided through weighed quantities of foods containing protein and phenylalanine.

Since it is evident that the elimination of natural food sources, as the AA-based on a low-*phe* diet, brings potential nutrient deficiencies, the increment of intake of vitamins and minerals must compensate for poor absorption and metabolism. The adherence to PKU foods reduces in diet those nutrients; calcium, iron, selenium, zinc, cholesterol, saturated and polyunsaturated fats, taurine, carnitine, and vitamins (C, B complex, A, D, and E). Therefore, it is crucial to monitor vitamin, mineral, and essential fatty acid status [47, 50].

According to Marcason [51], the Academy of Nutrition and Dietetics in 2013 [26, 27] recommends the following calculations to assess intake and nourishment for clients fully.

- Total energy intake and percentage of energy from formula/medical food and other foods
- Total protein intake and percentage of total protein from formula/medical food and other foods
- *Phe* intake from foods
- Tyrosine intake from medical foods/formula
- Vitamin and mineral intakes (including calcium, iron, vitamin D, and others) from formula medical foods and other foods.

The dietician nutritionist needs to compare the calculated *Phe* intake with the blood *Phe* levels and adjust *Phe* intake to bring its levels into the treatment range of 2 to 6 mg/dL or 120 to 360 mmol/L.

The PKU diet is also cumbersome for the patients and their families, which often leads to a lack of compliance starting in childhood. For these reasons, new medical formulas with improved nutritional quality and palatability developed to lower the volume of food and to improve compliance [2].

Supplementation with these special medical formulas that supply vitamins, minerals, and all essential fatty acids and amino acids except *Phe* is imperative. Dietitians should prescribe it and carefully monitor energy intake, physical activity, and weight. Moreover, there is a severe need for daily supplementation of micronutrients and long-time instructions for diet [50].

However, the medical foods industry avoids using some of these nutrients because of the food's palatability. This type of food must be improved in its nutrient composition to correct nutritional problems. It must be encouraged through the label the daily intake of these specific nutrients from vitamin and mineral supplements [47, 52 - 54].

Alternatively, the PAH deficiency or PKU disease in any of its classifications causes *Phe* to build up in the body. *Phe* principal metabolic pathway yields the amino acid tyrosine, which is involved in the production of melanin pigments.

Defects or absence of the enzymes responsible for the phenylalanine pathway of metabolites conversion is cause for PKU, albinism (melanin deficiency), and alkaptonuria (excess homogentisic acid HA) diseases. Consequently, the PKU individuals are deficient in tyrosine and for hence of DOPA (L-3, 4-dihydro-
-phenylalanine) with its subsequent products: p-hydroxyphenylpyruvate, 2,5dihydroxyphenyl-pyruvate, tyrosine, homogentisic acid (HA), maleyacetoacetic acid from tyrosine, and catecholamines, and melanin from DOPA.

DOPA is also the precursor to the neurotransmitters dopamine, norepinephrine (noradrenaline), and epinephrine (adrenaline), which are collectively known as catecholamines. Then, tyrosine is a relevant nutrient in diet and formulas.

DEVELOP AND INNOVATION OF FOOD FOR PKU

The original commercial formulas for inborn errors of metabolism were regulated as drugs, later as Foods for Special Dietary Use, and recently they have been named as medical foods [55]. FDA [56] defines medical foods as. "A food which is formulated to be consumed or administered enteral under the supervision of a physician and which is intended for the specific dietary management of a disease or condition for which distinctive nutritional requirements, based on recognized scientific principles, are established by medical evaluation"

Data from the survey applied by Vockley *et al.* [20] have shown that the individuals with PKU report.

* Difficulty managing their disease.
* They have problems maintaining their blood *Phe* within the recommended range.
* The ability to control blood-*Phe* worsens with age, and many of them desire new therapies and treatments with tolerable side effects.

According to a research survey performed by Brown and Lichter-Konecki [57] individuals with PKU are waiting for new treatments that would allow them new diet schemes. They want to increase their intake of natural protein, discontinue or reduce their intake of medical foods (medical formula and foods modified to be low in protein), improve their mental health (including a reduction in depression and anxiety), and a reduction of their blood *Phe* concentrations. Respondents preferred oral administration of any newly developed therapies. Consequently, an interesting focus for food scientists and industry shall be to manage challenges associated with PKU food that must be produced with low- or without protein. Among these targets are the individual's socioeconomic status, lifestyle and dietary preferences, raw material, food procedures, and control and assurance of its quality.

A variety of raw materials, methods, and procedures proposed for producing lowprotein or protein-free foods, are comparable with protein-containing counterparts.

There are few types of research conducted on producing PKU foods from meat and egg as sources of protein due to their high-fat content. However, seafood is prone to easy hydrolysis by proteases. Yamashita *et al.* [58] designed a method to obtain a tasteless and odorless plastein with 0.05% phenylalanine, 7.82% tyrosine, and 2.98% tryptophan content from fish proteins. In the method partially hydrolyzed fish protein concentrate with a low level of pepsin was exposed to pronase to liberate aromatic amino acids (AAA), which were absorbed by Sephadex G-15 and reacted with papain and ethyl esters of L-tyrosine and Ltryptophan to obtain the plastein.

Soltanizadeh and Mirmoghtadaie [50] have reviewed the current findings and the recent developments in the production of phenylalanine-free foods. The authors have also discussed the nutritional requirements and challenges encountered by PKU individuals and food technologists and report the list of companies and suppliers of PKU foods for infants, children, adolescents, and adults. The list includes baked goods, ready meals, suppliers of food protein, protein substitutes, breakfast cereals, mixed flours, desserts, among others. They also report 2 different ways to produce food for PKU.

(1) Some foods and beverages contain all nutritional supplements except

phenylalanine. These products are available in different forms, including some ready-to-consume items, bars, and powders to be mixed with some drinks such as water or juice.

(2) Some products are modified to decrease their phenylalanine content. Hydrolyzing the protein content or using protein substitutes with low phenylalanine produces these products. Modified foods can satisfactorily replace conventional products that PKU individuals should not consume, or their consumption is allowed only in minimal amounts in the daily diet. Examples of these products include meat and cheese substitutes; rice; pasta; baked goods such as cookies, bread, pizza crust, and crackers; flour; and "peanut butter" [52].

Pérez *et al.* [59] have verified in the pilot plant level, the feasibility of using nontraditional sources of local production in the manufacture of food products with consumer's acceptance, nutritious, and able to replace that conventional counterpart. The authors have developed, pasta (rice/amaranths), cake and pancake mix, and baby food. At this framework, the authors comment that there are in tropical areas pseudo-cereals, legumes, tuberous, and *Musaceae* plants yielding grains, roots, tubers, rhizomes, and fruit with enormous potential to be used as ingredients in food development.

All of them are sources of calories, carbohydrates, and healthy phytochemicals, ideal for the development of foods for PKU, due they can yield flours, and starches with low content or *Phe-* free, However, only a few of them are utilized [60 - 63].

Phenylalanine-low or free proteins and peptides in food must provide not only the essential aromatic amino acids but also the functional properties needed for manufacturing a wide food variety. A source of low or *Phe-* free protein is the glycomacropeptide (GMP) from whey [64].

GMP is a bioactive peptide with unique chemical properties (glycosylation, absence of aromatic amino acids, self-association) present in cheese or rennet whey. It is produced during cheese making when bovine kappa (κ)-casein is cleaved by chymosin into para-κ-casein, which remains with the cheese curd, and GMP, which remains with the whey. GMP consists of 64 amino acids and constitutes 15% to 20% of protein content in whey. GMP has a unique amino acid profile such that there are no aromatic AAs like tyrosine, tryptophan, and especially phenylalanine in the structure; however, threonine and isoleucine are in elevated amounts. Apart from the many biological and chemical properties, the peptide has several functional properties (emulsification and foaming properties, gel formation), making it an ingredient of choice.

Despite the high amount of these two amino acids, GMP is especially suitable to produce phenylalanine-free AA-based foods. Dairy ingredient companies have already realized GMP potential and are premium ingredients isolated from whey. Potential applications of GMP include its addition to the diet of hepatic and phenylketonuria patients [65 - 67].

Ney *et al.* [68] and Davisco Food International [69] define GMP as a natural whey protein produced during the cheese-making procedure. In the procedure kappa (K) casein is hydrolyzed by chymosin (renin) in para-K-casein which remains or forms part of the curd containing between 1-105 amino acid residues and the largest peptide, which contains between 106 to 169 amino acid residues, is soluble and forms part of the milk serum in these fractions is the GMP.

Lim *et al.*, in 2007 [65], have produced at lab-scale level foods such as strawberry pudding, strawberry fruit leather, chocolate beverage, snack cracker, and an orange sports beverage using the PURE-GMP™ (Davisco Foods International, Inc., LeSueur, MN) [69]. Authors have concluded that savory products containing a low level of phenylalanine could be manufactured with this GMP to provide a low-*Phe* protein source to the PKU diet.

Pérez *et al.* [70] pointed out the great potential for the production with high efficiency of macropeptides from non-conventional sources such as lentils (*Lens culinaris*), white beans (*Phaseolus vulgaris*), and amaranth panicle flours. They have produced, to lab-scale, hydrolysate by precipitation of its proteins using isoelectric point, and subsequent hydrolysis with protease enzymes from *Aspergillum oryzae*, and *Streptomyces griseus*. The amino acid profile in the hydrolysate from amaranth panicle flour is threonine-free and *Phe-* free, with low isoleucine content. Therefore, they are a potential source of PKU food development.

To produce glycomacropeptides, Villafuerte *et al.* [71] have elaborated a protein isolate from chachafruto (*Erythrina edulis* T.) and dry whey. The solubilization and precipitation of the protein from chachafruto flour produce the isolated protein (96.01% crude protein) while whey proteins (15.69% crude protein) are treated in their original matrix Whey and isolated proteins were enzymatically hydrolyzed with pepsin and *Streptomyces griseus* protease. The concentration of *Phe* was determined by fluorometry and by HPLC, and *Phe* separated by using charcoal activated as *Phe* captor. The results indicate a total reduction of the content of phenylalanine in the hydrolysates and the reduction of the concentration of other amino acids.

Anchundia and Pérez [72] have assayed the nutritional characteristics and sensory evaluation of a drink of sweet potato flour and glycomacropeptide elaborated on a pilot level with PKU consumers. The content of phenylalanine in the drink was 65.90- mg/100 ml; therefore, recommended for PKU children older than one year. The authors report that this drink also provides higher content of protein than those provided by a glass of milk (4.67%). Authors have concluded that the sweet potato flour autoclaved can be used, together with a protein source, in the elaboration of drink for the special regime and conventional diets.

On the other hand, Soltanizadeh and Mirmoghtadaie [50] have concluded that post hydrolysis procedures remove protein-rich foods like meat and milk hydrolyzed using appropriate enzymes before free phenylalanine and other cyclic AAs. Other foods could be restrictively consumed or applied for making formulated products after the elimination of protein. The development of this type of food is dependent on the greater communication between medical professionals, food scientists, processors, and nutritionists.

There is a challenge that food Scientifics and processors must face in the development and production of foods for PKU. Therefore, a subject for food scientists to cope with is overcoming the challenges associated with PKU food produced with low-protein or without protein. Despite each method of producing foods presents its limitations, there must be an equilibrium among its nutritional efficiency, functional properties, storage stability (shelf-life), and palatability (organoleptic properties).

Ruiz *et al.* [73] have performed research to evaluate the effect of banana flour (*Musa paradisiaca* L.) on pathological changes in mice with induced phenylketonuria. The authors have highlighted that banana flour with low phenylalanine content used in the study to feed mice with PKU is a key ingredient to the regulation of phenylalanine levels in the blood, helping to reduce the effects of the disease.

RECIPES

Peruvian Carrot Gnocchi in Spinach Sauce
Ingredients

500g	Peruvian carrot (*Arracacia xanthorrhiza*) roots
150g	Corn starch
1g	Salt
500g	Spinach leaves (without twigs).
10	Garlic cloves
15 ml	Olive oil
Pinch	Salt (to taste)
Pinch	White Pepper (to taste)

Preparation

Peel and chop the Peruvian carrot roots into 2-inch chunks, and then boil in salted water for 15 minutes or until soft. While the Peruvian carrot is boiling, clean the spinach, and pop it into a colander. Use the hot water from the boiled Peruvian carrot to wilt the spinach, drain off the water.

Whizz-cooked Peruvian carrot into a puree in a food processer, and mash it. Add the salt, and corn starch until you get a smooth dough. Sprinkle some starch over a clean work surface, take a ball of the dough and roll it into an elongated rope shape about 1.5 – 2cm wide.

Take the gnocchi rope and cut it into 1-1.5 cm square bites by using a knife or pastry cutter. Just try to keep them around 1.5 cm, as they inflate slightly in the water. Roll the gnocchi using a special wooden board to roll them. It made them have ridges on to soak up, as much sauce as possible when served.

When the gnocchi is ready, bring a pan of water to the boil and then pop in batches of the gnocchi. They should take approx. 2 minutes to float to the surface and done. Take them out with a slotted spoon into the serving bowl.

Spinach sauce. Whizz the wilted spinach into a puree in a food processer and mash it with garlic and olive oil. Add salt and white pepper to taste.

Note: Gnocchi elaboration is feasible by using the flour of any of the raw material dehydrated below. But to reach an excellent recipe, the solid content must be calculated from the raw material used. *e.g.*, if it is preparing from Peruvian carrot flour.

Beetroot and Carrot Cream

Ingredients

50g	Beetroot flour (See chapter 1)
8g	Carrot flour (See chapter 1)
9g	Corn starch
400 ml	Vegetable Broth (1 can of 14.5 oz. of vegetable broth)
1g	Onion powder
5g	Tomato paste
2g	Sugar
Pinch	Salt and black pepper to taste
Dash	Sour Cream to taste
Dash	Dill and Lemon wedges to taste

Preparation

Mix all dry ingredients in a premix. Place the vegetable broth in a saucepan and add the premix slowly, mixing until no lumps remain. Add the tomato paste, black pepper, and salt. Cook stirring the mix until it reaches 90°C (15 minutes). They are serving with the dill and a lemon wedge.

Note: Beetroot flour can be replaced by eggplant flour.

Cassava-Chocolate Chips Cookies

Ingredients

250g	Cassava flour (See chapter 1)
175 g	Ghee or grass-fed Butter
50g	Honey
4g	Sugar
20g	Glycomacropeptide (Davisco Food International)
3,5g	Baking soda (sodium bicarbonate)
3.5g	Baking powder
3,5g	Vanilla extract, pure
1.2g	Salt
250g	Chocolate chips, dark

Preparation

Preheat your oven to 350 °F (175 °C) and line a large cookie sheet (or 2) with parchment paper. Using an electric hand mixer, cream together the ghee (or butter), honey, sugar, and vanilla until smooth on medium speed Add in the glycomacropeptide and beat on low speed until combined. In a separate bowl, combine the dry ingredients, then add dry mixture to wet, beating on low speed until smooth. Stir in chocolate chips, then chill the dough for 10-15 minutes in the fridge. Using a medium cookie scoop, scoop dough onto a prepared cookie sheet about 2" apart since dough spread a bit while baking. Bake in the preheated oven for 10 minutes or until cookies are golden brown. Allow the cookies to cool completely on the baking sheet. Once completely cool to the touch, remove from sheet, and serve.

Cassava Bread
Ingredients

250g	Corn starch
100g	Cassava flour (see Chapter 1 recipes)
30g	Vegetable Oil
5g	Sugar
5g	Salt
5g	Baking powder
220 ml	Rice milk
10 g	Oregano (optional)

Preparation

Using an artisan stand mixer, mix on medium speed the dry ingredients. Add the oil, and the milk by adding one portion of each one, every time, and beat on low speed until combined and obtain the dough. To complete kneading the bread, bring the dough to a clean work surface, with sprayed cassava flour on it. Knead the dough by pressing it away with the heels of the hands, and then turn the dough 90 degrees, fold it over, and press again with the heels of the hands. Let the dough soak up all the cassava flour on the work surface and the hands. When it feels wet and sticky, add more flour to the hands and work surface. Keep up until the dough starts becoming elastic and smooth. The dough is ready when it does not become wet and sticky right after running out of flour, and the outside is smooth.

Divide the dough into enough portions to cover the six divisions of a baking pan. Spray the inside of each loaf pan with cooking spray and pop the dough piece inside. Once everything is ready, cover the bowl with a clean towel, place it in a warm place, and wander off for 30-45 minutes. Preheat the oven to 350 °F (175 °C), bake them for 40 minutes. The bake time depends on the oven. Getting the loaf out of the oven, turn it out of the baking pan, and leave it to cool on a baking rack.

CONSENT FOR PUBLICATION

Not Applicable.

CONFLICT OF INTEREST

The author confirms that this chapter contents have no conflict of interest.

ACKNOWLEDGEMENT

Declared none.

REFERENCES

[1]   Blau N, van Spronsen FJ, Levy HL. Phenylketonuria. Lancet 2010; 376(9750): 1417-27.
        [http://dx.doi.org/10.1016/S0140-6736(10)60961-0] [PMID: 20971365]

[2]   Strisciuglio P, Concolino D. New strategies for the treatment of phenylketonuria (PKU). Metabolites 2014; 4(4): 1007-17.
        [http://dx.doi.org/10.3390/metabo4041007] [PMID: 25375236]

[3]   PKU 612349. OMIM 261600. 2019. Available from: http://omim.org

[4]   Genetic home reference (GHR). Phenylketonuria. Your guide to understanding genetic condition. 2019. Available from. https://ghr.nlm.nih.gov

[5]   Gene Nomenclature Committee (HGNC). 2019. https://www.ncbi.nlm.nih.gov

[6]   Medline Plus Encyclopedia. Autosomal recessive 2019. https://medlineplus.gov

[7]   Kayaalp E, Treacy E, Waters PJ, Byck S, Nowacki P, Scriver CR. Human phenylalanine hydroxylase mutations and hyperphenylalaninemia phenotypes: a metanalysis of genotype-phenotype correlations. Am J Hum Genet 1997; 61(6): 1309-17.
        [http://dx.doi.org/10.1086/301638] [PMID: 9399896]

[8]   Kure S, Shintaku H. Tetrahydrobipterin-responsive phenylalanine hydroxylase deficiency. J Hum Genet 2019; 64(2): 67-71.
        [http://dx.doi.org/10.1038/s10038-018-0529-5] [PMID: 30504912]

[9]   Zurfluh MR, Zschocke J, Lindner M, Feillet F, Chery C, Burlina A, *et al.* Molecular genetics of tetrahydrobiopterin-responsive phenylalanine hydroxylase deficiency. Hum Mutat 2008; 29(1): 167-75.
        [http://dx.doi.org/10.1002/humu.20637]

[10]   Mahfoud A, de Lucca M, Domínguez CL, *et al.* Hallazgos clínicos y espectro mutacional en pacientes venezolanos con diagnóstico tardío de fenilcetonuria. Rev Neurol 2008; 47(1): 5-10.
        [http://dx.doi.org/10.33588/rn.4701.2007642] [PMID: 18592473]

[11]   Al Hafid N, Christodoulou J. Phenylketonuria: a review of current and future treatments. Transl Pediatr 2015; 4(4): 304-17.
[PMID: 26835392]

[12]   Milstien S, Abita J-P, Chang N, Kaufman S. Hepatic phenylalanine 4-monooxygenase is a phosphoprotein. Proc Natl Acad Sci USA 1976; 73(5): 1591-3.
[http://dx.doi.org/10.1073/pnas.73.5.1591] [PMID: 1064028]

[13]   Thöny B, Auerbach G, Blau N. Tetrahydrobiopterin biosynthesis, regeneration and functions. Biochem J 2000; 347(Pt 1): 1-16.
[http://dx.doi.org/10.1042/bj3470001] [PMID: 10727395]

[14]   Scriver CR, Kaufman S. Hyperphenylalaninemia:phenylalanine hydroxylase deficiency.The metabolic and molecular bases of inherited disease. 8th edn. New York: MacGraw-Hill Inc 2001; pp. 1667-724.

[15]   Sarodaya N, Suresh B, Kim K-S, Ramakrishna S. Protein Degradation and the pathologic basis of phenylketonuria and hereditary tyrosinemia. Int J Mol Sci 2020; 21(14): 4996.
[http://dx.doi.org/10.3390/ijms21144996] [PMID: 32679806]

[16]   Flydal MI, Martinez A. Phenylalanine hydroxylase: function, structure, and regulation. IUBMB Life 2013; 65(4): 341-9.
[http://dx.doi.org/10.1002/iub.1150] [PMID: 23457044]

[17]   Donlon J, Levy H, Scriver C. Hyperphenylalaninemia: Phenylalanine hydroxylase deficiency.Metabolic and Molecular Basis of Inherited Disease. New York: McGraw-Hill 2007.

[18]   Matthews DE. An overview of phenylalanine and tyrosine kinetics in humans. J Nutr 2007; 137(6) (Suppl. 1): 1549S-55S.
[http://dx.doi.org/10.1093/jn/137.6.1549S] [PMID: 17513423]

[19]   Jongkees BJ, Hommel B, Kühn S, Colzato LS. Effect of tyrosine supplementation on clinical and healthy populations under stress or cognitive demands--A review. J Psychiatr Res 2015; 70: 50-7.
[http://dx.doi.org/10.1016/j.jpsychires.2015.08.014] [PMID: 26424423]

[20]   Vockley J, Andersson HC, Antshel KM, *et al.* Phenylalanine hydroxylase deficiency: diagnosis and management guideline. Genet Med 2014; 16(2): 188-200.
[http://dx.doi.org/10.1038/gim.2013.157] [PMID: 24385074]

[21]   Maltzman S. My PKU Toolkit A transition guide to adult PKU management. New Jersey: Appl Nutr Corp. 2007; p. 5.

[22]   González Muñoz Y, Palomino Camargo C, Pérez Sira E, Mahfoud Hawilou A. Terapias nutricionales novedosas y otros enfoques utilizados en el tratamiento de pacientes con fenilcetonuria. SAN 2013; 14(3): 211-27.

[23]   Regier DS, Greene CL. Update 2017. Phenylalanine hydroxilase deficiency.GeneReviews®. Seattle, WA: University of Washington, Seattle 2000; pp. 1993-2019.https://www.ncbi.nlm.nih.gov [Internet]

[24]   Zhu M. The Guthrie Test for early diagnosis of phenylketonuria 2017.http://embryo.asu.edu

[25]   González I. Importancia del conocimiento de la enfermedad fenilcetonuria y su tratamiento, en los pacientes y familia. Buenos Aires, Argentina: Trabajo Final de Licenciatura en Nutrición. Facultad de Ciencias de la Salud. Universidad de Belgrano 2004.

[26]   Academy of Nutrition and Dietetics. Pediatric nutrition care manual 2019. http://www.nutrition caremanual.org

[27]   Academy of Nutrition and Dietetics. Pediatric nutrition care manual 2015. http://www.nutrition caremanual.org

[28]   Giovannini M, Verduci E, Salvatici E, Paci S, Riva E. Phenylketonuria: nutritional advances and challenges. Nutr Metab (Lond) 2012; 9(1): 7-12.
[http://dx.doi.org/10.1186/1743-7075-9-7] [PMID: 22305125]

[29]   The National PKU Alliance. 2017.Medical and dietary guidelines for PKU

[30]   Food and Drug Administration. 2007. https://wayback.archive-it.org http://www.fda.gov

[31]   Trefz FK, Belanger-Quintana A. Sapropterin dihydrochloride: a new drug and a new concept in the management of phenylketonuria. Drugs Today (Barc) 2010; 46(8): 589-600.
[http://dx.doi.org/10.1358/dot.2010.46.8.1509557] [PMID: 20830319]

[32]   BioMarin. BioMarin announces FDA approval for Kuva 2007. investor.biomarin.com

[33]   Hanley WB. Phenylketonuria (PKU) - What next? 2013. Mini-Review. J Genet Disord Genet Rep 2013; 2(2): 1-6.
[http://dx.doi.org/10.4172/2327-5790.1000108]

[34]   Harding CO, Gibson KM. Therapeutic liver repopulation for phenylketonuria. J Inherit Metab Dis 2010; 33(6): 681-7.
[http://dx.doi.org/10.1007/s10545-010-9099-1] [PMID: 20495959]

[35]   DiLella AG, Kwok SCM, Ledley FD, Marvit J, Woo SLC. Molecular structure and polymorphic map of the human phenylalanine hydroxylase gene. Biochemistry 1986; 25(4): 743-9.
[http://dx.doi.org/10.1021/bi00352a001] [PMID: 3008810]

[36]   Hofman KJ, Steel G, Kazazian HH, Valle D. Phenylketonuria in U.S. blacks: molecular analysis of the phenylalanine hydroxylase gene. Am J Hum Genet 1991; 48(4): 791-8.
[PMID: 2014802]

[37]   Guldberg P, Henriksen KF, Sipilä I, Güttler F, de la Chapelle A. Phenylketonuria in a low incidence population: molecular characterisation of mutations in Finland. J Med Genet 1995; 32(12): 976-8.
[http://dx.doi.org/10.1136/jmg.32.12.976] [PMID: 8825928]

[38]   Guldberg P, Rey F, Zschocke J, *et al.* A European multicenter study of phenylalanine hydroxylase deficiency: classification of 105 mutations and a general system for genotype-based prediction of metabolic phenotype. Am J Hum Genet 1998; 63(1): 71-9.
[http://dx.doi.org/10.1086/301920] [PMID: 9634518]

[39]   Hitzeroth HW, Niehaus CE, Brill DC. Phenylketonuria in South Africa. A report on the status quo. S Afr Med J 1995; 85(1): 33-6.
[PMID: 7784915]

[40]   Scriver CR, Hardelid P, Cortina-Borja M, Munro A, Jones H. Did phenylketonuria (PKU) arise after the Out-of-Africa migration? In: Program Nr: 995 for the 2006 ASHG Annual Meeting. 1995.

[41]   Loeber JG. Neonatal screening in Europe; the situation in 2004. J Inherit Metab Dis 2007; 30(4): 430-8.
[http://dx.doi.org/10.1007/s10545-007-0644-5] [PMID: 17616847]

[42]   Borrajo JCG. Epidemiologic view of phenylketonuria (PKU) in LatinAmerica. Acta Pediatr Mex 2012; 33(6): 279-87.

[43]   Li N, Jia H, Liu Z, *et al.* Molecular characterisation of phenylketonuria in a Chinese mainland population using next-generation sequencing. Sci Rep 2015; 5: 15769.
[http://dx.doi.org/10.1038/srep15769] [PMID: 26503515]

[44]   Dateki S, Watanabe S, Nakatomi A, *et al.* Genetic background of hyperphenylalaninemia in Nagasaki, Japan. Pediatr Int (Roma) 2016; 58(5): 431-3.
[http://dx.doi.org/10.1111/ped.12924] [PMID: 27173423]

[45]   Verbal Comunication Dr. Antonieta Mahfoud IDEA

[46]   Borrajo JCG. Newborn Screening for Phenylketonuria: Latin American consensus guidelines. JIEMS 2016; 4: 1-5.
[http://dx.doi.org/10.1177/2326409816682764]

[47]   Macleod EL, Ney DM. Nutritional management of phenylketonuria. Ann Nestle [Eng] 2010; 68(2): 58-69.
        [http://dx.doi.org/10.1159/000312813] [PMID: 22475869]

[48]   Waisbren SE, Noel K, Fahrbach K, *et al.* Phenylalanine blood levels and clinical outcomes in phenylketonuria: a systematic literature review and meta-analysis. Mol Genet Metab 2007; 92(1-2): 63-70.
        [http://dx.doi.org/10.1016/j.ymgme.2007.05.006] [PMID: 17591452]

[49]   Sullivan JE, Chang P. Review: emotional and behavioral functioning in phenylketonuria. J Pediatr Psychol 1999; 24(3): 281-99.
        [http://dx.doi.org/10.1093/jpepsy/24.3.281] [PMID: 10379143]

[50]   Soltanizadeh N, Mirmoghtadaie L. Strategies used in production of phenylalanine-free foods for PKU management. Compr Rev Food Sci Food Saf 2014; 13(3): 287-99.
        [http://dx.doi.org/10.1111/1541-4337.12057] [PMID: 33412654]

[51]   Marcason W. Is there a standard meal plan for phenylketonuria (PKU)? J Acad Nutr Diet 2013; 113(8): 1124.
        [http://dx.doi.org/10.1016/j.jand.2013.06.004] [PMID: 23885706]

[52]   Strisciuglio P, Concolino D, Moricca MT, Rivalta L, Parlato G. Normal serum levels of vitamin B12 and folic acid in children with phenylketonuria. Eur J Pediatr 1995; 154(10): 866-70.
        [http://dx.doi.org/10.1007/BF01959802] [PMID: 8529692]

[53]   Acosta PB, Yannicelli S, Singh R, *et al.* Nutrient intakes and physical growth of children with phenylketonuria undergoing nutrition therapy. J Am Diet Assoc 2003; 103(9): 1167-73.
        [http://dx.doi.org/10.1016/S0002-8223(03)00983-0] [PMID: 12963945]

[54]   Dobbelaere D, Michaud L, Debrabander A, *et al.* Evaluation of nutritional status and pathophysiology of growth retardation in patients with phenylketonuria. J Inherit Metab Dis 2003; 26(1): 1-11.
        [http://dx.doi.org/10.1023/A:1024063726046] [PMID: 12872834]

[55]   Camp K. Medical Foods for Inborn Errors of Metabolism: Issues in patient access Advisory Committee on Heritable Disorders in Newborns and Children NIH. National Instituto of Health 2016.

[56]   Food and Drug Administration (FDA). 2019.

[57]   Brown CS, Lichter-Konecki U. Phenylketonuria (PKU): A problem solved? Mol Genet Metab Rep 2015; 6(C): 8-12.
        [PMID: 27014571]

[58]   Yamashita M, Arai S, Fujimaki M. A low-phenylalanine, high-tyrosine plastein as an acceptable dietetic food. Method of preparation by use of enzymatic hydrolysis and resynthesis. J Food Sci 1976; 41(5): 1029-32.
        [http://dx.doi.org/10.1111/j.1365-2621.1976.tb14382.x]

[59]   Pérez EE, Mahfoud A, Domínguez CL, Guzmán R. Roots, Tubers, grains and bananas; flours and starches. Utilization in the development of foods for conventional, celiac, and phenylketonuric consumers. J Food Process Technol 2013; 4(3): 211.
        [http://dx.doi.org/10.4172/2157-7110.1000211]

[60]   Pérez Sira EE, Pacheco de Delahaye E. Capítulo 20. Almidones modificados de raíces y tubérculos tropicales. In: Lajolo FM, Wenzel de Menezes E, Ed. Carbohidratos en alimentos regionales Iberoamericanos. Ed. Córdoba, Argentina: CYTED Programa Iberoamericano de Ciencia y Tecnología para el Desarrollo 2005; pp. 467- 518

[62]   Pérez Sira EE. Pérez Sira EE. Raíces y Tubérculos. In: De tales harinas, tales panes. León AE, Rosell CM. Ed. Granos harinas y productos de panificación en Iberoamérica. Córdoba, Argentina: CYTED Programa Iberoamericano de Ciencia y Tecnología para el Desarrollo, (CYTED). 2007; pp., 363-401.

[62]   Ciarfella AT, Sívoli LJ, Pérez EE. Food products developed using cassava roots and its derivatives: A review.Cassava: Production, Nutritional Properties, and Health Effects. New York: Nova Publishers 2014; pp. 161-76.

[63]   Sívoli LJ, Ciarfella AT, Pérez EE. Functional and nutritional characterization of cassava flours for industrial applications.Cassava: production, nutritional properties, and health effects. New York: Nova Publishers 2014; pp. 25-50.

[64]   van Calcar SC, MacLeod EL, Gleason ST, *et al.* Improved nutritional management of phenylketonuria by using a diet containing glycomacropeptide compared with amino acids. Am J Clin Nutr 2009; 89(4): 1068-77.
[http://dx.doi.org/10.3945/ajcn.2008.27280] [PMID: 19244369]

[65]   Lim K, van Calcar SC, Nelson KL, Gleason ST, Ney DM. Acceptable low-phenylalanine foods and beverages can be made with glycomacropeptide from cheese whey for individuals with PKU. Mol Genet Metab 2007; 92(1-2): 176-8.
[http://dx.doi.org/10.1016/j.ymgme.2007.06.004] [PMID: 17644019]

[66]   Neelima SR, Sharma R, Rajput YS, Mann B. Chemical and functional properties of glycomacropeptide (GMP) and its role in the detection of cheese whey adulteration in milk: a review. Dairy Sci Technol 2013; 93(1): 21-43.
[http://dx.doi.org/10.1007/s13594-012-0095-0] [PMID: 23396893]

[67]   Patel S. Emerging trends in nutraceutical applications of whey protein and its derivatives. J Food Sci Technol 2015; 52(11): 6847-58.
[http://dx.doi.org/10.1007/s13197-015-1894-0] [PMID: 26884639]

[68]   Ney DM, Hull AK, van Calcar SC, Liu X, Etzel MR. Dietary glycomacropeptide supports growth and reduces the concentrations of phenylalanine in plasma and brain in a murine model of phenylketonuria. J Nutr 2008; 138(2): 316-22.
[http://dx.doi.org/10.1093/jn/138.2.316] [PMID: 18203898]

[69]   Davisco Food International. 2009. www.daviscofoods.com/fractions/gmp.cfm

[70]   Pérez E, Pérez L, Requena L, Mahfoud A, Domínguez CL, Rengel A, *et al.* Preparation of low-phenylalanine macro peptides and estimation of its phenylalanine content by fluorometric technique. J Nutr Ther 2013; 2: 145-53.
[http://dx.doi.org/10.6000/1929-5634.2013.02.03.2]

[71]   Villafuerte F, Pérez E, Mahfoud A, Valero Y, Pérez Martínez A. Obtaining protein products low in phenylalanine from milk whey and chachafruto (Erythrina edulis Triana). ALAN 2019; 69(1): 25-33.

[72]   Anchundia MA, Pérez E. Nutritional characteristics and sensory evaluation of a drink made with sweet potato flour for people with phenylketonuria. Agroindust Sci 2018; 8(1): 15-9.
[http://dx.doi.org/10.17268/agroind.sci.2018.01.02]

[73]   Ruiz A, Gahom D, Sívoli L, Zerpa H, Pradere D, Pérez E. Effect of banana flour (*Musa paradisiaca* L.) on pathological changes in mice with induced phenylketonuria. EC Nutr 2018; 13(12): 780-9.

CHAPTER 7

Foods for Celiac and Autistic Consumers

Elevina Pérez Sira[1,*]

[1] *Instituto de Ciencia y Tecnología de Alimentos, Facultad de Ciencias, Universidad Central de Venezuela, Caracas, Venezuela*

Abstract: Celiac disease (CD), non-celiac gluten sensitivity (NCGS), wheat allergy, and autism are associated with gluten intake. Although, there might be an overlap with the symptoms associated these conditions have distinct characteristics. The most concerning gluten-associated illnesses are celiac disease and autism: Celiac disease occurs in genetically predisposed subjects exposed to gluten-containing foods and other environmental factors. While autism has shown severe contradiction in regards to its control with a gluten-free diet. This chapter deals with this topic in a celiac and autism disease overview. The chapter compiles and discusses information concerning diagnosis and pathogenesis of both illnesses, the relationship between a gluten-free diet and these illnesses control, and substitutes of gluten flour. Gluten-free bakery products and pasta and some home recipes are also presented.

Keywords: Celiac and autism disease, Food development, Foods for celiac consumers, Gluten-free diet, Gluten-free flour, Gluten-free foods.

INTRODUCTION

Wheat Related Illnesses

There are three major cereal-related food illnesses: celiac disease (CD), non-celiac gluten sensitivity (NCGS), and wheat allergy. Although there might be an overlap with the symptoms associated with NCGS, wheat allergy, and CD, the conditions have distinct characteristics [1].

NCGS (non-celiac gluten sensitivity) is a term that refers to a spectrum of clinical phenotypes. In these phenotypes the ingestion of gluten or other wheat-related proteins produces gastrointestinal and other extra-intestinal symptoms that often overlap with symptoms seen in patients with CD (*e.g.*, abdominal pain, diarrhea, fatigue, rash, and depression). However, unlike CD, there are not in NCGS, hist-

---

[*] **Corresponding author Elevina Pérez Sira:** Instituto de Ciencia y Tecnología de Alimentos, Facultad de Ciencias, Universidad Central de Venezuela, Caracas, Venezuela; Tel: +58.212.751 4403; Fax: +58.212.751 3871; E-mail: elevina07@gmail.com

ologic or serologic abnormalities identified. Indeed, there is much disagreement as to what extent NCGS is a trustworthy clinical entity.

Wheat allergy is distinct from both CD and NCGS in that it is an IgE-mediated hypersensitivity response that occurs within minutes to hours of wheat ingestion or inhalation. The clinical spectrum of wheat allergy includes gastrointestinal and respiratory symptoms (also referred to as baker's asthma), exercise-induced anaphylaxis, and contact urticaria.

The only available treatment for these diseases is a lifelong gluten-free diet. Gluten is a complex mixture of hundreds of related but distinct proteins, mainly prolamins and glutelins [3].

Celiac Disease (CD) is an autoimmune disorder involving both an innate and adaptive immune response that occurs among genetically predisposed subjects exposed to gluten-containing foods and other environmental factors. Unlike food allergies, the pathogenesis of CD is not mediated by an immediate hypersensitivity reaction through an IgE-dependent mechanism [2].

CD is a systemic autoimmune disease triggered by the intake of gluten, more specifically to the protein fraction of prolamin found in cereals such as wheat (gliadin), rye (secalin), barley (hordein), and oats (avenine) [3]. It occurs in genetically susceptible and characterized individuals for a variable combination of clinical manifestations, specific antibodies, human leukocyte antigen (HLA) DQ2 and DQ8 haplotypes, and enteropathy [4 - 6]. The physiological role of HLA is to present antigenic peptides to T lymphocytes.

The ingestion of prolamin from wheat (gliadin) or related cereals by genetically predisposed individuals produces inflammatory injury of the small intestine mucosa and atrophy of the intestinal villi, preventing the correct absorption of nutrients [2, 7, 8]. Consequently, the prolamin is activated by the enzyme tissue transglutaminase (tTG), allowing its presentation to CD41 T cells in the lamina propria of the small intestine. The release of cytokines results in histologic changes in the intestinal mucosa (*e.g.*, intraepithelial lymphocytosis and villous atrophy) and a resulting variety of clinical manifestations (*e.g.*, abdominal pain, diarrhea, anemia, osteoporosis, and failure to thrive).

Autism is a disorder of neural development characterized by impaired social interaction and communication and by restricted and repetitive behavior. It is one of the three recognized autism spectrum disorders (ASDs).

The other two are:

Asperger's syndrome and pervasive developmental disorder.

Asperger's syndrome is impaired social interactions, restricted interests, desire for sameness, and distinctive strengths.

Pervasive developmental disorder (PDD-NOS) diagnosis is when the full set of criteria for autism or Asperger's syndrome did not meet [9].

ASDs eventually involve gastrointestinal issues, and gluten-restricted diets have become increasingly popular among parents seeking treatment for children diagnosed with autism. Some of the reported responses to celiac diets in children with autism may be related to the amelioration of nutritional deficiency resulting from undiagnosed gluten sensitivity and consequent malabsorption. However, an expert gastroenterologist should see the autistic patient with these symptoms before starting any treatments like the gluten-free diet.

Many research studies explore the biological basis of autism disorder, but the etiology remains unknown. Several publications describing upper gastrointestinal abnormalities and ileocolitis have focused attention on gastrointestinal function and morphology in autistic children. The authors highlight a high prevalence of histologic abnormalities in the esophagus, stomach, small intestine, and colon, and dysfunction of liver conjugation capacity, and intestinal permeability. Then a proposed solution is the treatment of the digestive problems that may have positive effects on their behavior [10].

Lau *et al.* [11] report that gastrointestinal symptoms are a common feature in children with autism, drawing attention to a potential association with celiac disease or gluten sensitivity. However, studies to date regarding the immune response to gluten in autism and its association with celiac disease have been inconsistent. Pavone *et al.* [12] completed an intervention study and did not report a celiac case among the group of autistic patients. The authors pointed out that although two of them had slightly increased levels of anti-gliadin antibody (AGA) IgG and antiendomysium antibody (AEMAb) subsequent antibody determinations and jejunal biopsies gave expected results. Moreover, none of the celiac patients had a positive DSM-III-R test for infantile autism [12].

Lau *et al.* [11] have concluded that a subset of children with autism displays increased immune reactivity to gluten, the mechanism of which appears to be distinct from that in celiac disease. The increased AGA response and its association with GI symptoms point to a potential mechanism involving immunologic and intestinal permeability abnormalities in affected children.

Furthermore, studies have not determined a direct link between celiac disease and autism [13].

Additionally, the Nga *et al.*, intervention study [14] found that children with autism had significantly higher levels of IgG antibodies to gliadin compared with the children in the study without autism (the control group). When researchers tested for a celiac-specific marker, the blood samples showed no statistically significant difference among the testing groups. Furthermore, when tested for the genetic markers of celiac disease (HLA-DQ2 and HLA-DQ8 alleles), researchers did not find an association between autism and celiac disease. They concluded that children with autism were more likely to have gluten-related antibodies present in their blood but did not show any indications of the presence of celiac disease.

Batista *et al.* [9] postulated that although studies report clinical and, especially, behavioral improvement with gluten-exclusion diets in patients with autism, it cannot ignore the difficulties for statistically demonstrate the association between autism spectrum disorder (ASD) and CD or between ASD and gluten sensitivity.

The reported deleterious effects on brain function, the behavior of children with ASD, consequent to gluten intake, and the frequently reported clinical improvement with restriction diets, if present, are possibly due to other and not wholly clarified mechanisms.

In the case of gluten sensitivity, in the absence of reliable biomarkers, the diagnosis is still dependent on establishing an exclusion diet in patients who experience distress when eating gluten-containing products. Buie [15] reported that currently, there is insufficient evidence to support instituting a gluten-free diet as a treatment for autism. While Ludvigsson *et al.* [16] reported that despite some cases suggest an association between autistic spectrum disorders (ASDs) and celiac disease (CD) or positive CD serologic test results, larger studies are contradictory.

On the other hand, patients with ASD treated with gluten- and casein-free diets have better intestinal permeability when compared to patients on an unrestricted diet [17].

Besides, Costa *et al.* [18] discussed the hypothesis that the symptoms of autism spectrum disorders could be affected by excluding foods containing gluten. The authors reported the thesis that gliadomorphins and casomorphins (exorphins released from the partial luminal digestion of dietary gliadin and casein, respectively) are absorbed through a leaky gut, enter into the central nervous system and interfere with normal brain function. However, they also concluded that only a few studies have experimentally assessed the potential effectiveness of a gluten- and casein-free diet for cases of autism, and the existing studies are based on small sample sizes and short-term treatment duration.

They highlighted that further controlled studies are required to clarify the role of a gluten- and casein-free diet for cases of autism spectrum disorder.

Far ahead in 2020, non-pharmacological approaches, such as dietary supplementations with certain vitamins, omega-3 polyunsaturated fatty acids, probiotics, some phytochemicals (*e.g.*, luteolin and sulforaphane), or overall diet interventions (*e.g.*, gluten-free and casein-free diets) are a proposal for the reduction of such comorbidities and the management of autism spectrum disorders [19].

Gluten

Gluten, the main storage protein of wheat grains, is a complex mixture of hundreds of related but distinct proteins [1 to 3].

From a structural point of view, gluten proteins in wheat according to its solubility include protein such as:

• Prolamin (gliadins) monomeric proteins, and

• Glutelin (glutenins), which are polymeric aggregated proteins.

Prolamin. It has been speculated that the potentially toxic components from the gluten are the prolamins present in different cereals, such as, wheat (gliadin), barley (hordein), rye (secalin), corn (zein), sorghum (kafirin), and oats (avenin), which are allergen because of their high proline and glutamine contents [20].

Gliadins (wheat prolamins) are alcohol-soluble and carry most of the gluten's well-described antigenic properties [8]. Gliadins are highly resistant to gastric, pancreatic, and intestinal proteolytic digestion in the gastrointestinal tract, escaping degradation in the human gut. This difficult digestion is due to gliadin's high content of amino acids, proline, and glutamine, which many proteases are unable to cleave. These proline-rich residues create tight and compact structures (epitopes) that can mediate the adverse immune reactions in coeliac diseases [3].

Besides gliadin, hordein, secalin, and avenin contain peptide sequences known as epitopes or antigen determinants. The amino acid composition of the surrounding epitope cores can influence the immunogenic capacity of a peptide regarding CD [21]. The epitopes are recognized by the immune system, mainly by antibodies, B cells, or T cells, due it is, as a function of its composition, a specific piece of the antigen to which the antibody binds.

Glutelins, which accumulate in the endosperm but not in the embryo, are insoluble in saline and soluble in dilute acidic and alkaline media and they are polymeric aggregated proteins.

From a functional point of view, gluten from grains such as wheat, rye, spelt, and barley has unusual rheological and functional properties.

These properties are crucial in determining the gluten viscoelasticity (entrapment of carbon dioxide released during bread leavening), and the quality of the final product.

The gluten formation begins once the water mixes with the wheat or rye flour. As water and flour start mixing the hydrated proteins (prolamins and glutelins) are brought together and begin to interact. They begin to stick to each other through the formation of chemical bonds (disulfide, ionic, and hydrogen bonds) called cross-links. Therefore, the chemical cross-linking of glutenin and gliadin in the wheat case forms the gluten, which is a very elastic substance as the mix continues, because more cross-links form between the proteins; until a large network of chemically linked proteins is formed (gluten).

In the bread elaboration, the formed gluten is inflated with the gas (CO_2) produced during the fermentation. By expanding, the bubbles strengthen gluten, increasing its cohesiveness and elasticity, producing in the bread a higher volume and finer crumb. Each one of the types of proteins has a function, for example, it has been pointed out that the purified, hydrated gliadins (wheat prolamin) contribute to the viscosity and extensibility of the dough, and the glutelin to dough elasticity [3].

CELIAC DISEASE DIAGNOSIS AND PATHOGENESIS

The evident symptoms of celiac disease include persistent diarrhea, abdominal pain, and involuntary weight loss. Besides, fatigue, malaise, anemia, hypoalbuminemia, vitamin deficiencies, and coexisting autoimmune disorders are perceived, as well as symptoms in other parts of the body, such as bone or joint pain, headaches. Moreover, they can include itching, hives, or anaphylaxis, a lifethreatening reaction [22 - 24].

Diagnosis is frequently established based on the following protocols: Serology (positive transglutaminase-IgA); biopsy (duodenal histology showing villous atrophy, crypt hyperplasia, and intraepithelial lymphocytosis); and clinical history during the gluten-free diet (by recording the clinical improvement of celiac patients, after the introduction of a gluten-free diet) [22, 25 - 27].

The pathogenesis of celiac disease is a T-cell driven process initiated by gluten, leading to increased intestinal permeability and villous atrophy. The process requires human leukocyte antigen (HLA) genotypes DQ2, DQ8, or both [28]. This disease is dependent on the interaction of a triad of genes, gluten, and environmental influences.

The genetic factor present in celiac individuals is due to two HLA classes of genes: HLA-DQ2 and HLA-DQ8. Other non-HLA genes are assumed to contribute to the development of celiac disease in different populations; however, HLA-DQ2 and HLA-DQ8 are present in virtually all patients with CD.

The body physiological response after exposure to gluten is explained through four sequentially steps:

1. Gluten digestion and formation of gliadin fragment:

The digestive tracts of the body have enzymatic machinery needed for gluten degradation. These proteases are commonly present in the human small intestine. Therefore, the gluten, once consumed, is partially digested into prolamin (gliadin, in the case of wheat) fragments by the digestive proteases (human elastase 3B, elastase 2A, and carboxypeptidase A1) [29].

To be absorbed by the body, the partially digested prolamin fraction must be digested by enzymes present in the luminal and brush border to minor molecules, such as amino acids. However, this prolamin fraction is poorly digested in the human gastrointestinal tract because they resist degradation by luminal and brush border endopeptidases. Prolamins degradation resistance is due to its high content of the alcohol-soluble proline and glutamine, peptides. Even more, a protein fraction from α2-gliadin; the c33-mer, called the most immunodominant gluten peptide, is resistant to cleavage by intestinal peptidases and remains intact after digestion [29 - 31].

Ciccocioppo *et al.* [32] pointed out that the gliadin, most studied, is an extremely heterogeneous mixture of proteins that contains at least 40 components. It is classified based on their electrophoretic mobility at acidic pH, in four groups (α-, β-, γ-, and ω-gliadins). According to these authors, all studied gliadins (α, β, γ, ω) possess immunogenic and toxic properties, and act under two pathways:

The direct effect on the epithelium involves the innate immune response.

The adaptive immune response involving CD4+ T cells in the lamina propria that recognize processed gluten epitopes.

Conveniently, Schalk *et al.* [33] review has shown that no all α-gliadins, from all species of wheat flour, contain the 33-mer. The authors showed that almost all the samples of wheat flour studied contained the 33-mer peptide at levels ranging from 91–603 µg/g flour. However, the 33-mer was absent (<limit of detection) in the tetra-, and diploid species (durum wheat, emmer, einkorn).

It is attributed most likely because of the absence of the D-genome, which encodes α2-gliadins in these species. They pointed out that due to the presence of the 33-mer in all common wheat and spelt flours analyzed in their study, the special focus in the literature on this most immunodominant peptide seems to be justified.

On the other hand, Gutierrez *et al.* [29] have reported that gliadin peptides derived from gastrointestinal digestion, especially the 33-mer, can potentially be used by commensal microbiota from both CD-positive and CD-negative individuals, and differences in bacterial hydrolysis can modify its immunogenic capacity.

2. Increment of the mucosal permeability and transport to capillary network:

Mucosal permeability increment: In the healthy intestinal epithelium, the intestinal barrier is impermeable to macromolecules, such as gliadin, due to competent paracellular tight junctions. However, Hollon *et al.* [34] demonstrated that the gluten-degraded products (gliadin) exposure induces an increase in intestinal permeability in all individuals, regardless of whether they have celiac disease. At that point, the production of interleukin-10 in non-celiac patients makes the difference.

The increment of mucosal permeability is due to: Intestinal exposure to gliadin (in the individual with genetic susceptibility) leads to zonulin upregulation and consequent disassembly of tight intercellular junctions and increased intestinal permeability [35].

Gliadin peptides may bind to the chemokine receptor, CXCR3, inducing the zonulin release from the tight junction region and causes a resultant increase in intestinal permeability [36].

The toxic gliadin peptide induces an innate immune response, which eventually leads to epithelial cell death and increased epithelial permeability.

Epithelial transport and immune recognition of gluten in celiac disease [32]: In celiac disease, gluten peptides may cross the intestinal epithelium either *via* the paracellular route or *via* the transcellular route. In the first case, the gluten peptide transportation occurs as a consequence of an increased permeability due to an upregulation of zonulin (which might be; gliadin-dependent or gliadin-independent). In the second case, it occurs by using enterocytic vesicles carrying the human leukocytes antigens (HLA) class II-peptides complex.

These vesicles can cross the basal membrane allowing intact gluten peptides to have access to the lamina propria. At this point, gluten peptides can activate both dendritic cells and lamina propria mononuclear cells to produce interleukin 15, which in turn causes an up-regulation of stress protein by enterocytes, which are recognized by the natural killer receptors present on intraepithelial lymphocytes.

Consequently, immunogenic gliadin peptide fragments entry through the epithelial barrier of the intestinal mucosa of celiac disease is in the setting of increased mucosal permeability. It has demonstrated that antigenic gliadin peptides, which are inherently resistant to intraluminal digestion, can cross the intestinal epithelium of celiac patients secondary to the gliadin mediated to reach the lamella propria [34].

3. Tissue transglutaminase (tTG) degradation and transformation of lymphocytes into a cytotoxic:

Inside of the lamella propria, tTG either deamidates or crosslinks the peptides to themselves. Human tissue transglutaminase (tTG) seems to be the target selfantigen for endomysial antibodies in celiac disease and to catalyze the critical deamidation of gliadin. Therefore, there are an external trigger, the gluten peptides, and an internal trigger, the autoantigen, the ubiquitous enzyme tissue transglutaminase (tTG).

The deamidation renders the gliadin as a more immunogenic molecule with effects on the adaptive immune system. In genetically predisposed individuals, the tTG enzyme converts the glutamine in a negatively charged amino acid or glutamic acid, and crosslinking with, forming a complex. The deamidated gliadin peptide or gliadin-tTG complexes are taken up by antigen-presenting cells (APCs), followed by DQ2-/DQ8-dependent activation of CD4+ T cells and the subsequent secretion of antibodies by mucosal plasma cells [37, 38].

The HLA-DQ2/8 receptor favors peptides that contain one or more amino acids with a negative charge. This data indicates that gliadins contain peptides able to activate, through a TCR/HLA class I interaction, CD8-mediated response in intestinal CD mucosa and to induce the enterocyte apoptosis [39 - 41].

Current understanding indicates that different gluten peptides are involved in the disease process; differently, some fragments being 'toxic' and others 'immunogenic.' The fragment defined as 'toxic' can induce mucosal damage, whereas a fragment defined as 'immunogenic' can specifically stimulate HLADQ2- or DQ8-restricted T cell lines and T cell clones derived from jejunal mucosa or peripheral blood of celiac patients.

On the other hand, peptides are also able to trigger two immunological pathways: one thought to be a rapid effect on the epithelium that involves the innate immune response, and the other represents the adaptive immune response involving CD4+T cells in the lamina propria that recognize gluten epitopes processed and presented by antigen-presenting cells [39].

4. Induction of the enterocyte apoptosis:

The subsequent stage is the identification of the gliadin epitopes by the T cells and the triggering of a cell and humoral response. The cell and humoral response induce the production of anti-tTG and anti-gliadin antibodies (AGA). Anti-tTG and AGA induce the release of inflammatory cytokines responsible for chronic inflammation of the intestinal mucosa.

The inflammatory cytokines, especially interferon-γ, induce the up-regulation of HLA-DQ expression, which enhances gluten–peptide binding. Cell damage caused by the inflammation releases intracellular tTG, which results in additional gluten modification, contributing to enhanced T-cell reactivity towards gluten.

Simultaneously, gluten can induce IL-15 production through an unknown mechanism, with activation of the memory T cells able to cause alterations of the enterocytes, ultimately resulting in their destruction. Villous atrophy, crypt hyperplasia, histologic changes, and severe inflammation characteristic of celiac disease.

Gluten plays a part in triggering some celiac disease-associated disorders, especially some forms of cerebellar ataxia. IgA- and IgG-type antigliadin antibodies (AGA) do not; however, they seem to play a part in the pathogenesis of the celiac disease [37, 42, 43].

Summary

After the non-digested and toxic gliadin peptides lead to epithelial cell death and increased epithelial permeability, the immunogenic gliadin peptides cross over to enter the lamina propria and meet the transglutaminase tissue (tTG) in the intestinal lumen. It is due to its high proline and glutamine content that makes them perfect substrates for the tissular transglutaminase reaction. This reaction renders an immunogenic molecule with effects on the adaptive immune system.

The innate immune response to toxic gliadin occurs in the epithelial component of the intestinal mucosa and involves increased production of cytokines, mainly IL15, which is proliferated by enterocytes, macrophages, and dendritic cells. This point is critical for the creation of active T-cell epitopes involved in celiac disease. Active T-cell epitopes are macromolecular complex, which can be recognized as antigens by antigen-presenting cells *via* allele of the major histocompatibility complex class II, namely HLA-DQ2 and HLA-DQ8 [21, 44]. Once activated, T cells produce cytokines and can help activate antibodyproducing B-cells.

Also, dendritic cells can directly activate B-cells to mature and produce highaffinity antibodies [45]. B-cell bind to a specific antigen, against which it initiates an antibody response. The celiac disease antibody effect includes inhibited epithelial cell differentiation, augmented epithelial cell proliferation, increased epithelial permeability, increased blood vessel permeability, defective angiogenesis [38]. The result is the differentiation of intraepithelial lymphocytes into cytotoxic CD81 T cells that express the natural killer cell marker NK-G2D. Furthermore, the production of IL-15 also promotes the upregulation of the epithelial ligand for NK-G2D, which is the MHC class I chain-related A molecule.

GLUTEN-FREE DIET

Nutrition plays a crucial role in patients with celiac disease. The treatment of celiac disease consists of a long-life gluten-free diet, with the elimination of gluten-based staples/foods, replacement with gluten-free substitutes, and naturally gluten-free foods. This diet must contain an appropriate amount of fiber, vitamins, and nutrients to guarantee good health and normal development. During the treatment, the celiac individual eventually must be assessed, and diet may require supplementation diagnosis by a medical and dietetic follow-up, with also a dietary education program [46].

Cereals containing gluten prolamins such as; wheat (all varieties and hybrids, such as; emmer, kamut, Khorosan wheat (Kamut®), spelt (sometimes called farro) and triticale (a combination of wheat and rye), rye, and barley are not allowed to the celiac patients.

An ingredient derived from a prohibited grain, previously processed to remove gluten only consumed, if the final food product contains less than 20 parts per million (ppm) of gluten. It must avoid other products such as semolina (durum wheat), einkorn, bulgur, and wheat derivatives (wheat germ, wheat bran, whole wheat, and cracked wheat). Additionally, all foods derived from gluten-containing cereals, including pasta, bread, and crackers are not allowed [47].

Malt is also toxic for celiac subjects because it is a partial hydrolysate of barley prolamins. Therefore, barley malt, malt syrup, malt extract, and malt flavoring cannot be part of this diet.

Beer usually contains appreciable quantities of hordein (barley gluten prolamin) [48]. However, some low gluten beers are in the market.

In 2007 and 2013, the FDA [49, 50] issued the final rule, which addressed the uncertainty in interpreting the results of gluten test methods for fermented and hydrolyzed foods. They have released the rule for labeling gluten-free food. Among the other criteria that met food labeled gluten-free is that they must contain less than 20 parts per million of gluten.

The review of Saturni *et al.* [47], demonstrated that 20-38% of celiac patients have some nutritional deficiencies such as calorie/protein, dietary fiber, minerals, and vitamins.

SUBSTITUTES OF GLUTEN FLOUR

As glucose in the body comes from foods that contain carbohydrates, the calories from rice [51 - 53] corn, and potatoes are usually used as the substitute for glutencontaining grains. Other non-conventional glucose sources that come from grains, pulses, minor cereals (fonio, teff, millet, teosinte, and Job's tears), and pseudocereals producing small grain-like seeds (buckwheat, Tartarian buckwheat, chia, quinoa, and amaranth grain) [53] roots and tubers [54] are available to be used in the gluten-free diet. All of them can produce flour and be an ingredient in the food development of gluten-free foods.

Rice (*Oryza sativa*)

Rice is a gluten-free natural and one of the few cereal grains consumed by people with celiac disease. Rice is a food staple, and because it has many different types, it lends itself to a limitless number of recipes. In the culinary sense, rice is often characterized by the length of its grain as long, medium, or short, or its texture as sticky or parboiled, by amylose content (waxy, normal, and amylotype), or color as white (polished), brown, black or wild (non-like botanically genus of *Oryza*, the wild rice is own to *Zizania* genus of grasses) or by its aroma: Basmati or Jasmine. Grains of rice transformed as flour from raw or thermally treated, which wide its functional properties. 100g of white rice unenriched cooked provide 97 calories, 21.09g of carbohydrates, and 2.02g proteins with a glycemic index of 73, without almost no fat in the dish, if it cooked without any oil or butter and 0 cholesterol. The serving of 100g contains moderate amounts of B vitamins, iron, and manganese (10–17% DV) [55 - 57].

Carbohydrates (amylose) and proteins (prolamin) are critical points to discuss in diet rice-based, even more to the celiac consumer. Carbohydrates are rice's most abundant constituents, with an approximate starch content of 80-85% (11-12%, moisture content).

The main components of starch are amylose and amylopectin. The relation amylose: amylopectin of rice starch varies among its varieties, and this variation has deep influences on its functional and metabolic properties. Amylose content predicts the texture of cooked rice; it is waxy (1-2% amylose), very low amylose content (2-12%), low amylose content (12-20%), intermediate amylose content (20-25%) and high amylose content (25-33%) [58, 59].

As postulated by Casagrande *et al.* [60], the amylose: amylopectin ratio significantly affects rice starch digestion in the gastrointestinal tract. The authors demonstrated that animals treated with rice with high amylose content presented lower feed intake, body weight gain and apparent digestibility, higher fecal water content and nitrogen excretion, reduced fecal pH, lower postprandial blood glucose response, total serum cholesterol, and triglycerides levels, and pancreas weight, and higher fasting serum glucose concentration and liver weight. The authors discussed that reduction in fecal pH and increment of fecal nitrogen excretion is an indication of increased fermentative activity.

From the results, Casagrande *et al* [60], hypothesized that the higher the amylose content in the diet, the more substrate available for fermentation. This available substrate when reaching the colon is fermented by the bacterial flora, resulting in the production of organic acids. The organism uses part of these acids, which is an important source of energy to the colon, besides being responsible for modulating the immune response and intestinal flora. Also, they pointed out that although not significant, the lower glycemic response in the treatments with high amylose content is especially important for patients with diabetes, helping in the maintenance of regular levels of blood glucose.

Casagrande *et al* [60], have concluded that amylose content, commonly used to evaluate some properties of product consumption, can aid in the choice of the grain to be used in the diet. To aim for controlling some biologically relevant parameters, such as blood glucose and triglycerides concentrations. In this context, Pérez *et al.* [61] have shown that rice grown in Venezuela has a mean of amylose content of 16.12±2%; and the imported polished rice showed a 12.62±5.22% of amylose content, with two types with very low amylose content, of 3.76 and 9.05%.

The usual value assigned to the protein content of milled rice is 7%; however, according to Juliano [55], the rice protein content can vary from 7-15%. They are nutritionally adequate for human health, with hypoallergenic properties and faster digestibility than other cereal proteins. Rice proteins are high in the sulphurcontaining amino acids, cysteine, and methionine, but low in lysine (essential amino acid).

They consist of four fractions, as a function of their solubility: water-soluble albumins, salt-soluble globulins, alkali-soluble glutelins (oryzenin), and alcoholsoluble prolamins. The storage proteins of rice seed differ from those of most cereals, other than oats, in that globulin rather than prolamin is the most abundant storage protein, which may constitute up to 75% of the grain protein. Rice prolamins are not a concern for the celiac consumer, and although they have a high content of proline and glutamine, and are not indigestible by nature, they are a smaller component of the storage proteins in rice [62]. Kubota *et al.* [63] have shown that rice prolamin is rendered digestible by cooking.

Rice prolamins have several characteristics that are different from the prolamins of most other cereals [62]. They that have molecular sizes of about 12 to 17 kD, as seen for other cereal prolamins, contain a high mole percentage of glutamine residues and low levels of lysine, histidine, cysteine, and methionine [64]. The prolamins in rice are in four different groups. The first one has a molecular weight of 10,000 Da and is very rich in sulfur amino acids. Second is a prolamin of 13,000 Da, which is into two types: A (major), consists of more than seven polypeptide groups and, B (minor), in more than five polypeptide groups. The last prolamin in this group exhibits a molecular weight of 16,000 Da and contains large amounts of sulfur-containing amino acids.

According to Wang *et al.* [65] with better digestibility, rice glutelin exhibits more excellent antioxidant capacity than rice prolamin. Their results suggest that digestibility is a critical factor in modifying the antioxidant ability of rice protein (globulin and glutelin) might play a dominant role in inducing antioxidant response to rice protein.

To elucidate the influence of methionine, which is an essential sulfur-containing amino acid, on the antioxidant activity of rice protein (RP), Li *et al.* [66] have suggested that the availability of methionine is a critical factor to augment the antioxidant ability of RP in the *in vitro* gastrointestinal tract.

Additionally, as reported by Chen *et al.* [67] rice prolamin is effective in activating human anti-leukemia immunity and may not induce unwanted inflammatory diseases.

Another significant value of rice is that its starch presents metabolic responses of glycemia and insulinemia different from the rest of cereals due to the different proportions of amylose: amylopectin. Thus, products with higher amylose content have a lower starch digestibility and, consequently, lower glycemic and insulinemic responses.

Corn (*Zea mays*)

Corn (maize), also known as maize, is one of the world's leading cereal grains along with rice and wheat [68]. Furthermore, corn (maize) grains (the edible and nutritive part of the maize plant) are an important source of protein, non-starch polysaccharides, and fat in human diets for those populations who consume corn as a staple. Starch is corn's main carbohydrate (61%to 78%, db), with a protein content varying as a function of its variety.

Normal corn kernels consist of 6% to 12% (db) protein with the majority located in the endosperm and germ and with essential amino acid deficiency. Zein belongs to the prolamin family, which is the major storage protein ($\approx$45–50%) of maize is exclusively found in the endosperm. Zein is composed of high amounts (> 50%) of hydrophobic amino acids (proline, glutamine, and asparagine) and deficient in lysine and tryptophan [69, 70]. Zein only could form the dough by transforming its structure [71, 72].

There are similarities and differences in the secondary structure of viscoelastic polymers of maize α-zein and wheat gluten proteins, some research has to test its functional and clinical interference in gluten-free foods.

From a functional point of view, Mejia *et al.* [73] have demonstrated that the stable β-sheet formation in the zein–viscoelastic polymer could increase the stability and relaxation time of the zein system and, thereby, create the possibility of zein dough with similar functionality to a viscoelastic wheat system.

Also, Schober *et al.* [74] prepared gluten-free bread by using commercial zein and maize starch. Later, Diatta [75] used corn zein, as a viscoelastic protein, to make better quality gluten-free bread. The objectives for using corn zein were to add chewiness and cohesiveness to the bread crumb and to maintain its integrity when sliced and used in sandwiches containing high moisture components.

Since corn is one of the most consumed grains in the gluten-free diet and celiac feeding concerns are the allergenic prolamins from cereals, it should be pertinent to analyzing the zein properties.

According to Several authors, zeins contain amino acid sequences that resemble the wheat gluten immunodominant peptides, and their integrity after gastrointestinal proteolysis is unknown [73, 76, 77]. To explain their integrity after gastrointestinal proteolysis, Green *et al.* [1] suggest that zein could have the same behavior as those shown by wheat gliadins once consumed. Therefore, the tissue transglutaminase enzyme (tTG) can modify prolamin present in foods containing wheat, barley, and rye, or also maize.

Cabrera-Chávez *et al.* [77] results, agree to indicate that the relative abundance of these zeins, along with factors affecting their resistance to proteolysis, may be of paramount clinical relevance. The authors pointed out the re-evaluation of the use of maize in the formulation and preparation of gluten-free foods in some cases of celiac disease.

Later, Ortiz-Sánchez *et al.* [78], highlight that, in spite, the low content of zeins in maize-containing foods, compared with that of gliadins in wheat-containing foods, maize could be responsible for persistent mucosal damage in a minimal subgroup of CD patients.

On the other hand, like many other cereal grains, corn proteins are deficient in lysine, which is the primary limiting amino acid. But it provides vitamin C, vitamin E, vitamin K, vitamin B_1 (thiamine), vitamin B_2 (niacin), vitamin B_3 (riboflavin), vitamin B_5 (pantothenic acid), vitamin B6 (pyridoxine), folic acid, selenium, N-p-coumaryl tryptamine, and N-ferrulyl tryptamine and potassium as major mineral [79, 80]. Ai and Jane [80], pointed out that despite the wellestablished enhanced protein nutritional value of high-lysine corn and improved energy value of high-oil corn, more research could help to understand their other physiological benefits. With many naturally existent mutations and affordable prices, corn is a promising crop for the development of functional food ingredients, and to produce high-quality and nutritious foods to meet consumer demands.

However, it is suggested that research must continue regarding the effect of corn prolamin in celiac disease. The use of maize in the formulation and preparation of gluten-free foods must be evaluated in some cases of celiac disease because uncontrolled celiac disease can lead to several malabsorption problems, osteoporosis, and other autoimmune diseases.

Besides, the use of cornflour in baking is limited because its proteins that make up the gluten are not functionally adequate. For this reason, the dough cannot reach the volume and texture quality obtained with wheat flour. To be introduced in the formulation of bread for special regimes must be introduced several additives.

Sorghum (*Sorghum bicolor* M)

Sorghum is one of the cereals that due to their agronomic and nutritional characteristics could contribute considerable benefits in humans, as well as, animal feeding, at the world, tropical and national level [81]. In developed countries, the consumption of sorghum, especially varieties with tannin, may promote the intake of low calories associated with high antioxidant, dietary fiber content, with the consequent benefits for celiac disease, obesity, and diabetesrelated health problems [82].

According to De Mesa-Stonestreet *et al.* [83, 84], sorghum grains and their proteins are safe for celiac patients and individuals with varying levels of gluten intolerances. However, the authors pointed out that the main sorghum proteins, kafirins, are resistant to digestion, and difficult to extract and modify in an industrial-scale process, limiting their use in foods. The same authors in 2006 [83] describe studies on kafirin extraction and methods for modifying sorghum proteins for improved nutrition and functionality, as well as food applications. The sorghum protein concentrate developed in this study can augment the nutritional value of gluten-free foods for individuals who have celiac disease and other forms of gluten and wheat intolerance.

Later, Ciacci *et al.* [85] highlight that sorghum protein digestion did not elicit any morphometric or immune-mediated alteration of duodenal explants from celiac patients. The authors' [85] studies with patients fed daily for 5 days with the sorghum-derived food product, showed that the patients did not experience gastrointestinal or non-gastrointestinal symptoms, and the level of antitransglutaminase antibodies was unmodified at the end of the 5-day challenge.

Since sorghum-derived products did not show toxicity for celiac patients in both *in vitro* and *in vivo* challenges, the authors considered sorghum safe for people with celiac disease. Moreover, Pontieri *et al.* [86] have provided molecular evidence for the absence of toxic gliadin-like peptides in sorghum. Its evidence confirming that sorghum can be definitively considered safe for consumption by people with celiac disease.

Fortified with this knowledge, scientists and technologists can enhance further the nutritional and functional value of sorghum proteins, to be used as gluten-free ingredients.

Potato (*Solanum tuberosum*)

Potato (*Solanum tuberosum*, from family *Solanaceae*), the most important tuber crop in terms of production, is the only major tuber crop that is grown in temperate regions. Due to their per capita consumption, potatoes have a valuable position as a source of carbohydrates, vitamins, minerals, and phytochemicals.

Potatoes have several kinds of proteins. Osborne and Campbell (1896) [87] reported that the major protein in potato tubers was globulin, which they termed 'tuberin.' Later, a fractionated potato protein showed the presence of globulin, prolamin, and glutelin. Potato proteins contain a minor proportion of prolamin. All the potato protein fractions, except prolamin, have a well-balanced essential amino acid profile, making it a potential nutritional source.

In 1980, researchers reported a glycoprotein named patatin (relative molecular mass (Mr) about 45 000) that represents 20-40% of the total protein content in potato. Patatin represents a group of immunologically identical glycoprotein isoforms with molecular mass ≈ 40–43 kDa (native conformation is a dimer) that serves as a storage protein but unlike most other plant storage proteins; it also has a surprising number of enzymatic activities [88 - 91]. Then the prolamin content in potatoes is quite low, and it does not represent a concern to celiac consumers.

Potato flour has plenty of potential for food development for celiac consumers. Potatoes are a good source of vitamin and minerals; potato also contains a complex variety of phytonutrients. These include polyphenols, flavonols, anthocyanins phenolic acids, carotenoids, polyamines, glycoalkaloids, tocopherols, calystegines, and sesquiterpenes. Potatoes are a well-known source of vitamin B6, C, folates in the diet due to the high level of consumption, more so than for its endogenous content.

They also are sources of different dietary minerals in less or mayor proportion, such as potassium, calcium, iron, phosphorus, magnesium, copper, and zinc [92, 93]. And they are also an important source of dietary phenolics, flavonols, anthocyanins, and kukoamines, and similarly contain lipophilic compounds that are dietarily desirable, such as carotenoids [92].

Navarre *et al.* [94] showed that there is a bunch of genetic diversity of potatoes mainly those wild-potato species available, that is, the latent to be nutritional powerhouses, mainly to develop food for celiac consumers.

Non-convectional Sources

Moreover, there are plenty of non-conventional sources of carbohydrates that have enormous potential to be used and transformed into native and modified starches and flour. They also increase variety, improved palatability, and high nutritional quality for the gluten-free diet.

In this context, numerous researches have formulated different types of foods [52, 54, 95 - 100] using non-conventional flour sources. These sources include fruit from the *Musaceae* family (unripe bananas), and other starch-containing foods that are naturally gluten-free such as, pulses and beans (soy, haricot bean, kidney bean, lima bean, French bean, common bean, lentil, chickpea), other grains and pseudocereals (millet, quinoa, amaranth, buckwheat groats (also known as kasha), teff, flax, chia, gluten-free oats, nut), roots and tubers (carrot, beet, cassava, arrowroot, sweet potato, different kind of yams), coconut and cocoa.

Sweet potato (*Ipomoea batatas*)

Ipomea batatas known as sweet potato, is native to Central America, is a source of energy, with contributions of pro-vitamin A and ascorbic acid, potassium (808.8 mg/100g), and iron (4.1mg/100g).

Yams (*Dioscorea* spp)

Dioscorea, known as yam, is grown in South America, India, and East Africa, showing a mineral profile with a high content of calcium (140.4 mg/100g) and potassium (864.8 mg/100g). Among other phytochemicals, yams may contain alkaloids, tannins, phytosterols, and steroid saponins. Diosgenin is obtained from the latter, serving as a precursor in the semisynthesis of steroid drugs (cortisone, sex hormones, contraceptive). Some species can cause convulsions or infertility in women who consume them. A few are threatened or endangered plants, whereas others are invasive species [101].

Cassava (*Manihot esculenta* C)

Cassava produces high-quality flour and starch used as a substitute for wheat flour, which is used in baking products, a binder in the meat industry, in the production of dehydrated soups, and the formulation of dietetic products.

Cassava starch is an ingredient useful in the production of baby food, sausages, sauces, and mayonnaise. Modified cassava starches are used in bakeries in the production of fillings and frozen products, because of the physicochemical characteristics they impart stability and provide a final product that stays fresh and of excellent texture.

Carrot (*Daucus carota* S), and Beetroot (*Beta vulgaris*)

Carrot and beet are the most consumed vegetables in the world. They are ideal for infant feeding, due to their nutritional value, and pleasant flavor. They are important in the diet because they are a source of sugar, fiber, folate, manganese, potassium, iron, and vitamin C and pro-vitamin A, phytochemicals (other carotenes, betanin, nitrate inorganic, and vulgaxanthine).

Beans

Legumes are an important source of macro and micronutrients, containing polyphenols, soluble fiber, β-galactosides, and the isoflavones that give it functional food properties. Flavonoids are attributed to antioxidant properties and as phytoestrogens. However, legume consumption is limited by different causes:

The flatulence produced to particular consumers, needs long periods for cooking, and the content of anti-nutritional factors (such as inhibitors of proteases, phytates, and certain phenolic compounds) that decrease the use by the body of nutrients like proteins, amino acids, carbohydrates, and minerals.

Pseudocereals

There are dicotyledonous seeds, from the Andean region, such as quinoa, amaranth, and chia that are rich in starch. They have several phytochemicals with important effects on consumer's health. They have high nutritional value and low glycemic index carbohydrates and offer high biological content proteins without the toxic prolamin that is not allowed to celiac consumers. Most of these sources can be milled into flour, flakes, or grits, or be starch sources. All of them are into different gluten-free specialty products. To offers celiac consumers versatility, there are increments in the range of processed gluten-free products.

OTHER DIETETIC CONSIDERATIONS

Proteins from other sources different from wheat and rye gluten, will not ever have the same functional properties to produce specific foods. A continuous gluten network is needed to elaborate on some bread and baked goods; therefore, it must be in formulation a gluten substitute. Gluten has a nutritional, toxic, or functional point of views:

Nutritionally gluten offers a caloric value of 4cal/g.

As a toxic component that affects celiac consumers, the prolamins are the main concern component of gluten [47, 102].

Functionally, these proteins have a specific purpose to develop a continuous network (gluten) that forms the structure of the different dough to produce baked goods like bread, cakes, cookies, biscuits, among others.

The marketplace offers several modified flour, hydrocolloids, and enzymes with functional properties that help to produce a continuous network of optimal results to obtain these products of high quality. Favorably, some flat cakes, wafers, and crepes, do not need the gluten network and, thus, their gluten-free counterparts are easily available.

An increment in the number of fruits and vegetables, avoid micronutrient deficiencies in celiac subjects. It recommends an intake of at least five portions of fruit or vegetable a day. Those individuals with clinical evidence of malabsorption should initially receive multivitamin preparations, supplemented for iron and folate deficiency.

Usually, the gluten-free diet induces the consumption of food rich in fat, sugar, and calories, resulting in excessive consumption of total and saturated fats.

Celiac patients need to pay attention to food labels, looking for words that involve gluten-free ingredients. The absence of gluten in natural and processed foods represents a key aspect of the food safety of the gluten-free diet.

According to Saturni *et al.* [47], the term "gluten-free" was introduced in food labels several years ago. The authors pointed out that the current Codex Standard for GF foods was adopted by the Codex Alimentarius Commission of the World Health Organization (WHO) and by the Food and Agricultural Organization (FAO) in 1976 and amended in 1983 (Codex Alimentarius Commission, 1983). The definition came under review in the 1990s [47].

As pointed out by several authors there have been significant increases in the adoption of the consumption of gluten-free foods, as a new strategy for the nonceliac population, despite proven benefits for them [103, 104]. The restriction of gluten from diets to improve gastrointestinal and non-gastrointestinal symptoms, as well as the perception that gluten is potentially harmful, represents a healthy lifestyle. As authors pointed out, a gluten-free diet promotion is by social and traditional media coverage, aggressive consumer-directed marketing by manufacturers and retail outlets, and reports in the medical literature and mainstream press of the clinical benefits of gluten avoidance. However, the authors addressed that as with other dietary interventions, a gluten-free diet is a rapidly evolving topic, and additional insight is needed to guide a complete discussion between patients and their health care providers.

Other authors have reported that the need for new therapies for celiac disease, because adherence to a gluten-free diet results in a reduced quality of life [8, 105]. Moreover, various studies have reported alarmingly high percentages of celiac patients being unable for various reasons to adhere to the diet sufficiently. Previously Osman *et al.* [106] had reported promising approaches that included:

Some strategies attempt to decrease the immunogenicity of gluten-containing grains by manipulating the grain itself or by using oral enzymes to break down immunogenic peptides that typically remain intact during digestion. In this context, there are preparations of endopeptidase enzymes that effectively cleave gliadin peptides and thereby circumvent gliadin-associated immune activation.

Vaccination for relevant gliadin epitopes to induce oral tolerance to gluten, resulting in a malabsorptive enteropathy histologically highlighted by villous atrophy and crypt hyperplasia. The University of Chicago Celiac Disease Center [107] has been working on an injectable vaccine called Nexvax2 that induces a measure of gluten tolerance and thus may counter gluten's ability to induce intestinal damage. Nexvax2 was developed to protect celiac disease patients, who carry the HLA-DQ2.5 immune recognition genes, from inadvertent gluten exposure. Patients with the HLA-DQ2.5 genes account for more than 90% of the celiac population.

Other strategies that focus on preventing the absorption of these peptides prevent tissue transglutaminase from rendering gluten peptides more immunogenic or inhibiting them from binding to CD-specific antigen-presenting molecules. Celiac patients develop IgA and IgG Abs directed against gluten peptides as well as an autoantigen, transglutaminase 2 (TG2). The use of transglutaminase inhibitors reduces the affinity of gliadin peptides for T cells, thereby might ameliorate the T-cell response to gluten.

Studies of Hollon *et al.* [34] report the presence, in non-celiac subjects, of intestinal mucosal secretion of interleukin 10 (IL-10) from the basolateral surface, as compared with its absence in gluten sensible individual. IL-10 may be protective, limiting tissue damage caused by inflammation, avoiding the exaggerated increase of intestinal permeability that is a central concern in celiac disease.

Research explores the strategies that limit T cell migration to the small intestine or that re-establish mucosal homeostasis and tolerance to gluten antigens. However, the authors also point out that, to date, it is unknown if the intestinal barrier is targeted directly or indirectly by these therapies.

The University of Chicago [107] work on other three strategies; A new class of orally delivered biopharmaceuticals (ActoBiotics) that use beneficial bacteria to induce tolerance to gluten, a protective agent (Bioniz) that tamps down the deleterious immune response induced by gluten, and a drug previously approved as safe and effective for asthma; Montelukast, that appears to alleviate inflammation in adults exposed to gluten.

GLUTEN-FREE BAKERY PRODUCTS AND PASTA

In gluten-free products, a mixture of flour and starch from different sources must replace wheat flour. Nevertheless, for products like bread, pasta, and some cookies, a gluten network development is required; in this case, a gluten substitute, usual hydrocolloids, is added in the formulation.

Gluten-free products are plenty in starch and contain few proteins and fibers. The addition of proteins and fibers as ingredients in these products overcomes deficiencies. Several gluten-free grains exist, such as the pseudo-cereals amaranth, quinoa, and buckwheat; all of them characterized by an excellent nutrient profile. Therefore, these gluten-free grains are alternatives for the formulation of highquality and healthy gluten-free products, such as bread and pasta [108].

Additives and enzymes added to gluten-free products, as well as and their functionality, needs analysis when are discrepancies in their function on wheatbased and gluten-free products. Nowadays, the most feasible treatment for celiac patients is to follow a gluten-free diet.

Avoiding gluten consumption, allows the celiac patient's intestine to heal, and the nutritional deficiencies and other symptoms are solved. Also, a gluten-free diet reduces the development of many other serious long-term complications related to untreated celiac disease. However, people that follow a gluten-free diet have to deal with difficult challenges, as it not only involves eliminating glutencontaining grains and all products that contain them, requiring constant vigilance, but there is also a sense of social isolation and pressure that accompanies the process.

Since most of the bread, biscuits, pasta, cakes, cookies, breakfast cereals, bagels, soups are from wheat, avoidance of all these indicates a complete change in lifestyle which might not be feasible for all (Due to all these reasons, the demand for gluten-free products (ready to cook or eat) is now on the rise [109]. Then the development of gluten-free food is a challenge to the food industry to provide and develop a wide spectrum of palatable and high-quality foods for celiac and nonceliac consumers.

In this context, the use of probiotics, genetic engineering to manipulate those crops with toxic gliadin, use of non-conventional free gluten crops such as Musaceae, legumes, roots, tubers, pseudo-cereals, additives, and technologies such as; fermentation and use of enzyme solve the problem.

RECIPES

Gluten-Free Pastas (Rigatoni and Fettuccini)

Table 1. Recipe for the elaboration of 200g gluten-free pasta (fettuccine or rigatoni) using the vegetal flour (see chapter 2 recipes).

Ingredients	Cassava/Eggplant	Cassava/ Carrot	Cassava/Cacao	Rice/Beetroot
Mañoco*	72	72	72	72
Rice flour	0	0	0	75
Ingredients	Cassava/Eggplant	Cassava/ Carrot	Cassava/Cacao	Rice/Beetroot
Cassava flour	63	63	105	0
Eggplant flour	62	0	0	0
Carrot flour	0	62	0	0
Beetroot flour	0	0	0	50
Cacao powder	0	0	20	0
Salt	1	1	1	1
CMC**	2	2	2	2
Egg	40	40	40	40
Water	120	135	129	112

*Mañoco: Casabe flour; casabe is a kind of cassava cookie **CMC: Carboxymethylcellulose. Rigatoni. Slightly curved, tube-shaped pasta. Fettuccine: Flat, thick noodles with a name meaning "little ribbons" in Italian.

Preparation

Weigh the flour, CMC, and salt according to the desired recipe from Table **1**. Add the flour mix to the mixing section of the paste extruder machine. Mix for 5 minutes. Mix the water with the egg (see Table **1**). Slowly add the water: egg mixture through the hole arranged in the extruder machine, mixing until smooth. Transfer the dough to the extrusion section and extrude with the fettuccine or rigatoni format. Once the extrusion is completely dry, the performed fettuccine or rigatoni in a dehydrator at 45°C for 3 hours (pre-drying) and 5 hours at 131 °F (55 °C.) Store in airtight plastic bags until use.

Microwavable Cupcake

Ingredients

50g	Microwavable cupcake pre-mix (see **Table 2**)
55g	Egg whole
15g	Vegetable Oil

Table 2. Recipe for the elaboration of one cupcake using the vegetal flour see chapter 1 recipes.

Ingredients	Rice/Pumpkin	Banana/Cocoa	Rice/Carrot	Rice /Beetroot
Rice flour	22,5	0	22,5	23
Banana flour	0	22,5	0	0
Pumpkin flour	10	0	0	0
Carrot flour	0	0	10	0
Beet root flour	0	0	0	10
Cocoa powder	0	10	0	0
Sugar	15,5	15,5	15,5	15, 5
Baking powder	1	1	1	1
Vanillin powder	0,5	0,5	0,5	0
Salt	0,5	0,5	0,5	0, 5
Total	50	50	50	50

Microwavable Flour Premix

Weigh the ingredients, according to the desired recipe from Table **2** and mix them to produce a premix.

Cupcake

Put the contents of the premix (50g) with egg and oil into a cup or container microwave-safe. Mix to obtain a homogeneous (without lumps) paste. Place the paste in the microwave for 1.30 minutes, at 100% power. Optional: Place nuts, colored sugar, or some other design ingredient on the cupcake dough before microwave treatment.

CONSENT FOR PUBLICATION

Not Applicable.

CONFLICT OF INTEREST

The author confirms that this chapter contents have no conflict of interest.

ACKNOWLEDGEMENT

Declared none.

REFERENCES

[1]   Green PH, Lebwohl B, Greywoode R. Celiac disease. J Allergy Clin Immunol 2015; 135(5): 1099-106,1107.

[2]   Biesiekierski JR. What is gluten? J Gastroenterol Hepatol 2017; 32 (Suppl. 1): 78-81.
[http://dx.doi.org/10.1111/jgh.13703] [PMID: 28244676]

[3]   Jabri B, Sollid LM. T cells in celiac disease. J Immunol 2017; 198(8): 3005-14.
[http://dx.doi.org/10.4049/jimmunol.1601693] [PMID: 28373482]

[4]   Lorenzo G, Zaritzky N, Califano A. Optimization of non-fermented gluten-free dough composition based on rheological behaviour for industrial production of "empanadas" and pie crusts. J Cereal Sci 2008; 48(1): 224-31.
[http://dx.doi.org/10.1016/j.jcs.2007.09.003]

[5]   Ortiz C, Valenzuela R, Lucero A Y. [Celiac disease, non celiac gluten sensitivity and wheat allergy: comparison of 3 different diseases triggered by the same food]. Rev Chil Pediatr 2017; 88(3): 417-23.
[http://dx.doi.org/10.4067/S0370-41062017000300017] [PMID: 28737204]

[6]   Online Mendelian Inheritance in Man (OMIM) # 212750. Celiac disease, susceptibility to, 1; celiac1. 2019. Available from: https://www.omim.org

[7]   Ali I, Mariasch N, Maurel S, Deschutter S. Enfermedad celíaca: formas de presentación clínica en la población pediátrica 2006.

[8]   Schumann M, Siegmund B, Schulzke JD, Fromm M. Celiac disease: Role of the epithelial barrier. Cell Mol Gastroenterol Hepatol 2017; 3(2): 150-62.
[http://dx.doi.org/10.1016/j.jcmgh.2016.12.006] [PMID: 28275682]

[9]   Batista IC, Gandolfi L, Nobrega YK, *et al.* Autism spectrum disorder and celiac disease: no evidence for a link. Arq Neuropsiquiatr 2012; 70(1): 28-33.
[http://dx.doi.org/10.1590/S0004-282X2012000100007] [PMID: 22218470]

[10]   Horvath K, Perman JA. Autistic disorder and gastrointestinal disease. Curr Opin Pediatr 2002; 14(5): 583-7.
[http://dx.doi.org/10.1097/00008480-200210000-00004] [PMID: 12352252]

[11]   Lau NM, Green PHR, Taylor AK, *et al.* Markers of celiac disease and gluten sensitivity in children with autism. PLoS One 2013; 8(6)e66155
[http://dx.doi.org/10.1371/journal.pone.0066155] [PMID: 23823064]

[12]   Pavone L, Fiumara A, Bottaro G, Mazzone D, Coleman M. Autism and celiac disease: failure to validate the hypothesis that a link might exist. Biol Psychiatry 1997; 42(1): 72-5.
[http://dx.doi.org/10.1016/S0006-3223(97)00267-9] [PMID: 9193744]

[13]   Genuis SJ, Bouchard TP. Celiac disease presenting as autism. J Child Neurol 2010; 25(1): 114-9.
[http://dx.doi.org/10.1177/0883073809336127] [PMID: 19564647]

[14]   Lau NM, Green PHR, Taylor AK, Hellberg D, Ajamian M, Tan CZ, *et al.* 2013.Gluten sensitivity linked to autism: findings are only a part of a very complicated puzzle https://celiac.org

[15]   Buie T. The relationship of autism and gluten. Clin Ther 2013; 35(5): 578-83.
         [http://dx.doi.org/10.1016/j.clinthera.2013.04.011] [PMID: 23688532]

[16]   Ludvigsson JF, Reichenberg A, Hultman CM, Murray JA. A nationwide study of the association
         between celiac disease and the risk of autistic spectrum disorders. JAMA Psychiatry 2013; 70(11):
         1224-30.
         [http://dx.doi.org/10.1001/jamapsychiatry.2013.2048] [PMID: 24068245]

[17]   Jackson JR, Eaton WW, Cascella NG, Fasano A, Kelly DL. Neurologic and psychiatric manifestations
         of celiac disease and gluten sensitivity. Psychiatr Q 2012; 83(1): 91-102.
         [http://dx.doi.org/10.1007/s11126-011-9186-y] [PMID: 21877216]

[18]   Costa C, Sampaio AS, Rodrigues I, Miranda M, Pinto E. Gluten- and casein-free diet as an
         Intervention for Autism Spectrum Disorders: A Review. Rev Nutr 2015; 24: 6-9.

[19]   Pistollato F, Forbes-Hernández TY, Calderón Iglesias R, *et al.* Pharmacological, non-pharmacological
         and stem cell therapies for the management of autism spectrum disorders: A focus on human studies.
         Pharmacol Res 2020; 152104579
         [http://dx.doi.org/10.1016/j.phrs.2019.104579] [PMID: 31790820]

[20]   Mills C, Johnson PE, Zuidmeer-Jongejan L, Critenden R, Wal J-M, Asero R, *et al.* Chapter fourteen
         Effect of Processing on the Allergenicity of Foods Risk Management for Food Allergy. New York:
         Academic Press 2014; pp. 227-51.
         [http://dx.doi.org/10.1016/B978-0-12-381988-8.00014-2]

[21]   Salentijn EMJ, Mitea DC, Goryunova SV, *et al.* Celiac disease T-cell epitopes from gamma-gliadins:
         immunoreactivity depends on the genome of origin, transcript frequency, and flanking protein
         variation. BMC Genomics 2012; 13: 277.
         [http://dx.doi.org/10.1186/1471-2164-13-277] [PMID: 22726570]

[22]   Nijeboer P, van Wanrooij RL, Tack GJ, Mulder CJJ, Bouma G. Update on the diagnosis and
         management of refractory coeliac disease. Gastroenterol Res Pract 2013; 2013518483
         [http://dx.doi.org/10.1155/2013/518483] [PMID: 23762036]

[23]   National Library of Medicine. 2017. https://medlineplus.gov/foodallergy.html

[24]   National Institute of Allergy and Infectious Diseases (NIAID). Characterizing food allergy &
         addressing related disorders 2019. niaid.nih.gov

[25]   Tonutti E, Bizzaro N. Diagnosis and classification of celiac disease and gluten sensitivity. Autoimmun
         Rev 2014; 13(4-5): 472-6.
         [http://dx.doi.org/10.1016/j.autrev.2014.01.043] [PMID: 24440147]

[26]   Felber J, Aust D, Baas S, *et al.* Ergebnisse einer S2k-Konsensuskonferenz der Deutschen Gesellschaft
         für Gastroenterologie, Verdauungs- und Stoffwechselerkrankungen (DGVS) gemeinsam mit der
         Deutschen Zöliakie-Gesellschaft (DZG) zur Zöliakie, Weizenallergie und Weizensensitivität. Z
         Gastroenterol 2014; 52(7): 711-43.
         [http://dx.doi.org/10.1055/s-0034-1366687] [PMID: 25026010]

[27]   Ludvigsson JF, Leffler DA, Bai JC, *et al.* The Oslo definitions for coeliac disease and related terms.
         Gut 2013; 62(1): 43-52.
         [http://dx.doi.org/10.1136/gutjnl-2011-301346] [PMID: 22345659]

[28]   Zhu J, Mulder CJJ, Dieleman LA. Celiac disease: Against the grain in gastroenterology. J Can Assoc
         Gastroenterol 2019; 2(4): 161-9.
         [http://dx.doi.org/10.1093/jcag/gwy042] [PMID: 31616857]

[29]   Gutiérrez S, Pérez-Andrés J, Martínez-Blanco H, *et al.* The human digestive tract has proteases
         capable of gluten hydrolysis. Mol Metab 2017; 6(7): 693-702.
         [http://dx.doi.org/10.1016/j.molmet.2017.05.008] [PMID: 28702325]

[30]   Shan L, Molberg Ø, Parrot I, *et al.* Structural basis for gluten intolerance in celiac sprue. Science 2002; 297(5590): 2275-9.
[http://dx.doi.org/10.1126/science.1074129] [PMID: 12351792]

[31]   Shan L, Qiao SW, Arentz-Hansen H, *et al.* Identification and analysis of multivalent proteolytically resistant peptides from gluten: implications for celiac sprue. J Proteome Res 2005; 4(5): 1732-41.
[http://dx.doi.org/10.1021/pr050173t] [PMID: 16212427]

[32]   Ciccocioppo R, Di Sabatino A, Corazza GR. The immune recognition of gluten in coeliac disease. Clin Exp Immunol 2005; 140(3): 408-16.
[http://dx.doi.org/10.1111/j.1365-2249.2005.02783.x] [PMID: 15932501]

[33]   Schalk K, Lang C, Wieser H, Koehler P, Scherf KA. Quantitation of the immunodominant 33-mer peptide from α-gliadin in wheat flours by liquid chromatography tandem mass spectrometry. Sci Rep 2017; 7: 45092.
[http://dx.doi.org/10.1038/srep45092] [PMID: 28327674]

[34]   Hollon J, Puppa EL, Greenwald B, Goldberg E, Guerrerio A, Fasano A. Effect of gliadin on permeability of intestinal biopsy explants from celiac disease patients and patients with non-celiac gluten sensitivity. Nutrients 2015; 7(3): 1565-76.
[http://dx.doi.org/10.3390/nu7031565] [PMID: 25734566]

[35]   Fasano A. Intestinal permeability and its regulation by zonulin: diagnostic and therapeutic implications. Clin Gastroenterol Hepatol 2012; 10(10): 1096-100.
[http://dx.doi.org/10.1016/j.cgh.2012.08.012] [PMID: 22902773]

[36]   Freeman HJ. Drug-induced sprue-like intestinal disease. Inter J Celiac Dis 2014; 2: 49-53.
[http://dx.doi.org/10.12691/ijcd-2-2-5]

[37]   Bizzaro N, Tonutti E. Anti-gliadin antibodies. 2007.
[http://dx.doi.org/10.1016/B978-044452763-9/50060-3]

[38]   Caja S, Mäki M, Kaukinen K, Lindfors K. Antibodies in celiac disease: implications beyond diagnostics. Cell Mol Immunol 2011; 8(2): 103-9.
[http://dx.doi.org/10.1038/cmi.2010.65] [PMID: 21278768]

[39]   Ciccocioppo R, Di Sabatino A, Ara C, *et al.* Gliadin and tissue transglutaminase complexes in normal and coeliac duodenal mucosa. Clin Exp Immunol 2003; 134(3): 516-24.
[http://dx.doi.org/10.1111/j.1365-2249.2003.02326.x] [PMID: 14632760]

[40]   Mazzarella G, Stefanile R, Camarca A, *et al.* Gliadin activates HLA class I-restricted CD8+ T cells in celiac disease intestinal mucosa and induces the enterocyte apoptosis. Gastroenterology 2008; 134(4): 1017-27.
[http://dx.doi.org/10.1053/j.gastro.2008.01.008] [PMID: 18395083]

[41]   Green PHR, Lebwohl B, Greywoode R. Celiac disease. Clinical reviews in allergy and immunology.USA. American Academy of Allergy, Asthma & Immunology 2015; pp. 1099-106.

[42]   Rowland LM, Demyanovich HK, Wijtenburg SA, Eaton WW, Rodriguez K, Gaston F, *et al.* Antigliadin antibodies (AGA IgG) are related to neurochemistry in schizophrenia. Front Psychiatry 2017; 19:8:104.

[43]   Shalimar DM, Das P, Sreenivas V, Gupta SD, Panda SK, Makharia GK. Mechanism of villous atrophy in celiac disease: role of apoptosis and epithelial regeneration. Arch Pathol Lab Med 2013; 137(9): 1262-9.
[http://dx.doi.org/10.5858/arpa.2012-0354-OA] [PMID: 23991739]

[44]   Cecilio LA, Bonatto MW. The prevalence of HLA DQ2 and DQ8 in patients with celiac disease, in family and in general population. Arq Bras Cir Dig 2015; 28(3): 183-5.
[http://dx.doi.org/10.1590/S0102-67202015000300009] [PMID: 26537142]

[45]   Amorim KNS, Rampazo EV, Antonialli R, *et al.* The presence of T cell epitopes is important for induction of antibody responses against antigens directed to DEC205⁺ dendritic cells. Sci Rep 2016; 6: 39250.
[http://dx.doi.org/10.1038/srep39250] [PMID: 28000705]

[46]   Ciacci C, Ciclitira P, Hadjivassiliou M, *et al.* The gluten-free diet and its current application in coeliac disease and dermatitis herpetiformis. United European Gastroenterol J 2015; 3(2): 121-35.
[http://dx.doi.org/10.1177/2050640614559263] [PMID: 25922672]

[47]   Saturni L, Ferretti G, Bacchetti T. The gluten-free diet: safety and nutritional quality. Nutrients 2010; 2(1): 16-34.
[http://dx.doi.org/10.3390/nu2010016] [PMID: 22253989]

[48]   Ellis HJ, Doyle AP, Day P, Wieser H, Ciclitira PJ. Demonstration of the presence of coeliac-activating gliadin-like epitopes in malted barley. Int Arch Allergy Immunol 1994; 104(3): 308-10.
[http://dx.doi.org/10.1159/000236683] [PMID: 7518270]

[49]   Food and Drug Administration FDA US. Federal Register Proposed Rule—72 FR 2795 January 23, 2007: Food Labeling; Gluten-Free Labeling of Foods. Available from: http://www.fda.gov.

[50]   Food and Drug Administration FDA US. Proposed rule for gluten-free labeling of fermented or hydrolyzed foods. In: Federal Register / 78 (150), August 5, 2013 / Rules and Regulations, 2013; pp., 1-26.

[51]   Rosell M, Moita C, Pérez E, Gularte M. Arroz.De tales harinas, tales panes Granos harinas y productos de panificación en Iberoamérica. Córdoba, Argentina: Programa Iberoamericano de Ciencia y Tecnología para el Desarrollo 2007; pp. 123-59. http://agro.unc.edu.ar

[52]   Pérez E, Baragaño-Mosqueda M, Arteaga M, Schroeder M. Proximal composition and categorization by the amylose content of rice (*Oryza sativa* L.) varieties. Rev Fac Agro UCV 2009; 35(3): 94-9.

[53]   Comino I, Moreno MdeL, Real A, Rodríguez-Herrera A, Barro F, Sousa C. The gluten-free diet: testing alternative cereals tolerated by celiac patients. Nutrients 2013; 5(10): 4250-68.
[http://dx.doi.org/10.3390/nu5104250] [PMID: 24152755]

[54]   Pérez Sira EE. Raíces y tubérculos.De tales harinas, tales panes Granos harinas y productos de panificación en Iberoamérica. Córdoba, Argentina 2007; pp. 363-401.http://agro.unc.edu.ar

[55]   Juliano BO. Rice in human nutrition Published with the collaboration of the International Rice Research Institute (INRA) and Food and Agriculture Organization of the United Nations. Rome: FAO 1993.

[56]   Nutrient Data Laboratory. United States Department of Agriculture 2019.
https://ndb.nal.usda.gov/ndb/search/list

[57]   United States Department of Agriculture (USDA). Agricultural Research Service National USDA Food Composition Databases. Nutrient Database for Standard Reference Legacy Release 2019.

[58]   Coffman WR, Juliano BO. Nutritional quality of cereal grains: Genetic and agronomic improvement.Rice. Madison: American Society of Agronomy 1987; pp. 101-31.

[59]   Suwannaporn P, Pitiphunpong S, Champangern S. Classification of rice amylose content by discriminant analysis of physicochemical properties. Starke 2007; 59(3-4): 171-7.
[http://dx.doi.org/10.1002/star.200600565]

[60]   Casagrande Denardin C, Boufleur N, Reckziegel P, Picolli da Silva L, Walter M. Amylose content in rice (*Oryza sativa*) affects performance, glycemic and lipidic metabolism in rats. Cienc Rural 2012; 42(2): 381-7.
[http://dx.doi.org/10.1590/S0103-84782012005000002]

[61]　Pérez Sira E, Sívoli L, Guzmán R. Procesos de obtención de harina de maíz no-nixtamalizada y sus usos.Alternativas tecnológicas para la elaboración y la conservación de productos panificados. Editorial Facultad de Ciencias Exactas, Físicas y Naturales, Universidad Nacional de Córdoba 2009; pp. 207-34.

[62]　Muench DG, Ogawa M, Okita T. The Prolamins of Rice. In: Shewry R, Casey R, Eds Seed Proteins, Springer. Nature. 1999.
[http://dx.doi.org/10.1007/978-94-011-4431-5_5]

[63]　Kubota M, Saito Y, Masumura T, Watanabe R, Fujimura S, Kadowaki M. *In vivo* digestibility of rice prolamin/protein body-I particle is decreased by cooking. J Nutr Sci Vitaminol (Tokyo) 2014; 60(4): 300-4.
[http://dx.doi.org/10.3177/jnsv.60.300] [PMID: 25297621]

[64]　Kim WT, Okita TW. Structure, expression, and heterogeneity of the rice seed prolamines. Plant Physiol 1988; 88(3): 649-55.
[http://dx.doi.org/10.1104/pp.88.3.649] [PMID: 16666363]

[65]　Wang Z, Li H, Liang M, Yang L. Glutelin and prolamin, different components of rice protein, exert differently *in vitro* antioxidant activities. J Cereal Sci 2016; 72: 108-16.
[http://dx.doi.org/10.1016/j.jcs.2016.10.006]

[66]　Li H, Wang Z, Liang M, Cai L, Yang L. Methionine augments antioxidant activity of rice protein during gastrointestinal digestion. Int J Mol Sci 2019; 20(4): 868.
[http://dx.doi.org/10.3390/ijms20040868] [PMID: 30781587]

[67]　Chen Y-J, Chen YY, Wu C-T, Yu C-C, Liao H-F. Prolamin, a rice protein, augments anti-leukaemia immune response. J Cereal Sci 2010; 51(2): 189-97.
[http://dx.doi.org/10.1016/j.jcs.2009.11.011]

[68]　Nuss ET, Tanumihardjo SA. Maize: a paramount staple crop in the context of global nutrition. Compr Rev Food Sci Food Saf 2010; 9(4): 417-36.
[http://dx.doi.org/10.1111/j.1541-4337.2010.00117.x] [PMID: 33467836]

[69]　Krishnana HB, Coe EH Jr. Seed storage proteins Encyclopedia of Genetics 2001. Academic Press 2014; pp. 1782-7.

[70]　Elzoghby AO, Elgohary MM, Kamel NM. Implications of protein- and Peptide-based nanoparticles as potential vehicles for anticancer drugs. Adv Protein Chem Struct Biol 2015; 98: 169-221.
[http://dx.doi.org/10.1016/bs.apcsb.2014.12.002] [PMID: 25819280]

[71]　Arvanitoyannis IS, Dionisopoulou NK. Irradiation of edible film of plant and animal origin. Iradiation of foods commodities, Elsevier Inc., 2010, pp., 15-19.

[72]　Luo Y, Wang T. Pharmaceutical and cosmetic applications of protein by-products.Protein byproducts transformation from environmental Burden into value-added products. Academic Press 2016; pp. 147-60.
[http://dx.doi.org/10.1016/B978-0-12-802391-4.00009-4]

[73]　Mejia CD, Mauer LJ, Hamaker BR. Similarities and differences in secondary structure of viscoelastic polymers of maize α-zein and wheat gluten proteins. J Cereal Sci 2007; 45(3): 353-9.
[http://dx.doi.org/10.1016/j.jcs.2006.09.009]

[74]　Schober TJ, Scott R, Bean SR, Boyle DL, Parka S-H. Improved viscoelastic zein–starch doughs for leavened gluten-free breads: Their rheology and microstructure. J Cereal Sci 2008; 48(3): 755-67.
[http://dx.doi.org/10.1016/j.jcs.2008.04.004]

[75]　Diatta A. Using corn zein to improve the quality of gluten-free bread 2018.

[76]   Cabrera-Chávez F, Rouzaud-Sández O, Sotelo-Cruz N, Calderón de la Barca AM. Transglutaminase treatment of wheat and maize prolamins of bread increases the serum IgA reactivity of celiac disease patients. J Agric Food Chem 2008; 56(4): 1387-91.
[http://dx.doi.org/10.1021/jf0724163] [PMID: 18193828]

[77]   Cabrera-Chávez F, Iametti S, Miriani M, de la Barca AM, Mamone G, Bonomi F. Maize prolamins resistant to peptic-tryptic digestion maintain immune-recognition by IgA from some celiac disease patients. Plant Foods Hum Nutr 2012; 67(1): 24-30, 30.
[http://dx.doi.org/10.1007/s11130-012-0274-4] [PMID: 22298027]

[78]   Ortiz-Sánchez JP, Cabrera-Chávez F, de la Barca AM. Maize prolamins could induce a gluten-like cellular immune response in some celiac disease patients. Nutrients 2013; 5(10): 4174-83.
[http://dx.doi.org/10.3390/nu5104174] [PMID: 24152750]

[79]   Rouf Shah T, Prasad K, Kumar P. Maize-A potential source of human nutrition and health: A review. Cogent Food Agric 2016; 21166995
[http://dx.doi.org/10.1080/23311932.2016.1166995]

[80]   Ai Y, Jane J-L. Macronutrients in corn and human nutrition. Compr Rev Food Sci Food Saf 2016; 15(3): 581-98.
[http://dx.doi.org/10.1111/1541-4337.12192] [PMID: 33401819]

[81]   Pérez A, Saucedo O, Iglesias J, *et al.* Caracterización y potencialidades del grano de sorgo (Sorghum bicolor L. Moench). Pastos Forrajes 2010; 33(1): 1-26.

[82]   Chavez DW, Ramirez Ascheri JL, Martins A, Piler Carvalho WC, Oliveira Bernardo C, Teles A. Sorghum, an alternative cereal for gluten free products. Rev Chil Nutr 2018; 45(2): 169-77.
[http://dx.doi.org/10.4067/S0717-75182018000300169]

[83]   De Mesa-Stonestreet NJ. Processing and characterization of sorghum protein concentrates using extrusion-enzyme liquefaction 2006.

[84]   de Mesa-Stonestreet NJ, Alavi S, Bean SR. Sorghum proteins: the concentration, isolation, modification, and food applications of kafirins. J Food Sci 2010; 75(5): R90-R104.
[http://dx.doi.org/10.1111/j.1750-3841.2010.01623.x] [PMID: 20629895]

[85]   Ciacci C, Maiuri L, Caporaso N, *et al.* Celiac disease: *in vitro* and *in vivo* safety and palatability of wheat-free sorghum food products. Clin Nutr 2007; 26(6): 799-805.
[http://dx.doi.org/10.1016/j.clnu.2007.05.006] [PMID: 17719701]

[86]   Pontieri P, Mamone G, De Caro S, *et al.* Sorghum, a healthy and gluten-free food for celiac patients as demonstrated by genome, biochemical, and immunochemical analyses. J Agric Food Chem 2013; 61(10): 2565-71.
[http://dx.doi.org/10.1021/jf304882k] [PMID: 23432128]

[87]   Osborne TB, Campbell GF. Proteins of the potato. J Am Chem Soc 1896; 18: 575-92.
[http://dx.doi.org/10.1021/ja02093a002]

[88]   Lindner J, Jaschik S, Korpaczy J. Amino acid composition and biological value of potato protein fractions. Qual Pl Mater Veg 1960; 7(3): 290-4.

[89]   Lim T.K. Solanum tuberosum. In: Edible Medicinal and Non-Medicinal Plants. Springer, Cham. 2016, pp., 12 – 23.
[http://dx.doi.org/10.1007/978-3-319-26065-5_2]

[90]   Bárta J, Bártová V. Patatin, the major protein of potato (*Solanum tuberosum* L.) tubers, and its occurrence as genotype effect: processing *versus* table potatoes. Czech J Food Sci 2008; 26: 347-59.
[http://dx.doi.org/10.17221/27/2008-CJFS]

[91]   Gambuti A, Rinaldi A, Moio L. Use of patatin, a protein extracted from potato, as alternative to animal proteins in fining of red wine. Eur Food Res Technol 2013.

[92]   True RH, Ho Gan JM, Augustin J, Johnson SJ, Teitzel C, Toma RB, *et al.* Mineral composition of freshly harvested potatoes. Am J Potato Res 1979; 56(7): 339-50.
[http://dx.doi.org/10.1007/BF02853849]

[93]   Mahamud MA, Chowdhury MAH, Rahim MA, Mohiuddin KM. Mineral nutrient contents of some potato accessions of USA and Bangladesh. J Bangladesh Agril Univ 2015; 13(2): 207-14.
[http://dx.doi.org/10.3329/jbau.v13i2.28781]

[94]   Navarre DA, Goyer A, Shakya R. Chapter 14-Nutritional value of potatoes: vitamin, phytonutrient, and mineral content. In Advances in Potato Chemistry and Technology; Singh, J., Kaur, L.B.T.-A., Eds.; Academic Press: San Diego, CA, USA, 2009; pp. 395–424. ISBN 978-0-12-374349-7.

[95]   Pérez E, Pacheco de Delahaye E. Características químicas, físicas y reológicas de la harina y el almidón nativo aislado de Ipomoea batatas Lam. Acta Científica, 2005; 56(1):12-20.

[96]   Pérez EE, Mahfoud A, Domínguez CL, Guzmán R. Roots, tubers, grains and bananas; flours and starches. Utilization in the development of foods for conventional, celiac, and phenylketonuric consumers. Food Proc Tech 2013; 4(3): 1-6.

[97]   Pérez E, Sivoli L, Cueto D, Pérez L. Cassava flour an alternative to producing gluten-free baked goods and pasta.Cassava: Production, Consumption, and Potential Uses Plant Science Research and Practice. NOVA Science Publisher 2017; pp. 87-104.

[98]   Sívoli LJ, Ciarfella AT, Pérez EE. Functional and nutritional characterization of cassava flours for industrial applications.Cassava: Production, Nutritional Properties, and Health Effects. New York: NOVA Publishers 2014; pp. 25-50.

[99]   Ciarfella AT, Sívoli LJ, Pérez EE. Food products developed using cassava roots and its derivatives: A review.Cassava: production, nutritional properties, and health effects. New York: NOVA Publishers 2014; pp. 161-76.

[100]   Anchundia MA, Pérez E. Nutritional characteristics and sensory evaluation of a drink made with sweet potato flour for people with phenylketonuria. Agro Sci 2018; 8(1): 15-9.

[101]   Waizel-Bucay J. El uso tradicional de las especies del género *Dioscorea*. Rev Fitoterapia 2009; 9(1): 53-67.

[102]   San Mauro Martín I, Garicano Vilar E, Collado Yurrutia L, Ciudad Cabañas MJ. ¿Es el gluten el gran agente etiopatogenico de enfermedad en el siglo XXI? Nutr Hosp 2014; 30(6): 1203-10.
[PMID: 25433099]

[103]   Kohout P. Nutrition in celiac disease. International Journal of Celiac Disease 2014; 2(3): 115-7.
[http://dx.doi.org/10.12691/ijcd-2-3-2]

[104]   Niland B, Cash BD. Health benefits and adverse effects of a gluten-free diet in non–celiac disease patients. Gastroenterol Hepatol (N Y) 2018; 14(2): 82-91.
[PMID: 29606920]

[105]   Francavilla R, Cristofori F, Stella M, Borrelli G, Naspi G, Castellaneta S. Treatment of celiac disease: from gluten-free diet to novel therapies. Minerva Pediatr 2014; 66(5): 501-16.
[PMID: 24938882]

[106]   Osman AA, Günnel T, Dietl A, *et al.* B cell epitopes of gliadin. Clin Exp Immunol 2000; 121(2): 248-54.
[http://dx.doi.org/10.1046/j.1365-2249.2000.01312.x] [PMID: 10931138]

[107]   University of Chicago Medicine Celiac Disease Center. 2019.http://www.cureceliacdisease.org

[108]   Alvarez-Jubete L, Arendt EK, Gallaghera E. Nutritive value of pseudo-cereals and their increasing use as functional gluten-free ingredients. Trends Food Sci Technol 2010; 21(2): 106-13.
[http://dx.doi.org/10.1016/j.tifs.2009.10.014]

[109] Jnawali P, Kumar V, Tanwar B. Celiac disease: Overview and considerations for development of gluten-free foods. Food Sci Hum Wellness 2016; 5(4): 169-76.
[http://dx.doi.org/10.1016/j.fshw.2016.09.003]

CHAPTER 8

Dyslipidemia and Foods

Elevina Pérez Sira[1,*]

[1] *Instituto de Ciencia y Tecnología de Alimentos, Facultad de Ciencias, Universidad Central de Venezuela, Caracas, Venezuela*

Abstract: Dyslipidemia is a disorder of lipoprotein metabolism. Among the several causes of this disorder, there are secondary causes (mainly in adults), such as a sedentary lifestyle with excessive dietary intake of saturated fat, cholesterol, and *Trans* fats, alcohol overuse, and cigarette smoking. The chapter compiles and discusses as an overview, the types of dyslipidemia, clinical pathologies, and its causes. The chapter addresses fatty foods, and their fatty acid profile, the essential fatty acids, fat replacers, and some practical hints for fat-free foods including some home recipes.

Keywords: Cholesterol, Dyslipidemia, Essential fatty acids, Fat, Fatty acids, Foods for consumers with dyslipidemia.

INTRODUCTION

Dyslipidemia is a medical condition or disorder of lipoprotein metabolism; It includes lipoprotein overproduction (hyperlipidemia or high lipid levels) or lipoprotein deficiency (hypolipidemia or low lipid levels). The disorder produces alterations in plasma cholesterol; mainly in the high-density lipoprotein cholesterol (HDL-c) and in low-density lipoprotein cholesterol (LDL-c), and plasma triglycerides [1].

The dyslipidemia classification provides a useful determination method to the underlying cause of dyslipidemia in patients. Dyslipidemia has been classified by Fredrickson using patterns of lipoprotein abnormalities. The Fredrickson classification [2] based on the pattern of lipoproteins on electrophoresis or ultracentrifugation profile varying from I to V is as follows:

Type I. Hyperchylomicronemia that presents and VLDL (pre-/3-lipoproteins) normal or only slightly increased.

[*] **Corresponding author Elevina Pérez Sira:** Instituto de Ciencia y Tecnología de Alimentos, Facultad de Ciencias, Universidad Central de Venezuela, Caracas, Venezuela; Tel: +58.212.751 4403; Fax: +58.212.751 3871; E-mail: elevina07@gmail.com

Type II. Hyper-p-lipoproteinemia presents an abnormal increase in LDL (β) concentration. This type pertains to additional treatment *i.e.*, IIa and IIb. In both, the criterion for type II, an increase in LDL (pre β), is present, but in one (IIb), an increase in VLDL.

Type III. "Floating β "or "Broad β" Pattern. Presence of VLDL having abnormally high cholesterol content and abnormal electrophoretic mobility ("floating-β"; "β-VLDL").

Type IV. Hyperpre-g-lipoproteinemia presents increased VLDL (pre-β), no increase in LDL (β), and chylomicrons absent.

Type V. Hyperpre-β-lipoproteinemia and chylomicronemia that present: VLDL increased and chylomicrons present.

Fredrickson's classification was somewhat controversial, but it is still a reference.

There is another alternative method for classifying dyslipidemia, which divides conditions into primary or secondary hyperlipidemia and characterizes the conditions by the characteristic serum lipid pattern (elevated cholesterol or triglycerides or both). This alternative method has advantages over the Fredrickson classification (which is based primarily on the observed phenotype) because, in some inherited hyperlipidemias, the same genotype expresses more than one phenotype and in some secondary hyperlipidemias the phenotypes can vary [3].

Hyperlipidemia, also called hyperlipoproteinemia, is a disorder of excess fatty substances, mainly cholesterol and triglycerides, in the blood. Chemical forces, different from the covalent, attach these fatty substances to specific proteins making the lipoproteins. Then, they can remain dissolved while in circulation [4].

According to Nirosha *et al.* [4], hyperlipidemia can be divided into two subcategories

1. Hypercholesterolemia, or a high level of cholesterol.

2. Hypertriglyceridemia, or a high level of triglycerides.

HYPERCHOLESTEROLEMIA

Cholesterol

Cholesterol is a fat-like substance found in the bloodstream and bodily organs and nerve fibers and required for numerous vital functions in the body. Cholesterol is vital for the synthesis of bile acids, and many hormones such as testosterone, estrogen, dehydroepiandrosterone, progesterone, and cortisol, and sun exposure to produce vitamin D. It is also cell membranes support, antioxidant element, transporter or conductor of nervous impulses, especially at the synapse level [5].

However, cholesterol is not an essential nutrient because the body can make it. The liver makes most of the cholesterol in the body from a wide variety of foods, but especially from saturated fats, especially animal products such as meats, poultry, fish, eggs, and dairy products. Furthermore, several causes such as genetic, lifestyle, or diseases could influence an individual's level of cholesterol [6].

Lipoproteins

Cholesterol, triglycerides, and other lipids (fats) move as lipoproteins around the body in particles that include [7]

Low-density lipoprotein cholesterol (LDL-C, which carries most of the blood cholesterol)

IDL-C, intermediate-density lipoproteins cholesterol

Very low-density lipoprotein cholesterol (VLDL-C, which carry most of the blood triglycerides)

High-Density Lipoprotein Cholesterol (HDL-C)

Chylomicrons (recently absorbed fat)

Low-Density-Lipoprotein cholesterol (LDL-C) is the most considerable portion of circulating cholesterol [8] because it consists of more cholesterol than triglycerides and protein. It is a spheroidal particle of about 220-275 Å in diameter that contains a cholesteryl ester-rich core surrounded by a phospholipidrich shell attached to apolipoprotein B-100 (apoB-100) in a single unit per lipoprotein particle [9, 10]. LDL-C transports 3,000 to 6,000 fat molecules by particles and varying in size according to the number and mix of fat molecules contained within them [9]. The carried lipids include all fat molecules with cholesterol, phospholipids, and triglycerides dominant, amounts of each varying considerably. Epidemiologic investigations have validated LDL-C as an independent predictor of CV risk [11]. Excess of LDL-C contributes to the blockage of arteries, which eventually leads to heart attack, and it has now largely replaced total cholesterol as the primary lipid measurement for evaluation of risk due to atherogenic lipoproteins [11]. LDL-C goes up if the diet is high in saturated and "trans" fat, also called Trans fatty acid, and an increase in blood triglyceride level typically accompanies its levels.

IDL intermediate-density lipoproteins are the first cholesterol-enriched species from VLDL in the process of LDL formation. VLDL is converted by lipoprotein lipase and cholesteryl ester transfer protein (CETP) into more cholesterolenriched species, first IDL, and then LDL [11].

VLDL-C (very low-density lipoprotein) is a large plasma lipoprotein rich in triglycerides, and the major cholesterol carrying in human plasma. VLDL-C transports the triglycerides from the sites of absorption and synthesis to the sites of storage and utilization [12]. Primarily the liver produces VLDL-C with lesser amounts contributed by the intestine [13]. These lipoproteins circulate through the blood, giving up their triglycerides to fat and muscle tissue. The VLDL remnants are modified and converted into LDL, leaving a residue of cholesterol in the tissues during the process of conversion to LDL. In this way, VLDL-C helps cholesterol build up on the walls of arteries [14].

High-Density-Lipoprotein cholesterol (HDL-C) particles range in diameter from 70 and 100 Å, and their molecular mass varies from 200 to 400 x103 Daltons. HDL-C synthesized in the liver, and the intestines have a higher density as compared to the VLDL-C and LDL-C. They have less amount of cholesterol and more protein content, which makes them densest [14]. HDL-C is the site of the plasma cholesterol esterification and the machinery for that significant reaction [12].

The cholesterol esterification mediated by the enzyme lecithin-cholesterol acyltransferase plays a critical role in the reverse cholesterol transport pathway [12, 14]. The mechanism is esterifying free cholesterol derived from the peripheral tissues and driving the cholesterol efflux forward [12, 15]. The enzyme activity is positively correlated with the HDL levels and is essential not only in lipoprotein metabolism but also in atherogenesis [16]. Besides the reverse transport involvement, the HDL-C has the function as anti-inflammatory, antithrombotic, and anti-oxidative functions, many studies have shown HDL-C to be an independent adverse risk factor for atherosclerosis [14].

Chylomicrons are relatively large immediately following a meal, and easily separated from smaller, denser VLDL [13]. Chylomicrons and VLDL are lipoproteins that carry triglycerides from sites of absorption and synthesis to sites of storage and utilization [12]. The chylomicron is dependent on dietary intake, and they are the basis for the formation of VLDL and LDL cholesterol. Chylomicrons assembled in intestines have triglyceride, cholesterol, phospholipid, and Apolipoprotein (Apo) B 48, a truncated version of Apo B 100, under the influence of microsomal triglyceride transfer protein [14].

Evidence has been reported that the smaller particles have greater access to arterial subendothelial space and, hence, greater ability to accelerate the atherosclerotic process [14].

High levels of serum cholesterol, mainly the chylomicrons, VLDL, LDL cholesterol are related to all-cause mortality and coronary heart disease.

Several trials have confirmed that cholesterol-lowering reduces the future risk of coronary disease. Risk reduction is not back to zero, but to that risk predicted by the resulting cholesterol level [7].

Although the focus in treating lipid disorders is on reducing LDL-cholesterol concentrations, additional lipid-related independent risk factors, such as triglyceride, HDL-cholesterol, and lipoprotein (a) levels should be used clinically to assess cardiovascular risk [17].

Foods high in saturated and trans-fat induce hypercholesterolemia saturated and trans fats are found mainly in fatty meats, full cream dairy products (*e.g.*, milk, cream, cheese, and butter), deep-fried take-away foods, baked products (*e.g.*, biscuits and pastries) [18].

Certain saturated vegetable fats and oils, including coconut fat and palm oil, are cholesterol-free but cause an increase in blood cholesterol [19]. Some foods that do not contain animal products may contain trans-fats, which also cause the body to make more cholesterol. Fruit, vegetables, and cereals do not contain cholesterol.

Hypertriglyceridemia

Hypertriglyceridemia (HTG) (hyperlipidemia) is a commonly encountered lipid abnormality frequently associated with other lipids and metabolic derangements [19]. This abnormality has primary and secondary subtypes. Primary (familiar) is due to genetic causes (such as a mutation in a receptor protein), while secondary or acquired arises due to other causes; such as diabetes. Usually, hyperlipidemia is classified as primary when there are no secondary causes identified.

It is vital to treat HTG to prevent pancreatitis by reducing triglyceride levels to <500 mg/dL. Therapeutic lifestyle changes are the first line of treatment for it. These changes include low saturated fat, carbohydrate-controlled diet, combined with alcohol reduction, smoking cessation, and regular aerobic exercise. High doses of omega-3 fatty acids are obtained from fish and fish oil supplements low triglyceride levels significantly [20].

As causes *hyperlipidemia* is account as part of the metabolic syndrome product of several genetic mutations and can be secondary to several diseases and drugs. Very severe or chylomicronemia syndrome results from rare mutations in the lipoprotein lipase complex. Indeed, multifactorial chylomicronemia syndrome develops as a result of the co-existence of genetic and secondary forms of HTG. Some but not all causes of mild to moderate HTG are associated with an increased risk of premature cardiovascular disease, while very severe HTG can lead to pancreatitis and other features of the chylomicronemia syndrome [21].

Hypotriglyceridemia

Hypotriglyceridemia (hypolipidemia) is a decrease in plasma lipoproteins caused by primary (genetic) or secondary factors. It is usually asymptomatic and diagnosed incidentally on routine lipids screening [22]. Treatment of secondary hypolipidemia involves treating underlying disorders. Treatment of primary hypolipidemia is often unnecessary, but patients with some genetic disorders require high-dose vitamin E and dietary supplementation of fats and other fatsoluble vitamins. Hypolipidemia is defined as total cholesterol (TC) < 120 mg/dL (< 3.1 mmol/L) or low-density lipoprotein (LDL) cholesterol < 50 mg/dL (< 1.3 mmol/L) [22].

DYSLIPIDEMIA CAUSES

Causes of dyslipidemias are multifactorial; they may be the primary cause of single or multiple gene mutations, which result in either overproduction or defective clearance of triglycerides and LDL, or underproduction or excessive clearance of HDL [23]. The use of drugs, such as thiazides, beta-blockers, retinoids, highly active antiretroviral agents, cyclosporine, tacrolimus, estrogen and progestins, glucocorticoids, and anabolic steroids also are causing of low levels of HDL cholesterol.

As secondary causes (mainly in adults) of dyslipidemia should be a sedentary lifestyle with excessive dietary intake of saturated fats, cholesterol, and trans fats, alcohol overuse, and cigarette smoking [23, 24]. The secondary causes also could be derived from *Diabetes mellitus*, chronic kidney disease, hypothyroidism, primary biliary cirrhosis, and other cholestatic liver diseases HIV infection [24 - 26].

Nutrition is an important treatment for dyslipidemia, coronary heart disease (CHD) risk factors, and the prevention and treatment of cardiovascular disease (CVD). Several studies have established the relationship between diet, serum lipids, inflammation, and CVD, including CHD and stroke [27].

The risk for dyslipidemia increased by a variety of factors, including family history, aging, weight gain, physical inactivity, and menopause. Other factors are insulin resistance diseases such as type 2 diabetes mellitus, and hypothyroidism, and diets high in saturated fats, *Trans* fats, and cholesterol.

According to the 2018 guideline of blood cholesterol management published in the Journal of the American College of Cardiology (JACC) [28], these are the acceptable, borderline, and high measurements for adults (Table **1**).

Table 1. Guideline on the management of blood cholesterol and triglyceride [29].

	Total (mg/dL)	HDL (mg/dL)	LDL (mg/dL)	Triglyceride
Optimum/desirable/normal	<200	-	< 100	< 150
Near-optimal/above optimal	-	-	100-129	-
Low	-	< 40	-	-
Borderline high	200-239	-	130-159	150-199
High	≥240	≥60	160-189	200-499
Very high	-	-	≥190	≥500

Dyslipidemia and atherosclerosis

The biggest contributing factor to the development of atherosclerosis and subsequent cardiovascular diseases is dyslipidemia, mainly hyperlipoproteinemia. There exists a relationship between diet, serum lipids, inflammation, and cardiovascular disease, including coronary heart disease and stroke [30]. Dietary treatment is a successful control in the management of hyperlipidemia. It has been argued that elevated levels of plasma low-density lipoprotein and very lowdensity lipoprotein cholesterol, as seen in hypercholesterolemia or hypertriglyceridemia, are primarily caused by a diet high in saturated fat, cholesterol, and calories, and by excessive intake of alcohol [29].

The world prevalence of dyslipidemia increased noticeably according to the income level of the country. Low-income countries around a quarter of adults had raised total cholesterol; in lower-middle-income countries, this rose to around a third of the population for both sexes. In high-income countries, over 50% of adults had raised total cholesterol, more than double the level of the low-income countries [31].

Several studies have shown the effectiveness of certain foods in reducing the risk of dyslipidemia [32]. In this context, there are specific ingredients, which are potential in the formulation and production of ready-to-eat and cook foods, as adjuvant strategies in the reduction of the risk of this disease.

Since world dyslipidemia prevalence has increased, the market offers of food of easy consumption help to the prevention and control of this disease. Therefore, it must be done intense research to formulate and produce processed foods. However, there is not yet a commitment from food research and processing of easy consumption food for consumers with dyslipidemia disease.

FATTY FOODS AND FATTY ACID PROFILE

The lipids are classified in regards to their melting points, like fats or oils, being the physical state for fat, a solid-state, and oil liquid. Fats and oils are glycerolipids, which are essentially composed of triglycerides (TG). Minor amounts of phospholipids, monoacylglycerols, diacylglycerols, and sterols/sterol esters are with lipids. One TG comprises three fatty acids esterified with a glycerol backbone. 'Triacylglycerols' is the correct chemical name, but more commonly known as triglycerides, they are the principal representative of dietary fat.

Dietary fat includes all the lipids in plant and animal tissues eaten as food. The fatty acid profile is a measure of the number and amount of its fatty acids, and it is the essential nutritional information of fats.

The fatty acids constitute the main components of lipids entities required in human nutrition as a source of energy, and for metabolic and structural activities [33]. Fatty acids are carbon chains with a methyl group at one end of the molecule (designated as omega, Ω) and a carboxyl group at the other end. The fatty acids represent 30–35% of total energy intake for consumers in many industrial countries. The most important dietary sources of fatty acids are vegetable oils, dairy products, meat products, grain, and fatty fish, or fish oils [34].

As a function of the degree of unsaturation and isomeric configuration, the most common dietary fatty acids are: saturated, monounsaturated, polyunsaturated, and *Trans* fat [33].

Saturated fats are rich in saturated fatty acids. They are found in higher proportions in animal products and are usually solid at room temperature.

Monounsaturated and polyunsaturated fats (rich in mono and polyunsaturated fatty acids in different proportions) are found in higher proportions in plants and are usually liquid at room temperature.

Trans-fat (a type of unsaturated fat) found primarily in partially hydrogenated oils, foods containing these oils, and in small amounts in some animal products.

The *Trans* fatty acids are geometric isomers of monounsaturated and polyunsaturated fatty acids having at least one carbon-carbon double bond with hydrogen on opposite sides of the double bond (trans configuration) [35], which makes the molecule kinked [36]. The Trans fatty acids have physical properties generally resembling saturated fatty acids, and their presence tends to harden oils [35].

Food rich in unsaturated fat is considered healthy, and contrarily those fats with high proportions of saturated fatty acids are called unhealthy foods. At the same time, *Trans*-fat has detrimental health effects due to the correlation between diets high in *Trans*- fats, and diseases like atherosclerosis and coronary heart disease.

Stencel and Dobbins [37] recommended that the *Trans* fatty acids must be on nutrition labels. The authors concluded that because *Trans* fatty acids are not essential and provide no known health benefit, however, and there is no safe level of them. Therefore, people should eat as little of them as possible while consuming a nutritionally adequate diet. Indeed, due to *Trans* fatty acids occur in so many types of food, an all-out ban is impractical and would make it extremely difficult to get a nutritionally adequate diet [31].

Doell [38]. pointed out that although the overall intake of industriallyproduced *Trans*- fatty acids (IP-TFA) in US population has decreased, as a result of the implementation of labeling requirements, individuals with certain dietary habits may still consume high levels of IP-TFA through certain choose brands or types of food products.

ESSENTIAL FATTY ACIDS

An essential nutrient is a nutrient required for normal physiological functions, which cannot be synthesized by the body. Among them, there are polyunsaturated fatty acids (PUFAs) [34]. PUFAs are fatty acids that contain more than one double bond in their backbone. The PUFA type includes many essential compounds, such as; essential fatty acids (EFAs), and those that give frying oils their characteristic [34].

The human body is capable to synthesizes all the fatty acids needed, except for the linoleic acid (LA, 18:2, Ω-6) an omega-6 fatty acid, and alpha-linolenic acid (ALA, 18:3, Ω-3) an omega-3 fatty acid. LA and ALA are used by the body to make other essential fatty acids, which the body cannot produce [39 - 41]. For example; arachidonic acid (ARA, 20:4, Ω-6), which is from LA, and the eicosapentaenoic acid (EPA, 20:5, Ω-3), docosapentaenoic acid (DPA, 22:5, isomers: Ω-6 and Ω-3), and docosahexaenoic acid (DHA, 22:6, Ω-3), which come from ALA. There exists an omega-3 fatty acid limited conversion in the body, which leads to include them in the diet. Moreover, not all vertebrates can convert stearic acid (C18 PUFA) to the higher arachidic acid (C20) and behenic acid (C22); consequently, the C20 and C22 are essential fatty acids for these species [34, 39 - 41].

The essential fatty acids are considered functional food and nutraceuticals because several studies have documented their significant roles in biochemical pathways [42]. It is a cardio protector because of its considerable antiatherogenic, antithrombotic, anti-inflammatory, antiarrhythmic, hypolipidemic effects. They also have the potential to reduce the risk of serious diseases, especially cancer, osteoporosis, diabetes, and others [42]. Their health promotion activities following from their complex influence on concentrations of lipoproteins, the fluidity of biological membranes, the function of membraned enzymes and receptors, modulation of eicosanoids production, blood pressure regulation, and the metabolism of minerals [42].

As the higher organisms, including mammals and fish, cannot synthesize all PUFAs, they are essential fatty acids [43]. The essential fatty acids are linoleic acid (LA), alpha-linolenic acid (ALA), arachidonic acid (ARA), eicosapentaenoic acid (EPA), and docosahexaenoic acid (DHA) [39]. ALA and LA are found in plant and seed oils, and EPA and DHA come only from fish (salmon, mackerel, and herring, among others) [42]. Although the levels of LA are usually higher than those of ALA, the rapeseed and walnut oils are excellent sources of ALA. ALA comes from animal sources, such as meat and egg yolk [44].

LA is a major fatty acid in plant lipids and is in higher plants (soybean and rapeseed oils) and algae. ARA is a significant component of the phospholipid's membrane in the animal kingdom, but very little is found in the diet. EPA and DHA are the major fatty acids of marine algae, fatty fish, and fish oils. DHA is found in high concentrations, especially in phospholipids in the brain, retina, and testes [43].

Humans have high requirements of Ω-6 than Ω-3 fatty acids [42]. However, according to several authors, at this time, diets are deficient in Ω-3 fatty acids as compared with the diet on which humans evolved. Consequently, a balanced $\Omega6$ /Ω-3 ratio in the diet is essential for normal growth and development and should lead to decreases in cardiovascular disease and other chronic diseases and improve mental health [39, 45].

The ratio of membrane Ω-3 to Ω-6 fatty acids influences neurotransmission and prostaglandin formation. These processes are vital in the maintenance of normal brain function [46]. However, the Simopoulos studies [47] have indicated that the optimal ratio may vary with the disease under consideration, which is consistent with the fact that chronic diseases are multigenic and multifactorial. Therefore, the authors concluded that the therapeutic dose of omega-3 fatty acids might depend on the degree of severity of the disease resulting from the genetic predisposition. By way of a lower ratio of omega-6/omega-3 fatty acids should more desirable in reducing the risk of many of the chronic diseases of high prevalence in the world.

As was reported, Ω-3s play an important role in cognition, behavioral function, mood, circulation, and skin and heart health and have anti-inflammatory properties [48, 49].

The fatty acids influence inflammation through a variety of mechanisms; many of these are mediated by, or at least associated with, changes in the fatty acid composition of cell membranes. EPA and DHA give rise to newly discovered resolving which is anti-inflammatory and inflammation resolving.

Increased membrane content of EPA and DHA (and decreased arachidonic acid content) results in a changed pattern of production of eicosanoids and probably also of resolvins [50]. Resolvins are metabolic byproducts of omega-3 fatty acids that are involved in promoting the restoration of normal cellular function following the inflammation that occurs after tissue injury [50, 51].

On the other hand, Ω-6s are pro-inflammatory and are necessary for normal growth and development, maintaining the reproductive system, and contributing to the synthesis of hair, skin, and bones. The inflammation is part of the normal host response to infection and injury. However, excessive or inappropriate inflammation contributes to a range of acute and chronic human diseases.

Studies indicate that a high intake of n−6 fatty acids shifts the physiologic state to one that is prothrombotic and pro-aggregatory, characterized by increases in blood viscosity, vasospasm, and vasoconstriction and decreases in bleeding time, Ω−3 Fatty acids, however, have anti-inflammatory, antithrombotic, antiarrhythmic, hypolipidemic, and vasodilatory properties [48]. The beneficial effects of Ω −3 fatty acids have in the secondary prevention of coronary heart disease, hypertension, type 2 diabetes, and, in some patients with renal disease, rheumatoid arthritis, ulcerative colitis, Crohn disease, and chronic obstructive pulmonary disease [52, 53].

Most of the studies carried out with fish oils [eicosapentaenoic acid (EPA) and docosahexaenoic acid (DHA)]. However, α-linolenic acid, found in green leafy vegetables, flaxseed, rapeseed, and walnuts, desaturates and elongates in the human body to EPA and DHA, and by itself may have beneficial effects in health and the control of chronic diseases [42, 53, 54]. Therefore, the food industry is already taking steps to return Ω-3 essential fatty acids to the food supply by enriching various foods with Ω-3 fatty acids. It is necessary to consider the issues involved in enriching the food supply with n-3 PUFA in terms of dosage, safety, and sources of n-3 fatty acids [39].

Most vegetable oils (from corn, soybean, and cottonseed), nuts, and animal products are sources of omega-6 fats. The alpha-linolenic acid (ALA) an omega-3 fat is found in vegetable sources such as walnuts, flaxseeds, and chia seeds. EPA and DHA can be obtained directly from marine sources, such as cold-water fatty fish (*e.g.*, salmon, sardines, herring, albacore tuna, lake trout, mackerel, and sardines) and algae [42, 43].

There are reports that the adequate intakes of linoleic acid (18:2 Ω-6) and alinolenic acid (18:3 Ω-3) should be 2% and 1% of total energy, respectively [54]. Present evidence suggests that 0.2–0.3% of the energy should be derived from pre-formed very-long-chain Ω-3 PUFAs (EPA and DHA) to avoid signs or symptoms of deficiency. These percents correspond to approximately 0.5 g of these Ω-3 fatty acids per day. It stressed that this is the minimum intake to avoid clinical symptoms of deficiency (Table **2**), and the ratio between Ω-3 and Ω -6 fatty acids should be 1:4 [34, 47].

Table 2. The recommended intake of essential PUFAs [34].

	Intake (as % of energy)		Intake (mg/day)	
	Ω-3	Ω-6	Ω-3	Ω-6
Minimum	0.2-0.3	1-3	400-600	2400-7200
Optimum	1-2	3-5	2400-4800	7200-12000

Excessive amounts of omega-6 polyunsaturated fatty acids (PUFA) and a very high omega-6/omega-3 ratio promote the pathogenesis of many diseases, whereas increased levels of omega-3 PUFA (a low omega-6/omega-3 ratio) exert suppressive effects [47].

MUFA may have an advantage over PUFA because the enrichment of lipoprotein lipids with MUFA increases their resistance to oxidation [55]. The excessive intake of PUFAs in the diet also can cause damage because of their high peroxidability index. The double carbon bonds of PUFAs increase their susceptibility to reacting with oxygen, resulting in harmful compounds responsible for oxidation and inflammation involved in the aging process and the development of the following chronic conditions [55].

Examples of food with monounsaturated and polyunsaturated fats:

Avocado

According to the fatty acid profile results of different investigations, the avocados have a high proportion of monounsaturated oleic acid ranging from 40-65% followed by saturated palmitic acid (18-20%, monounsaturated palmitoleic acid (10-16%), and polyunsaturated linoleic (11-16%) acid [56 - 58].

The composition of the fatty acids in avocado fruit did not change when ripened without chilling, during chilling or when ripened after a chilling exposure. This resistance to treatment is in contrast to reported changes associated with ripening and chilling for other chilling sensitive fruit, but they show variation concerning the grown latitude and extraction methods.

Margarine, mayonnaise, oil, salad dressing

In its composition, the mayonnaise must contain at least 65% vegetal oil by weight (usually from soybean), salad dressings must contain 30-40% vegetable oil, and margarine must contain no less than 80% fat. Margarine, mayonnaise, cooking oil, oil-based salad dressings, food service fat and oil, and shortening are usually from canola or soybean oils. These oils are the principal food sources of the n-3 fatty acid alpha-linolenic acid [59].

Naturally, rapeseed (canola) oil contains palmitic (4%), stearic (2%), oleic (62%; Ω-9), linoleic (22%; Ω-6), and linolenic (10% Ω-3) acids and has low total saturated acid than any other commodity oil. In rapeseed (canola) oil, the triacylglycerol profiles were: OOO (22%), LOO (22%), LnOO (10%), LLO (9%), and LnLO (8%) [60]. The unsaturated soybean oil has 51% linoleic (18:2 n-6), 23% oleic 18:1 n-9, and 7% linolenic 18:3 n-3. Partial hydrogenated soybean oil has 81% unsaturated (including 14% trans) that are subdivided in 35% linoleic (18:2 n-6), 43% oleic (18:1 n-9) and 3% linolenic 18:3 n-3 [61].

Orsavova *et al* [42] studied the fatty acids composition of fourteen vegetable oils considered as functional foods and used as an important part of healthy diets. Samples produced as virgin oils with a sustentative content of monounsaturated (MUFAs) and polyunsaturated (PUFAs) fatty acids. Table **3** shown, the significant contribution of omega-3 is from olive, rapeseed, and wheat germ oils.

Table 3. The nutritional profile of fatty acids from fourteen oils [42].

FA	Safflower	Grape	Cardus marianus	Hemp	Sunflower	Wheat Germ	Pumpkin Seed
SFAs	9.3	10.4	15.1	9.2	9.4	18.2	19.6
MUFAs	11.6	14.8	20.7	28.1	28.3	20.9	26.1
PUFAs	79.1	74.9	64.2	62.8	62.4	61.0	54.3
Ω - 3	0.2	0.2	0.9	0.4	0.2	1.2	0.1
Ω -6	79.0	74.7	63.3	62.4	62.2	59.7	54.2
	Sesame	Rice Bran	Almond	Rapeseed	Peanut	Olive	Flaxseed
SFAs	16.9	22.5	9.3	6.3	10.7	19.4	36.2
MUFAs	42.0	44.0	67.9	72.8	71.1	68.2	7.5
PUFAs	41.2	33.6	22.8	20.9	18.2	18.0	28.7
Ω - 3	0.2	0.5	0.0	1.2	0.0	1.6	22.8
Ω - 6	40.9	33.1	22.8	19.6	18.2	16.4	5.9
SFAs= Saturated Fatty Acids; MUFAs =Monosaturared Fatty Acids; PUFAsPolyosatured Fatty Acids							

Over 50% of the omega 6 is in 7 of the oil of the table, less contribution of sesame, rice bran, almond, rapeseed, peanut, olive. Coconut shows a high concentration of saturated fatty acids.

Frying in vegetable oils is one of the simplest methods of turning raw food ingredients into palatable meals. Oils are refined before use to remove components that might adversely affect the quality of the oil. During this process, some unwanted side reactions may occur. Similarly, during frying, changes can occur in the frying oil, including hydrolysis oxidation, cis/trans-isomerization, and cyclization.

These have the potential to affect the taste and produce undesirable nutritional effects in consumers [60, 62]. According to Jokić [63], some oil extraction procedures could improve its nutritional profile; as an example, the authors assayed the supercritical carbon dioxide to fractionate soybean oil to decrease palmitic, linoleic, and linolenic fatty acids concentrations and to increase stearic and oleic acids concentrations.

Nuts (Almonds, Hazelnuts, Peanuts, and Pecans)

The nut is one of the natural plant foods richest in fat after vegetable oils. Except for chestnuts (which are relatively low in calories and fats; 1.5 - 2%), their total fat content ranges from 46 to76% [55]. Fats from nuts are rich in unsaturated fatty acids.

As can see in Table **4**, they contain a substantial amount of MUFA and other such, as walnuts are especially rich in both n-6 and n-3 PUFA. MUFA, mainly oleic acid, is predominant in almonds, cashews, hazelnuts, macadamia nuts, peanuts, pecans, and pistachios. Brazil nuts and pine nuts contain similar proportions of MUFA and PUFA (linoleic acid), and walnuts are rich in both linoleic acid and alinolenic acid. These kinds of fat contribute to their beneficial effects in the prevention of coronary heart disease, diabetes, and sudden death and cholesterollowering, LDL resistance to oxidation, and improved endothelial function [56]. Macadamia nuts (Macadamia integrifolia) grown in Venezuela have shown an average total fat content of 70% [64]. The oleic acid (18:1) was the main monounsaturated fatty acid (MUFA) (51.3%), followed by palmitoleic acid (16:1, 22.6%).

The content of polyunsaturated fatty acids (PUFAs), C18:2, and C18:3 represented 5.4%. Thus, MUFAs and PUFAs together constituted more than 80% of the total fatty acids present. Trans-vaccenic acid was also present (3%). As regards other phytochemical compounds, tocopherols and tocotrienols were not in the sample, but the presence of squalene was detected. The phytochemicals present produced the antioxidant activity (44.2%) of the extract [64].

Fish (Such as Herring, Mackerel, Salmon, Trout, and Tuna)

Fish fatty acids and particularly poly-unsaturated fatty acids (PUFAs) play an important role in human health [65]. Fish is an excellent source of the omega-3s EPA and DHA. Therefore, the consumption of fish should routinely take place in human nutrition [65].

Since fish species vary for their Ω-3 long-chain PUFA contents, eating a variety of fish is desirable. High Ω-6 PUFA containing pre-fried fish supports the imbalance of Ω-3/Ω-6 ratio in the Western diet. Thus, the consumption of pure fish fillets is to be favored [65].

The higher fat content can offset the lower Ω-3 PUFA portion in farmed fish, however, with an undesirable fatty acid distribution compared to wild fellows [65]. Lipid content in fish can vary significantly, in wild fish, seasonal changes, sexual maturity, reproduction period, and the nutrients they consume; in farmed fish, the feed content and quality directly affect their lipid content [61].

Table 4. Average fat content and fatty acid composition (g/100g) [55].

Nuts	Total Fat	SFA	MUFA	PUFA	Ω - 6	Ω - 3
Almonds	50.6	3.9	32.2	12.2	12.2	0.0
Brazil nuts	66.4	15.1	25.5	20.6	20.5	0.05
Cashews	46.4	9.2	27.3	7.8	7.7	0.15
Hazelnuts	60.8	4.5	45.7	7.9	7.8	0.09
Macadamia nuts	75.8	12.1	58.9	1.5	1.3	0.21
Peanuts	49.2	6.8	24.4	15.6	15.6	0.00
Pecans	72.0	6.2	40.8	21.6	20.6	1.00
Pine nuts (dried)	68.2	4.9	18.8	34.1	33.2	0.16
Pistachios	44.4	5.4	23.3	13.5	13.2	0.25
Walnuts	65.2	6.1	8.9	47.2	38.1	9.08
SFA=Satured Fatty Acid; MUFA=Monounsaturated Fatty Acid; PUFAs Polyunsaturated Fatty Acid; Ω-6= linoleic acid; Ω–3= α-linolenic acid						

However, realistically at food concerns, it has been divided into three categories according to its fat composition [66].

Lean fish (less than 2% fat), which include cod, haddock, flounder/sole, and tuna, tilapia, halibut, ocean perch, and salmon (chum, pink).

Mid-fat fish (2–10% fat) among them are bluefish, catfish, rainbow trout, and swordfish.

Fatty fish (10–35% fat) such as herring, mackerel, sardines, and salmon (Atlantic, sockeye, coho, and chinook).

Table **5** is a summary of relevant data of the fat composition and fatty acid profile of the edible part of selected fish species. As can be seen, the fatty fish have higher cholesterol and Ω-3 fatty acid content as compared with the lean and medium fat fish. Halibut fish shown the optimal Ω-6/Ω-3 ratio, followed by the anchovies and Alaska pollock. Eel and sardines have high cholesterol content.

Table 5. Fat in the edible part of selected fish species [66].

Fish species	Fat (%)	Ω-3 (%)	Ω6/Ω3 ratio	Cholesterol (mg)
Lean fish				
Haddock [67].	0.8-1	0.34	1:1	49
Cod [67].	0.7-1	0.23	1:6	50
Saithe/Coalfish	0.3	0.1	1:1	49
Tusk	1.3	4.1	-	53
Medium fat fish				
Snapper	2	0.5	0.5:1	50
Alaska pollock	3.71	0.29	5:1	70
Atlantic wolffish	2.7	0.66	1:1	46
European Plaice	2.6	0.5	-	68
Halibut	3.9	0.69	4:1	32
Rainbow trout	6.8	1.48	1:2.5	72
Spotted wolfish	4.8	1.1	2.2:1	46
Tilapia	2.7	0.115	-	53
Tuna	5	0.28	1:31	42
Fatty Fish				
Anchovies	6.21	0.93	3:1	85
Greenland Halibut	22	1.9	1:0.2	46
Salmon	7	2.65	1:11.7	60
Mackerel broiled	24.4	4.64	1:13.9	79
Herring (summer)	14.5	1.85	1:9.8	60
Herring (winter)	19	4.68	1:9.8	60
Eel	31.5	3.34	1:1.5	125
Sardines	10.5	2.58	2.4:1	142

Seeds (pumpkin, chia, flax, hemp nigella, and sesame seeds)

Although seeds from many vegetables are garbage, several of them are edibles; some are byproducts (pumpkins and hemp seeds), oily (sesame, sunflower), or are seeds from the plants (chia, flax, hemp nigella).

Some researchers have shown that these seeds are sources of several healthy fats, vitamins, and minerals, which could provide proper help to health to consumers. Each 100 g of these seeds could provide 14 grams of fat mostly (mono and polyunsaturated) not accompanied by cholesterol.

Chia (*Salvia hispanica*) seeds contain 32% of fat (17 of which are omega-3s).

Hemp (*Cannabis sativa*) seeds provide 50% of fat with are a great source of essential fatty acids, such as alpha-linolenic acid (ALA), which is an omega-3.

Flax (*Linum usitatissimum*) seeds contain 42% fats, which are mainly monounsaturated (7.53) and polyunsaturated (28.73). Among them are the fatty acids omega-3 (22.81g.) and omega-6 (5.9g).

Nigella (*Nigella sativa*) seeds have 15% fats which are mainly monounsaturated (10g) and polyunsaturated (1.7g).

Pumpkin (*Cucurbita maxima*) seeds, provide 0.17% of fat and 0% cholesterol, and more than 10% of the dietary requirement of vitamin E.

Sesame (*Sesamum indicum*) seeds, provide 50% of total fat, which consists of 7% saturated fat, 22% polyunsaturated fat, and 19% monounsaturated fat with zero cholesterol. The Oil resulting from sesame seeds is mainly linoleic and oleic acids, gamma-tocopherol, and other isomers of vitamin E.

Sunflower (*Helianthus annuus*) seeds shown 51% fat distributed as; 4.5 saturated fat, 23% polyunsaturated fat, and 19% monounsaturated fat with zero cholesterol.

Other Foods

Olive's fruits shown 11-15% of fat, mainly monounsaturated (7.89) with 0.06 omega-3 and 0.85 omega-6. Tofu cheese 4% fat content with 2.5% of polyunsaturated fatty acids with an omega 6/omega 3 ratios of 7:1. Fat-free milk, also called skim milk or non-fat milk is declared as 0% of total fat, with only a trace of saturated fat (0.08%). However, skimmed milk has 2% de cholesterol. There is in the market organic skimmed milk supplemented with 32 mg of DHA Omega-3 per serving.

Examples of Food with Saturated Fats

Saturated fats are a type of fat-containing a high proportion of fatty acid molecules without double bonds. Consequently, foods with saturated fats are those that contain a high content of saturated fats. The foods with saturated fats are less healthy in the diet than those with unsaturated fat.

Excessive consumption of saturated fat can cause cholesterol to build up in body arteries (blood vessels). Saturated fats also raise body LDL cholesterol.

High LDL cholesterol increases body risk for heart disease and stroke. Among these foods, there are high-fat cheeses, high-fat cuts of meat, whole-fat milk and cream, butter ice cream and ice cream products, palm and coconut oils.

Examples of Foods *Trans* Fats

Trans fatty acids (TFA) are unsaturated fatty acids with at least one double bond in the *Trans* (hydrogen on opposite sides) position. Most TFA found in foods are produced commercially *via* the hydrogenation of unsaturated fatty acids found in vegetable oils. Hydrogenation and partial hydrogenation result in a semi-solid or solid product with a higher melting point, increased stability, resistance to oxidation, and shelf life [68]. There is also a small amount of *Trans* fat that occurs naturally in some meat and dairy products [69]. *Trans* fat is a liquid oil turned into solid fats during food processing, but those found in processed foods tend to be the most harmful to body health.

There is also a small amount of *Trans* fat that occurs naturally in some meat and dairy products [69].

Hydrogenated oils can be sold directly but also used in the food industry in the manufacture of many foodstuffs. The use of hydrogenated oils helps to prolong the shelf life of the food and maintain flavor stability. Among the food manufactured with hydrogenated oils are cookies, pastries, and desserts, savory snacks and crackers, bread, and refrigerated dough products, frozen pizza, fast food, margarine, and refrigerated spreads [69].

FAT REPLACERS

High dietary fat intake, implicated in the etiology of fatness and certain cancers, has an increased prevalence of obesity and overweight in the world. Obesity, in turn, is a risk factor for Type 2 diabetes and hypertension. Furthermore, a high intake of saturated fats elevates total blood cholesterol levels, in particular, LDLcholesterol. High total and LDL-cholesterol levels are key risk factors for coronary heart disease and ischaemic stroke [70, 71].

The use of fat replacers may be useful in helping to meet dietary guidelines to reduce fat intake and, in conjunction with other lifestyle and dietary changes, useful in improving public health status [70].

Fat replacer is a carbohydrate, protein, or fat-based compound that replaces one or more of the functions of fat to reduce calories in foods [72]. Fat replacers are emulsifiers or surface-active agents, starch derivatives, maltodextrins, hemicelluloses, B-glucans, bulking agents, microparticles, composites, and functional blends [72].

Today, the use of fat replacers has facilitated the development of reduced-fat and fat-free foods that have the taste and texture of high-fat foods with less fat fewer calories. The actual use of reduced-fat foods by the population is due to dietary advice and recommendations, individual health concerns, sensory characteristics of products, usefulness in the dietary pattern, and willingness to accept fat substitutes [73].

Fat replacers are classified as: fat substitutes, fat mimetic, fat analogous, and fat extenders [70, 72].

Fat substitutes are molecules that possess the physical and functional characteristics of the conventional fat molecules (*e.g.*, triglycerides), and they can replace conventional fat molecules in foods on a weight-for-weight basis. They are typically synthetic molecules, usually having a similar chemical structure to fat, but resistant to hydrolysis against digestive enzymes [70]. They provide no energy calories, or structured lipid molecules, which provide reduced energy calories.

Fat substitutes can successfully maintain the palatability of foods as they can reproduce the texture and mouthfeel of fat. They are generally heat stable and suitable for high-temperature cooking and frying applications [70]. They may not reproduce the taste properties of fat as fat itself provides a flavor to foods and is a carrier of other fat-soluble flavor compounds in foods.

Fat mimetics are substances (typically protein, or carbohydrate-based molecules), which can mimic some of the organoleptic and physical properties of conventional fat molecules. However, they cannot replace fat molecules in food on a weight-for-weight basis. Their energy contribution to the diet ranges from 0 to 4 kcal g−1. Referred as "texturing agents," they are generally not suitable for high-temperature applications, such as frying, being susceptible to denaturation, or caramelization [70].

Fat mimetics are generally polar, water-soluble compounds. Thus, they cannot replace some of the non-polar functional characteristics of fats, such as lipidsoluble flavor carrying capacity. However, their polar nature facilitates waterbinding water, which helps generate a sense of creaminess and lubricity in foods similar to that found in full-fat products. It requires a high-water content to achieve its functionality.

Fat analogs: are compounds with many of the characteristics of fat but have an altered digestibility and altered nutritional value.

Fat extenders: They optimize the functionality of fat, thus allowing a decrease in the usual amount of fat in the product. It is a system in which, besides the standard fats, there are other accompanying compounds.

PRACTICAL HINTS FOR FAT-FREE FOOD

Dietary Fibers

Obesity is the accumulation of fat in the human body, beyond the amount of fat required for its normal function. The continuous body accumulation of fat leads to weight gain or obesity [74].

A high dietary fat intake implicated in obesity etiology is a cause for the development and worsening of many diseases.

A fiber-rich diet is low in energy density and often has low-fat content, being larger in volume and rich in micronutrients. Therefore, a high fiber, sugar low, and low-fat diet should protect consumer's health. Dietary fiber is not digested or absorbed by the intestinal tract after ingestion for the body, and it is desirable a fiber intake of 30 to 40 g/d; one-half derived from cereal bran and the other half from fruits and vegetables [75]. High-fiber diets may also reduce the risk of developing some types of cancer, especially colon cancer. High-fiber diets may be useful for people to lose weight. Fiber itself has no calories yet provides a "full" feeling because of its water-absorbing ability [74]. Dietary fiber also protects against inflammatory bowel diseases, such as Crohn's disease and ulcerative colitis, by increasing the production of short-chain fatty acids (SCFAs). SCFAs act as immunomodulators in the inflamed intestine and by also increasing the proportions of beneficial, rather than pathogenic bacteria that make up the gastrointestinal microflora [74]. However, it may be broken down by bacteria in the lower gut.

From a point of view, nutritional for fibers, there are two terms: dietary fiber and crude fiber. Dietary fiber refers to the total amount of non-digestible material naturally occurring in foods and mainly of plant origin. It includes fiber from foods such as whole legumes, vegetables, fruits, seeds and nuts, undigested products, and undigested biosynthetic polysaccharides, whereas crude fiber is the material that in chemical analysis remains after vigorous treatment with acids and alkalis [76].

The type and quantity of fibers vary among the foods. Based on its solubility, they are two dietary fiber types: soluble and insoluble [77].

1-Soluble or water-soluble/well-fermented fibers comprise pectin, gums, and mucilage.

2-Non-soluble dietary fiber or water-insoluble/less fermented fibers, which include cellulose, hemicellulose, and lignin.

The soluble dietary fiber (SDF) is generally used to modify texture, influence the colligative properties of the food systems, and improve the marketability of the food product as a health-promoting or functional product in food and animal feeding [76]. Besides these functional properties, a dietary fiber performs certain critical physiological functions in the body, acting as a prebiotic and improving host health, and reducing the postprandial glucose response. It is also associated with protective effects against C-reactive protein (CRP), a marker of acute inflammation recognized as an independent predictor of future cardiovascular disease and diabetes [78].

The consumption of water-soluble fiber binds to bile acids resulting in increased excretion of cholesterol. Most of the water-soluble fibers have hypocholesterolemic properties, possibly due to inhibition of fat digestion and absorption and inhibition of cholesterol synthesis in the liver by propionate or other bacterial products and the action of viscous non-starch polysaccharides on insulin and other hormone secretions [76].

The main effect of SDFs is associated with viscous polysaccharides such as pectin and gums, which decrease the assimilation of nutrients. The bacterial mass formed from the high fermentable substances (pectin), the residues of the less fermentable polymers (cellulose and hemicelluloses), and the water retained by them is responsible for the increase of the fecal bulk [76].

Insoluble dietary fiber primarily consists of cellulose and some hemicelluloses, resistant starch, and lignin [79]. As general function insoluble dietary fiber moves bulk through the intestines, controls, and balances the pH (acidity) in the intestines, therefore prevent constipation, speed up the passage of food through the digestive tract, removing fast waste toxic substance through the colon, prevents colon cancer (by pH balance and by restriction of cancer producer microorganisms). Therefore, it is helpful in the treatment and prevention of constipation, hemorrhoids, and diverticulosis.

Wheat bran and whole grains contain the highest amounts of insoluble fiber, but vegetables and beans also are good sources.

In a summary, the fiber in foods can change foods' functional properties and sensory characteristics. The occurrence of new sources of fibers has offered new opportunities in their use in food development. Due to dietary fiber's beneficial health effects, on functional food development dietary fiber plays an important role. Among the foods enriched with dietary fiber are breakfast cereals and bakery products such (integral bread and cookies), drinks, milk and meat products, ground beef, and pork sausage products, among others [77].

Li *et al.* [80] completed a study, as a part of the continuous efforts of the Nutrient Data Laboratory, Agricultural Research Service (ARS) of USDA in updating and expanding the carbohydrate data in its database. In this study, several foods were selected based on dietary fiber content and frequency of consumption. The authors concluded that most baked products contained fructose, glucose, maltose, and no sucrose; cereal grains and pasta contained mainly sucrose, though in low levels compared to all other food groups. Almost all fruits contained fructose, glucose, and sucrose.

Legumes contained mostly sucrose and no detectable maltose; vegetables eaten cooked can contain more sucrose than those eaten raw. Overall, fruits contain the most sugar and cereal grains/pasta the least. Almost all the foods may be considered good sources of dietary fiber.

The proportion of soluble dietary fiber to insoluble dietary fiber varied across the food groups and even within each food group. The results of this study support evaluating foods on a case-by-case basis rather than developing generalizations on the relative proportions of fiber fractions according to food groups.

There exists a need for the strengthening of collaborative efforts between the food science and nutritionist disciplines. The goal between these fields should be to increase the likelihood that dietary fiber is added to foods in effective quantities without deleterious effects on the sensory appeal of the food.

This collaborative effort would allow for the creation of many additional fiberrich food products with the high potential to positively impact consumer health by combatting obesity, cardiovascular disease, and type II diabetes.

Sugars

According to the results from [81] large scale survey applied to American's consumers, Welsh *et al.* [82], have postulated concerning sugars consumption "Generally, the higher the consumption, the more unfavorable the lipid levels," Sugar is calorie-dense with no nutritional value and can come in many different forms. On the label must distinguish ingredients like glucose, fructose, sucrose, maltose, lactose, dextrose, starch, corn syrup, fruit juice, raw sugar, and honey, or a combination of them. It can contribute to diabetes; affect the pH of blood, and impact brain and heart health.

Despite the number of studies that are not enough to compare the associations between obesity or dyslipidemia-related diseases and the intake of nutrients such as sodium, fat, and sugar, there is a consensus that low intake of sugars and fat could reduce the risk of several disorders including dyslipidemia.

It has been reported the effects of sustained consumption of dietary fructose compared with those of sustained glucose consumption on circulating apoCIII and large triglyceride (TG)-rich lipoprotein particles [83]. It was concluded that 10 weeks of fructose consumption increased the circulating apoCIII and postprandial concentrations of large triglyceride (TG)-rich lipoproteins particles compared with glucose consumption [83, 84].

They have pointed out that fructose consumption promoted lipid dysregulation, while glucose consumption did not. Compared with glucose, the consumption of fructose increased the circulating concentrations of postprandial triglycerides (TG), remnant-like particle lipoprotein (RLP)-TG, and RLP-cholesterol (chol), as well as those of fasting total chol, low-density lipoprotein (LDL)-chol, apolipoprotein B (apo B), small dense LDL-chol (sdLDL-chol), and oxidized LDL.

Subjects consuming fructose also exhibited increased postprandial hepatic de novo lipogenesis (DNL) and decreased insulin sensitivity compared with subjects consuming glucose.

RECIPES

Zucchini Spaghetti

Ingredients

3	Zucchini's spaghetti-like strands, large (made using spiralizer)	6g	Garlic Clove, minced
500g	Beef (97% lean/3% fat) ground	3,5g	Oregano dried
7g	Black Pepper ground	1.5g	Salt
450g	Tomato juice	180g	Tomato paste
500g	Tomatoes peeled and minced	-	-
15g	Basil dried	-	-
100g.	Onion, fresh and peeled and minced	-	-
50g	Red Pepper flakes	-	-

Preparation with beef meat

Heat a large skillet over medium-high heat. Cook and stir beef and black pepper in the hot skillet until browned and crumbly, 5 to 7 minutes; drain and discard grease. Mix tomato juice, tomatoes, salt, basil, oregano, garlic powder, onion powder, thyme, and red pepper flakes into ground beef; cook and stir until sauce is warmed through, about 2 minutes. Stir tomato paste into the sauce. Mix zucchini "noodles" into the sauce, pressing down to submerge them fully; simmer over medium-low heat until zucchini is tender, about 10 minutes.

Preparation as marinara sauce

Heat a large skillet over medium-high heat. Cook the mix of tomato juice, tomatoes, salt, basil, oregano, garlic powder, onion powder, thyme, and red pepper flakes; stir until the sauce is warmed through, about 10 minutes. Stir tomato paste into the sauce. Mix zucchini "noodles" into the sauce, pressing down to submerge them fully; simmer over medium-low heat until zucchini is tender, about 10 minutes.

Hawaiian Chicken Kabobs

Ingredients

8	Chicken breast; skinless, boneless, halves cut into 2 inches pieces.	3.5g	Ginger ground
510g	Pineapples; fresh chunks	3.5g	Garlic powder
30g	Sherry	45g	Soy sauce

Preparation

In a shallow glass dish, mix the soy sauce, sherry, ginger, and garlic powder. Stir the chicken pieces and pineapple into the marinade until well coated. Cover and marinate in the refrigerator for at least 2 hours. Preheat grill to medium-high heat. Lightly oil the grill grate. Thread chicken and pineapple alternately onto skewers.

Grill 15 to 20 minutes, turning occasionally, or until, chicken juices run clear.

Homemade Beef Broth

Ingredients

1.5kg	Meat boneless	300g	Carrots cut into 1-inch pieces
500 g	Beef bones (meaty)	300g	Celery, cut into 1-inch pieces
100g	Onion; white, halved	1	Leek, white part only, cut into 2-inch pieces
1tbsp.	Black Peppercorns	1	Bouquet Garni*
3liters	Water		*(1 rosemary sprig, 5 thyme sprigs, 1 bay leaf, 5 parsley stems), wrapped inside a leek leaf and tied together with kitchen twine.

Preparation

Bring a large pot of water to a boil, and blanch the soup meat and bones in the heavily boiling water for 2-3 minutes to remove excess scum. Drain the meat and bones, and set aside. Heat a sauté pan over medium-high heat, and without adding any oil place the halved onions, cut side down on the pan surface. Let them sit for 3-4 minutes until they are slightly charred. Take the onions out of the pan and turn the heat down to the lowest setting.

Add the black peppercorns and toast them for 1-2 minutes until they smell fragrant. Add all the soup ingredients into a large stockpot and add just enough cold water to cover all the ingredients, about 3.2 quarts.

Bring the water to a simmer, and then turn the heat to the lowest setting, strain off any impurities that might rise to the top. Cover your stockpot and let the broth lightly simmer for 4 hours. When the broth is ready, discard the bones, vegetables, herbs, and black peppercorns.

Take out the meat and let it cool down and drain off the superficial fat. Pass the broth through a fine-mesh sieve or cheesecloth. Let the strained broth cool down entirely and discard all of the fat that solidifies on top of your broth after chilling it in the fridge.

Broccoli/Green Beans Beef

Ingredients

30g	Flour all-purpose	3.5g	Ginger root fresh (chopped)
300ml	Beef (homemade broth; defatted)	200g	Broccoli (chopped)
15g	Soy sauce	200g	Green Beans
500g	Steak, boneless round; cut into bite pieces	-	-

Preparation

In a small bowl, combine flour, broth, and soy sauce. Stir until flour dissolve. In a large skillet or wok over high heat, cook and stir beef 2 to 4 minutes, or until browned. Stir in broth mixture, ginger, garlic, and broccoli.

Bring to a boil, and then reduce heat. Simmer 5 to 10 minutes, or until sauce thickens.

Salmon Avocado Salad

Ingredients

4	Wild Salmon fillets, 120g each	20g	Vinegar (apple cider
15g.	Dijon Mustard, divided	2g	Garlic powder
6g	Parsley (dried)	200g	halved Cherry Tomatoes
10g	Salt	225g	Avocado, diced (from 2 small)
Pinch	Black Pepper, fresh to taste	200g	Romaine Lettuce, chopped
50g	Red Onion (chopped)	300g	Cabbage, red, shredded
60g	Olive oil; extra virgin	-	-

Preparation

Season salmon with ¾ Dijon mustard, ½ portion of dried parsley, ½ portion of salt, and black pepper.

Adjust the oven on the second rack. Broil salmon 6 to 7 minutes, until cooked through. In a large bowl, combine the red onion with olive oil, ½ portion of apple cider vinegar, garlic powder, the remaining Dijon and salt, and pepper to taste; let it sit about 5 minutes, so the flavor of the onion mellows.

Add the tomatoes, avocado, and toss. When ready to serve, toss in chopped lettuce and cabbage, finish with the remaining portion of vinegar, and taste for salt and pepper.

Yacón/Fruit Salad

Ingredients

250g	Yacón (peeled, chunk)
250g	Pineapple (chunks)
250g	Papaya (chunks)
250g	Mango (chunks)
150g	Orange juice
1	Lemon (medium)

Preparation

Combine the yacón with the chunks of pineapple, papaya, and mango and dress in freshly squeezed orange juice and a spritz of lemon.

CONSENT FOR PUBLICATION

Not Applicable.

CONFLICT OF INTEREST

The author confirms that this chapter contents have no conflict of interest.

ACKNOWLEDGEMENT

Declared none.

REFERENCES

[1]   Michael HD. Dyslipidemia (Hyperlipidemia). In MSD Manual. Professional version. Available from https://www.msdmanuals.com/professional/endocrine-and-metabolic-disorders/li-id-disorders/dyslipidemia.

[2]   Beaumont JL, Carlson LA, Cooper GR, Fejfar Z, Fredrickson DS, Strasser T. Classification of hyperlipidaemias and hyperlipoproteinaemias. World Health Organization (WHO). Bull World Health Organ 1970; 43(6): 891-915.http://ahajournals.org
[PMID: 4930042]

[3]   Guha N. Classification of dyslipidaemia. 2019. Available from: https://doi.org

[4]   Nirosha K, Divya M, Vamsi S, Sadiq M. A review on hyperlipidemia. Int J Novel Trends Pharm Sci 2014; 4(5): 81-92.

[5]   Colpo A. LDL cholesterol: "Bad" cholesterol, or bad science? J Am Phy Surg 2005; 10(3): 83-9.

[6]   Lawes CC, Vander Hoorn S, Law MR, Rodgers A. High cholesterol.Comparative quantification of health risks: Global and regional burden of disease attributable to selected major risk factors. Geneva: WHO 2004; pp. 1651-801.

[7]   Simons LA. Lipids & cardiovascular disease 2019.

[8]   Mahan KL, Escott-Stump S. Krause's food, nutrition, and diet therapy. 10th ed., Philadelphia, Pa: W.B. Saunders 2000.

[9]   Segrest JP, Jones MK, De Loof H, Dashti N. Structure of apolipoprotein B-100 in low density lipoproteins. J Lipid Res 2001; 42(9): 1346-67.
[http://dx.doi.org/10.1016/S0022-2275(20)30267-4] [PMID: 11518754]

[10]   Johs A, Hammel M, Waldner I, May RP, Laggner P, Prassl R. Modular structure of solubilized human apolipoprotein B-100. Low resolution model revealed by small angle neutron scattering. J Biol Chem 2006; 281(28): 19732-9.
[http://dx.doi.org/10.1074/jbc.M601688200] [PMID: 16704977]

[11]   Wadhera RK, Steen DL, Khan I, Giugliano RP, Foody JM. A review of low-density lipoprotein cholesterol, treatment strategies, and its impact on cardiovascular disease morbidity and mortality. J Clin Lipidol 2016; 10(3): 472-89.
[http://dx.doi.org/10.1016/j.jacl.2015.11.010] [PMID: 27206934]

[12]   Eisenberg S. High density lipoprotein metabolism. J Lipid Res 1984; 25(10): 1017-58.
[http://dx.doi.org/10.1016/S0022-2275(20)37713-0] [PMID: 6392459]

[13]   German JB, Smilowitz JT, Zivkovic AM. Lipoproteins: When size really matters. Curr Opin Colloid Interface Sci 2006; 11(2-3): 171-83.
       [http://dx.doi.org/10.1016/j.cocis.2005.11.006] [PMID: 20592953]

[14]   Tomkin GH. Triglyceride and high-density lipoprotein metabolism in diabetes. J Diabetes Metab Disord Control 2018; 5(5): 158-65.
       [http://dx.doi.org/10.15406/jdmdc.2018.05.00157]

[15]   Kaiser T, Kinny-Köster B, Bartels M, *et al.* Cholesterol esterification in plasma as a biomarker for liver function and prediction of mortality. BMC Gastroenterol 2017; 17(1): 57-60.
       [http://dx.doi.org/10.1186/s12876-017-0614-9] [PMID: 28427335]

[16]   Subbaiah PV, Jiang X-C, Belikova NA, Aizezi B, Huang ZH, Reardon CA. Regulation of plasma cholesterol esterification by sphingomyelin: effect of physiological variations of plasma sphingomyelin on lecithin-cholesterol acyltransferase activity. Biochim Biophys Acta 2012; 1821(6): 908-13.
       [http://dx.doi.org/10.1016/j.bbalip.2012.02.007] [PMID: 22370449]

[17]   Burnett JR. Lipids, lipoproteins, atherosclerosis and cardiovascular disease. Clin Biochem Rev 2004; 25(1): 2.
       [PMID: 18516207]

[18]   Povey K. Developing food products, which help consumers to lower their cholesterol level in Developing Food Products for Consumers with Specific Dietary Needs 2016.
       www.sciencedirect.com/topics/agricultural-and-biological-sciences/saturated-fat

[19]   Sun Y, Neelakantan N, Wu Y, Lote-Oke R, Pan A, van Dam RM. Palm Oil Consumption Increases LDL Cholesterol Compared with Vegetable Oils Low in Saturated Fat in a Meta-Analysis of Clinical Trials. J Nutr 2015; 145(7): 1549-58.
       [http://dx.doi.org/10.3945/jn.115.210575] [PMID: 25995283]

[20]   Pejic RN, Lee DT. Hypertriglyceridemia. J Am Board Fam Med 2006; 19(3): 310-6.
       [http://dx.doi.org/10.3122/jabfm.19.3.310] [PMID: 16672684]

[21]   Chait A, Subramanian S, Brunzell JD. Genetic disorders of triglyceride metabolism.South Dartmouth (MA): MDTextcom, Inc 2000. Feingold, KR 2000.

[22]   Goldberg AC. Goldberg, A.C. Hypolipidemia. 2019. Available from: https://www.msdmanuals.com

[23]   Kinosian B, Glick H, Garland G. Cholesterol and coronary heart disease: predicting risks by levels and ratios. Ann Intern Med 1994; 121(9): 641-7.
       [http://dx.doi.org/10.7326/0003-4819-121-9-199411010-00002] [PMID: 7944071]

[24]   Gerber J. Dyslipidemia.WSCC clinics conservative care pathways. Western States Chiropractic College 2006.

[25]   Vodnala D, Rubenfire M, Brook RD. Secondary causes of dyslipidemia. Am J Cardiol 2012; 110(6): 823-5.
       [http://dx.doi.org/10.1016/j.amjcard.2012.04.062] [PMID: 22658245]

[26]   John W, McEvoy RS, Blumenthal L. Dyslipidemia.Hypertension: A companion to braunwald's heart disease. 3rd ed., 2018.

[27]   Houston M. Dyslipidemia.Integrative medicine. 4th ed., New York: Elsevier 2018.
       [http://dx.doi.org/10.1016/B978-0-323-35868-2.00027-X]

[28]   American College of Cardiology. 2018 Guideline of blood cholesterol management. J Am Coll Cardiol 2019; 73(24): e285-350.
       [http://dx.doi.org/10.1016/j.jacc.2018.11.003] [PMID: 30423393]

[29]   Kuo PT. Hyperlipoproteinemia and atherosclerosis: dietary intervention 1983.
       [http://dx.doi.org/10.1016/S0002-9343(18)30277-8]

[30]   Wickramasinghe M, Weaver JU. 10. Lipid Disorders in Obesity. In Weaver JU Ed, Practical Guide to Obesity Medicine, 2018 pp., 99-108. Available from: https://www.sciencedirect.com/science/article/pii/B9780323485593000105.
[http://dx.doi.org/10.1016/B978-0-323-48559-3.00010-5]

[31]   Herningtyas EH, Ng TS. Prevalence and distribution of metabolic syndrome and its components among provinces and ethnic groups in Indonesia. BMC Public Health 2019; 19(1): 377.
[http://dx.doi.org/10.1186/s12889-019-6711-7] [PMID: 30943932]

[32]   Rosa CdeO, Dos Santos CA, Leite JI, Caldas AP, Bressan J. Impact of nutrients and food components on dyslipidemias: what is the evidence? Adv Nutr 2015; 6(6): 703-11.
[http://dx.doi.org/10.3945/an.115.009480] [PMID: 26567195]

[33]   Food and Agriculture Organization of the United Nations (FAO). Fats and fatty acids in human nutrition. 2010.

[34]   Rustan AC, Drevon CA. Fatty acids: Structures and properties. Encyclopedia of Life Sciences & , John Wiley & Sons, Ltd., 2005; pp, 1-7. Available from: www.els.net

[35]   Iqbal MP. Trans fatty acids - A risk factor for cardiovascular disease. Pak J Med Sci 2014; 30(1): 194-7.
[PMID: 24639860]

[36]   Sánchez-Muniz FJ, Bastida S, Márquez-Ruiz G, Dobarganes C. Effect of heating and frying on oil and food fatty acids.Fatty Acids in Foods and their Health Implications. 3rd ed., Boca Raton: CRC, Press 2007.

[37]   Stencel C, Dobbins C. Report offers new eating and physical activity targets to reduce chronic disease risk. New from National Academics 2002.

[38]   Doell D, Folmer D, Lee H, Honigfort M, Carberry S. Updated estimate of trans fat intake by the US population. Food Addit Contam Part A Chem Anal Control Expo Risk Assess 2012; 29(6): 861-74.
[http://dx.doi.org/10.1080/19440049.2012.664570] [PMID: 22439632]

[39]   Simopoulos AP. Human requirement for N-3 polyunsaturated fatty acids. Poult Sci 2000; 79(7): 961-70.
[http://dx.doi.org/10.1093/ps/79.7.961] [PMID: 10901194]

[40]   Sargent JR, Bell JG, Bell MV, Henderson RJ, Tocher DR. Requirement criteria for essential fatty acids. Applied Ichthyology 1995; 11(3-4): 18-198.

[41]   Brenna JT, Salem N Jr, Sinclair AJ, Cunnan SC. Prostaglandins, leukotrienes, and essential fatty acids α-linolenic acid supplementation and conversion to n-3 long-chain polyunsaturated fatty acids in humans. Prostag Leukotr Ess 2009; 80(2-3): 85-91.
[http://dx.doi.org/10.1016/j.plefa.2009.01.004]

[42]   Orsavova J, Misurcova L, Ambrozova JV, Vicha R, Mlcek J. Fatty acids composition of vegetable oils and its contribution to dietary energy intake and dependence of cardiovascular mortality on dietary intake of fatty acids. Int J Mol Sci 2015; 16(6): 12871-90.
[http://dx.doi.org/10.3390/ijms160612871] [PMID: 26057750]

[43]   Shanab SMM, Hafez RM, Fouad AS. A review on algae and plants as potential source of arachidonic acid. J Adv Res 2018; 11: 3-13.
[http://dx.doi.org/10.1016/j.jare.2018.03.004] [PMID: 30034871]

[44]   Alagawany M, Elnesr SS, Farag MR, *et al.* Omega-3 and Omega-6 Fatty Acids in Poultry Nutrition: Effect on Production Performance and Health. Animals (Basel) 2019; 9(8): 573.
[http://dx.doi.org/10.3390/ani9080573] [PMID: 31426600]

[45]   Hibbeln JR, Nieminen LR, Blasbalg TL, Riggs JA, Lands WE. Healthy intakes of n-3 and n-6 fatty acids: estimations considering worldwide diversity. Am J Clin Nutr 2006; 83(6) (Suppl.): 1483S-93S.
[http://dx.doi.org/10.1093/ajcn/83.6.1483S] [PMID: 16841858]

[46]   Haag M. Essential fatty acids and the brain. Can J Psychiatry 2003; 48(3): 195-203.
[http://dx.doi.org/10.1177/070674370304800308] [PMID: 12728744]

[47]   Simopoulos AP. The importance of the ratio of omega-6/omega-3 essential fatty acids. Biomed Pharmacother 2002; 56(8): 365-79.
[http://dx.doi.org/10.1016/S0753-3322(02)00253-6] [PMID: 12442909]

[48]   Calder PC. n-3 polyunsaturated fatty acids, inflammation, and inflammatory diseases. Am J Clin Nutr 2006; 83(6) (Suppl.): 1505S-19S.
[http://dx.doi.org/10.1093/ajcn/83.6.1505S] [PMID: 16841861]

[49]   Calder PC. Omega-3 fatty acids and inflammatory processes. Nutrients 2010; 2(3): 355-74.
[http://dx.doi.org/10.3390/nu2030355] [PMID: 22254027]

[50]   Balta MG, Loos BG, Nicu EA. Emerging concepts in the resolution of periodontal inflammation: a role for resolvin E1. Front Immunol 2017; 8: 1682.
[http://dx.doi.org/10.3389/fimmu.2017.01682] [PMID: 29312286]

[51]   Moro K, Nagahashi M, Ramanathan R, Takabe K, Wakai T. Resolvins and omega three polyunsaturated fatty acids: Clinical implications in inflammatory diseases and cancer. World J Clin Cases 2016; 4(7): 155-64.
[http://dx.doi.org/10.12998/wjcc.v4.i7.155] [PMID: 27458590]

[52]   Simopoulos AP. Essential fatty acids in health and chronic disease. Am J Clin Nutr 1999; 70(3) (Suppl.): 560S-9S.
[http://dx.doi.org/10.1093/ajcn/70.3.560s] [PMID: 10479232]

[53]   Russo GL. Dietary n-6 and n-3 polyunsaturated fatty acids: from biochemistry to clinical implications in cardiovascular prevention. Biochem Pharmacol 2009; 77(6): 937-46.
[http://dx.doi.org/10.1016/j.bcp.2008.10.020] [PMID: 19022225]

[54]   Vannice G, Rasmussen H. Position of the academy of nutrition and dietetics: dietary fatty acids for healthy adults. J Acad Nutr Diet 2014; 114(1): 136-53.
[http://dx.doi.org/10.1016/j.jand.2013.11.001] [PMID: 24342605]

[55]   Ros E, Mataix J. Fatty acid composition of nuts--implications for cardiovascular health. Br J Nutr 2006; 96 (Suppl. 2): S29-35.
[http://dx.doi.org/10.1017/BJN20061861] [PMID: 17125530]

[56]   Eaks IL. Change in the fatty acid composition of avocado fruit during ontogeny, cold storage and ripening. In: Paull RE. Ed. 1990 Symposium on Tropical Fruit in International Trade. Acta Hortic 1990; pp. 141-152.
[http://dx.doi.org/10.17660/ActaHortic.1990.269.19]

[57]   Reddy M, Moodley R, Jonnalagadda SB. Fatty acid profile and elemental content of avocado (*Persea americana* Mill.) oil--effect of extraction methods. J Environ Sci Health B 2012; 47(6): 529-37.
[http://dx.doi.org/10.1080/03601234.2012.665669] [PMID: 22494376]

[58]   Carvalho CP, Bernal J, Velásquez MA, Cartagena JR. Fatty acid content of avocados (*Persea americana Mill. cv. Hass*) in relation to orchard altitude and fruit maturity stage. Agron Colomb 2015; 33(2): 220-7.
[http://dx.doi.org/10.15446/agron.colomb.v33n2.49902]

[59]   Hunter JE. n-3 fatty acids from vegetable oils. Am J Clin Nutr 1990; 51(5): 809-14.
[http://dx.doi.org/10.1093/ajcn/51.5.809] [PMID: 1970702]

[60]   Gunstone FD. Rapeseed (canola) oil. 2013. Availñable from: http://lipidlibrary.aocs.org

[61]   Anonymous . 2019.Typical fatty–acid compositions of some common fats http://web.pdx.edu

[62]   Dobarganes MC. Formation of new compounds during frying - general observations. 2013. Available from: http://lipidlibrary.aocs.org

[63] Jokić S, Sudar R, Svilović S, Vidović S, Bilić M, Jurkovic V. Fatty acid composition of oil obtained from soybeans by extraction with supercritical carbon dioxide. Czech J Food Sci 2013; 31(2): 116-25.
[http://dx.doi.org/10.17221/8/2012-CJFS]

[64] Rengel A, Pérez E, Piombo G, Ricci J, Servant A, Tapia MS, *et al.* Lipid profile and antioxidant activity of macadamia nuts (*Macadamia integrifolia*) cultivated in Venezuela. Nat Sci 2015; 7: 535-47.

[65] Strobel C, Jahreis G, Kuhnt K. Survey of n-3 and n-6 polyunsaturated fatty acids in fish and fish products. Lipids Health Dis 2012; 11(11): 144.
[http://dx.doi.org/10.1186/1476-511X-11-144] [PMID: 23110317]

[66] Taşbozan O, Gökçe MA. Fatty acids in fish. INTECH 2017.https://www.intechopen.com
[http://dx.doi.org/10.5772/68048]

[67] Duan Z, Kangsen M, Qinghui A, Milley JE, Lall SP. Lipid and fatty acid compositions of cod (Gadus morhua), haddock (Melanogrammus aeglefinus), and halibut (Hippoglossus hippoglossus). J Ocean Univ China 2010; 9(4): 381-8.
[http://dx.doi.org/10.1007/s11802-010-1763-4]

[68] Valenzuela A, Morgado N. Trans fatty acid isomers in human health and in the food industry. Biol Res 1999; 32(4): 273-87.
[http://dx.doi.org/10.4067/S0716-97601999000400007] [PMID: 10983247]

[69] Jones AM, Fetter D, Zidenberg-Cherr S. Center for nutrition in schools 2016.https://cns.ucdavis.edu

[70] O'Connnors TP, O'Brien NM. Butter and other milk fat products Fat replacer. Encyclopedia in Dairy Science 2011; pp. 528-32.

[71] Briggs MA, Petersen KS, Kris-Etherton PM. Saturated fatty acids and cardiovascular disease: Replacements for saturated fat to reduce cardiovascular risk. Healthcare (Basel) 2017; 5(2): 29. [Review].
[http://dx.doi.org/10.3390/healthcare5020029] [PMID: 28635680]

[72] Chavan RS, Khevas CD, Bhatt S. Fat replacer. The Encyclopedia of Food and Health 2016; 2:589-595.
[http://dx.doi.org/10.1016/B978-0-12-384947-2.00271-3]

[73] Miller J, Jonnalagadda S. The use of fat replacer for weight loss and control. 2005.
[http://dx.doi.org/10.1201/9781439823590.ch14]

[74] Polikandrioti M, Stefanou E. Obesity disease. Health Sci J 2009; 3(3): 132-8.

[75] Nayak SK, Pattnaik P, Mohanty AK. Dietary fiber: a low-calorie dairy adjunct. Indian Food Ind 2000; 19(4): 268-74.

[76] Chawla R, Patil GR. Soluble dietary fiber. Compr Rev Food Sci 2010; 9(2): 178-96.
[http://dx.doi.org/10.1111/j.1541-4337.2009.00099.x]

[77] Dhingra D, Michael M, Rajput H, Patil RT. Dietary fibre in foods: a review. J Food Sci Technol 2012; 49(3): 255-66.
[http://dx.doi.org/10.1007/s13197-011-0365-5] [PMID: 23729846]

[78] Ma Y, Griffith JA, Chasan-Taber L, *et al.* Association between dietary fiber and serum C-reactive protein. Am J Clin Nutr 2006; 83(4): 760-6.
[http://dx.doi.org/10.1093/ajcn/83.4.760] [PMID: 16600925]

[79] Perry JR, Ying W. A review of physiological effect of soluble and insoluble dietary fibers. J Nutr Food Sci 2016; 6(2): 476-82.

[80] Li BW, Andrews KW, Pehrsoon PR. Individual sugars, soluble, and insoluble dietary fiber contents of 70 high consumption foods. J Food Compos Anal 2002; 15(6): 715-23.
[http://dx.doi.org/10.1006/jfca.2002.1096]

[81]   Grant LJ. More added sugars, more dyslipidemia? 2010. Available from: https://www.researchgate.net/publication/311470707_More_Added_Sugars_More_Dyslipidemia.

[82]   Welsh JA, Sharma A, Abramson JL, Vaccarino V, Gillespie C, Vos MB. Caloric sweetener consumption and dyslipidemia among US adults. JAMA 2010; 303(15): 1490-7.
[http://dx.doi.org/10.1001/jama.2010.449] [PMID: 20407058]

[83]   Hieronimus B, Griffen SC, Keim NL, *et al.* Effects of fructose or glucose on circulating ApoCIII and triglyceride and cholesterol content of lipoprotein subfractions in humans. J Clin Med 2019; 8(7): 913-29.
[http://dx.doi.org/10.3390/jcm8070913] [PMID: 31247940]

[84]   Stanhope KL, Schwarz JM, Keim NL, *et al.* Consuming fructose-sweetened, not glucose-sweetened, beverages increases visceral adiposity and lipids and decreases insulin sensitivity in overweight/obese humans. J Clin Invest 2009; 119(5): 1322-34.
[http://dx.doi.org/10.1172/JCI37385] [PMID: 19381015]

CHAPTER 9

Covid-19 And Food: An Immunological Strategy

Elevina Pérez Sira[1,*]

[1] *Instituto de Ciencia y Tecnología de Alimentos, Facultad de Ciencias, Universidad Central de Venezuela, Caracas, Venezuela*

Abstract: The chapter is an overview of the relationship COVID 19-nutrition, it focuses on the relation of diet and the disease, some non-conventional raw material used as non-traditional medicine with properties to enhancement the body immunological systems. The chapter also recommends some home recipes for consumers.

Keywords: Coronavirus, COVID-19, Immunological system, Nutrition, SARS-CoV-2.

INTRODUCTION

According to WHO, 2003 [1] severe acute respiratory syndrome (SARS) has been recognized as the first severe infectious disease to emerge in the twenty-first century. SARS poses a serious threat to global health security, the livelihood of populations, the functioning of health systems, and the stability and growth of economies. SARS is an infectious disease with a high potential for transmission to close contacts associated with coronavirus.

A coronavirus is a group of viruses categorized into alpha-coronavirus and betacoronavirus often causing cold and other mild upper respiratory tract infections in the human body [2]. A coronavirus is a kind of common virus that causes an infection in your nose, sinuses, or upper throat. There are many coronavirus serotypes, most of them are not dangerous, however, and a kind of coronavirus, which has been identified in twenty early in patients with (SARS) has produced a dangerous pandemic until yet with more than 5 million contagious and over 300.000 deaths.

---

* **Corresponding author Elevina Pérez Sira:** Instituto de Ciencia y Tecnología de Alimentos, Facultad de Ciencias, Universidad Central de Venezuela, Caracas, Venezuela; Tel: +58.212.751 4403; Fax: +58.212.751 3871; E-mail: elevina07@gmail.com

The World Health Organization has identified SARS-CoV-2 as a new type of coronavirus [2]. Severe acute respiratory syndrome coronavirus 2, shortened to SARS-CoV-2, is the virus that causes COVID-19 (the disease). As was announced on 11 February 2020 by the Director-General of the WHO in 2020 Dr. Tedros Adhanom Ghebreyesus, as general public terminology it is used for the new disease the term COVID-19; where 'CO' stands for 'corona,' 'VI' for 'virus,' 'D' for disease and 19 indicates the year it was discovered. SARS-CoV-2 is genetically related to the SARS-associated coronavirus (SARS-CoV) that caused an outbreak of severe acute respiratory syndrome (SARS) in 2002-2003 [3 - 6], however, it is not the same virus. The coronavirus strains over time are becoming more aggressive to humans, so it is important to study the ways to eradicate from humanity.

SAR-CoV2 is an enveloped, non-segmented, positive-sense beta-virus, containing single strands of RNA and provided with crown-like spikes on the outer surface [7]. Since the SARS-CoV-2 virus has several complex immune-evasion components that contribute to its virulence, it does not ease, and on time to produce a vaccine for the prevention of the diseases caused by this virus.

Typically, the process of developing vaccines takes five to 10 years, and a significant amount of funding is needed to get vaccines ready for testing. Moreover, it has been demonstrated the fast and easy mutation of the virus, due to its RNA composition [8]. Viruses are biological systems with the widest variation in mutation rates, the largest differences being found between RNA and DNA viruses. According to several authors [9], the RNA viruses mutate faster than DNA viruses, single-stranded viruses mutate faster than a double-strand virus, and genome size appears to correlate negatively with mutation rate. Higher mutation rates lead to higher genetic diversity. Therefore, it looks that the SAR-CoV2 is a good candidate for fast mutation these premises: -there is not yet a vaccine for SARS-CoV-2, -and there are still concerns over safety for a COVID-19 vaccine, and the virus complex immune-evasion components; it is important to have another way to prevent the world pandemic.

The Covid-19 outbreak is quickly spreading around the world affecting the health system and economies of each country in more or less intensity. Since there are world areas less affected, it can be a hypothesis that other different factors of the usual prevention solutions applied (detection, quarantine, and strict corporal hygiene) be affecting the virus. The outbreak of SARS in several countries has led to the search for active antiviral vegetable raw material to treat this disease. Therefore, there is a scientific commitment to search for antiviral active food components to prevent the disease.

Consequently, for prevention by reinforcement of the human immunological system, the vegetable's food science and technology could be one of the solutions. The green belt of Mother Nature is the richest source of bioactive phytochemicals that act as natural nutraceuticals [10], which produce physiological actions on the human body. They are also sometimes added to food for medicinal purposes. Medicinal plants are of great importance to the health of individuals and communities. The medicinal value of these plants lies in some chemical substances that produce a definite physiological action on the human body [11]. Research strongly suggests that consuming foods rich in phytochemicals provides health benefits, but not enough information exists to make specific recommendations for phytochemical intake.

Its original function is to protect plants from disease and damage and also contribute to the plant's color, aroma, and flavor. Phytochemicals are defined in the strictest sense, as chemicals produced by plants. However, the term is generally used to describe chemicals from plants that may enhance the health status of organisms. In general, the plant chemicals that protect plants from environmental hazards such as pollution, stress, drought, UV exposure, and pathogenic attack are called phytochemicals.

Phytochemicals are found in fruits, vegetables, whole grains, legumes, beans, herbs, spices, nuts, and seeds. They can be nutrient or non-nutrient and are classified according to their chemical structures and functional properties. Phytochemicals include compounds such as salicylates, phytosterols, saponins, glucosinolates, polyphenols, protease inhibitors, monoterpenes, phytoestrogens, sulphides, terpenes, lectins, and many more [12].

Depending on their role in plant metabolism they are primary metabolites, which include the common sugars, amino acids, proteins, purines, and pyrimidines of nucleic acids, chlorophylls among others. The secondary metabolites are the remaining plant chemicals such as alkaloids, terpenes, flavonoids, lignans, plant steroids, curcumin, saponins, phenolics, and glucosides [13, 14]. The phenolics are the most common and structurally most diverse plant chemicals.

In the context of the use of vegetables as a preventive function to fight against viruses, some researchers mention some phytochemicals from plants. A significant number of traditional herbal medicine have been used as a chemotherapeutic treatment for inhibition and replication of SAR-Cov [15, 16]. However, to prevent viral infection, some of these medicinal herbs should be included in the dietary regimes of the consumers as a strategy for reinforcement of their immunological systems.

The immune response is often weakened by inadequate nutrition in many model systems, as well as, in human studies [17]. Indeed, these authors suggest that the nutritional interventions with vitamins: A, D, E, C, and those from the B complex, the omega-3, and the minerals: selenium, zinc, and Fe, as promising option for the treatment of this novel coronavirus and the prevention of lung infection.

On the other hand, It has been shown that the herbal extracts from *Gentianae Radix* (lóng dǎn; the dried rhizome of *Gentiana scabra*), *Dioscoreae* Rhizoma (shān yào; the tuber of *Dioscorea batatas*), *Cassiae Semen* (jué míng zǐ; the dried seed of *Cassia tora*) and *Loranthi Ramus* (sāng jì shēng; the dried stem, with a leaf of *Taxillus chinensis*), and two from Rhizoma *Cibotii* (gǒu jǐ; the dried rhizome of *Cibotium barometz*) are potent inhibitors of SARS-CoV at concentrations between 25 and 200 µg/ml [18].

Keeping in mind these assay cell-based that measured SARS-CoV-induced cytopathogenic effect *in vitro*, and the effect of the vitamins, mineral and omega 3; it is no difficult to assume that a dietary regime, which includes these raw materials will be a good way to reinforce the consumer's immunological body system. However, it is important to be clear that there are foods that can help strengthen the immune system, which does not guarantee that they prevent or prevent the spread of Covid-19, nor that a person who consumes these foods is safer than another who does not. But having a healthy body is something that improves the body's response to any threat, but does not prevent the infection.

Some of the herbal used as medicine could be not recommended as food because of their non-accepted taste and toxicity for the consumers. For example, despite the multiples, *Gentiana lutea* health benefices, including its anti-obesity properties, and elevation of secretory immunoglobulin levels capacity, their dried, fragmented underground organs have a characteristic odor and a strong and persistent bitter taste, due to the gentiamarine and gentiopicrine, and low amount of amarogentine [19 - 21].

Cibotium barometz is an evergreen fern with a creeping rhizome, producing fronds up to 2 meters tall. The rhizome is very thick, woody, and covered by long soft, golden-yellow hairs. Moreover, it was reported that the rhizome is edible [22]. Although there are no reports of toxicity for this species, several ferns contain carcinogens so some caution is advisable. Many ferns also contain thiaminase, an enzyme that binds the vitamin B complex. In small quantities, this enzyme will not harm people eating an adequate diet that is rich in vitamin B, though large quantities can cause severe health problems. However, the enzyme is destroyed by heat or thorough drying, so cooking the plant will remove the thiaminase [23].

Dioscorea batatas Decne (Chinese yam) has been widely cultivated in East Asia for food and medicinal uses for centuries. Its root has been extensively investigated in association with phytochemicals such as allantoin, flavonoids, saponins, and phenanthrenes. Phenanthrenes are especially considered the standard marker chemicals of the Chinese yam for their potent bioactivity. However, the whole yams must be dried and powdered for food used, because of the high value of the discarded peel [24].

The *Dioscorea batatas* tubers are usually eaten cooked. This is a top-quality root crop, very suitable for use as a staple food. They have a very pleasant flavor that is rather like a potato; as with other yams, they are boiled, baked, fried, mashed, grated, or added to soups. The root contains about 20% starch. 75% water, 0.1% vitamin B1, 10 - 15 mg% vitamin C. Its starch is not as good as binding as starches from other starchy foods [25].

Dioscorin, the extractable, water-soluble protein of yams (*Dioscorea* sp.), has been reported as playing a role as an antioxidant. In the Venezuelan Amazon, varieties of yams grow with differing sizes and colors that have not been completely identified. Pérez *et al.* [26], study estimate the dioscorin protein from *Dioscorea* sp., gathered from crops of the "Piaroa" community of the Amazonas state, Venezuela. By analyzing the results from the characteristic fingerprint obtained by MALDI-TOF MS FPP, it was concluded that the white yam is *Dioscorea japonica*. The yam protein crude content was 3.75% with an estimated concentration of dioscorin of 42.1%.

Cassia obtusifolia is a miraculous medicinal plant that is one of the most widely grown species of the family *Leguminosae*. Their roasted seeds are used as a coffee substitute and the dried leaves are eaten as vegetables to control undernutrition especially against kwashiorkor and anemia. Leaves are a well-known source of protein vitamin-A and minerals like iron and calcium [27].

Licorice, *Glycyrrhiza glabra* L. belongs to the Family Fabaceae; Tribe Astragaleae. The name Glycyrrhiza is of Greek origin which means "sweet wood". Glycyrrhizin is the major active constituent of licorice root (Glycyrrhiza glabra) and has been used in traditional medicine to alleviate bronchitis, gastritis, and jaundice (Ramos-Tovar and Muriel, 2019). Besides being a potent inhibitor of replication of viruses (Cinatl *et al.*, 2003), it is 50–100 times sweeter than sucrose and has a slow onset of sweetness followed by a lingering licorice-like aftertaste [28, 29]. According to this last author, it exhibits a sweet woody flavor, which limits its use as a pure sweetener. Glycyrrhizin enhances food flavors, masks bitter flavors, and increases the perceived sweetness level of sucrose. It has the potential for providing functional characteristics, including foaming, viscosity control, gel formation, and possibly antioxidant characteristics. It is mainly used as a coating for candies and chewing tobacco. Ingestion of large amounts of these foods may cause headaches, lethargy, and body retention of sodium, and water, excessive excretion of potassium, high blood pressure, and sometimes heart failure. Hence it behaves like a mineralocorticoid [30]. Licorice is widely used as a flavoring agent especially in the tobacco industry. In combination with sugar, the sweetness increased by 100 times. In pharmaceuticals and medicinal tea, it not only acts as a flavoring agent but also reduces the unpleasant taste of other constituents. It is used as a sweetener and flavoring agent in low caloric and noncariogenic food. It gives sparkle and aroma to confectionary products and beer respectively. Licorice serves as a preservative in the food industry. Excessive consumption, however, leads to harmful consequences.

Black tea, green tea, red wine, and cocoa are high in phenolic phytochemicals, among which theaflavin, epigallocatechin gallate, resveratrol, and procyanidin, respectively, have been extensively investigated due to their possible role as chemopreventive agents based on their antioxidant capacities [31]. According to their results, the authors suggest that cocoa is more beneficial to health than teas and red wine in terms of its higher antioxidant capacity, moreover, when it is unfermented [32].

Euterpe Olearacea (azaí, huasaí, murrapo, naidí, or açaí palm) is a palm native to northern South America, prized for the nutritional properties of its fruit. The study of Sanabria and Sangroni [33] on the proximal composition, fatty acid profile, the content of minerals, tannins, polyphenols, anthocyanins, antioxidant capacity, and the color of the acai pulp (*Euterpe oleracea* Mart) collected from Venezuelan Amazons at two harvest periods of the 2005 year concluded that the acai has a high nutritional value and contains antioxidant compounds which suggest the need to industrialize it to take advantage to the maximum of its properties. The fruit of acai has given great benefits to the health sector due to its anticancer, antioxidant, and anti-inflammatory properties, which explains the increase in the demand for açaí worldwide in recent years [34, 35].

Recently investigation in SARS-CoV-2 infected individuals have associated deficiencies of Vitamin D with severity/mortality of COVID-19, highlighting the need for interventional studies on Vitamin D supplementation [36].

In each chapter of the book, there are several recipes, which help to the reinforcement of the body's immunological system in different ways. However, to add something more, we will give some recipes with the raw materials discussed in this chapter.

RECIPES

Chicken Wing with Licorice Sauce

Ingredients

1 kg	Chicken wings	100 g	Light Cream Milk
25 gr	Sugar	2g	White Pepper and
18 g	Licorice (2 stick)	2g	Salt
200 ml	Chicken broth	-	Vegetable oil to fry
75g	Onion (chopped)	-	-
100g	Wheat flour, all-purpose	-	-

Preparation

Mix flour, salt, white pepper together in a wide, shallow bowl. Press wings into flour mixture to coat and arrange onto a large plate so they do not touch. Refrigerate coated wings for 15 to 30 minutes. Dredge wings again in flour mixture and return to the plate. Refrigerate wings again for 15 to 30 minutes.

Heat oil in a deep-fryer or large saucepan to 375 degrees F (190 °C). Fry chicken wings in hot oil until crisp and no longer pink at the bone and the juices run clear, 9 to 12 minutes. An instant-read thermometer inserted into the thickest part of the meat, near the bone should read 165 degrees F (74 °C).

Transfer fried wings to a large stainless-steel bowl.

Drizzle licorice sauce over the wings and toss to coat.

Licorice Sauce

Prepare the sauce in the same pan where the chicken was fried.

Put the sugar into the pan and let it take on color and texture until it almost becomes a caramel, incorporate the cream and start mixing.

This ingredient will make the sauce thicken a little more.

Next, add the chicken broth and onion and introduce the licorice sticks. Let everything cook until it takes cream texture.

Licorice Extract

Ingredients

Licorice stick	Vodka or grain alcohol

Preparation

Place the licorice roots into a clean canning jar, filling it approximately two-thirds full. Cover the licorice root with vodka or grain alcohol. Place a square of plastic wrap over the mouth of the jar and tightly screw on the lid.

The plastic wrap will help prevent rusting. Shake well and store in a dark place for six weeks. Shake the jar at least twice a week.

Strain the contents of the jar by placing the cheesecloth over a bowl. Squeeze the licorice root in the cheesecloth to extract as much of the liquid as possible.

Transfer the liquid in the bowl to a clean canning jar or another container. Store in a dark place. The extract should be good for about three years.

Licorice Syrup

Ingredients

150g	Molasses Sugar	5g	Fennel seeds
15g	Licorice root, powdered	50g	Sugar
5g	Aniseeds (*Pimpinella anisum* L)	500ml	Water
	-	30 ml	Vodka

Preparation

Slightly roast aniseed and fennel in a pan without oil. Put the roasted seeds in a teabag and make a tea. Add the infusion to a pot and turn on the heat.

Add the molasses and sugar, stirring in the licorice root. Bring to boil and remove from heat.

Strain through a tea strainer or use a coffee filter fill into a clean bottle and add the vodka.

Chinese Yam with Star Anise, Ginger, and Lime

Ingredients

500g	Chinese Yam, scrubbed and cut into 1 1/2-inch piece	1	Ginger (1-inch) piece fresh, finely grated
15 ml	Olive oil	1	Lime, zested, and juiced
1	Star Anise, finely crushed	2.5g	Salt
	-	Pinch	Pepper; fresh, ground

Preparation

Preheat oven to 425°F. Toss the cut yam with brown sugar and in a large bowl arrange the tossed yam in a single layer on a baking sheet. Roast for 10 minutes, then shake or flip the yam pieces over.

Continue roasting for 10 minutes or until tender and slightly browned, then add the ginger, lime zest, and juice to the olive oil mixture, toss them with the yam after roasting for a hotter and zestier flavor.

Serve warm or at room temperature.

Citrus Salad with Licorice Vinaigrette

Ingredients

	Salad	-	Dressing
3	Oranges	15 ml	Licorice syrup salty
2	Grapefruits (pink)	30 ml	Balsamic dark espresso
2	Lemons (pink)	-	-
2	Tunisian Blood Orange	-	-
	Olive oil to sprinkle	-	-
1 handful	Italian Parsley, chopped	-	-
2 tbsp	Shallots, finely chopped	-	-

Preparation

Whisk the licorice syrup with the balsamic, set it aside. Peel oranges, lemons, and grapefruits and slice them thinly. Arrange the slices in a platter and sprinkle them with olive oil and salt. Drizzle the dressing on top, and sprinkle with onion and parsley.

Dark Chocolate-Acai Chips Cookies

Ingredients

150g	Salted Butter* softened	270g	Wheat flour all-purpose
100g	Acai pulp	5 g	Baking Soda
225g	Sugar white (granulated)	2.5g	Baking Powder
225	Sugar packed light brown	6g	Salt (coarse)
4 g	Vanilla extract (pure)	200g	Dark Chocolate (80%) chips (or chunks, or chopped chocolate)
110 g	Eggs (whole)	-	-

Preparation

Preheat oven to 375 °F. Line a baking pan with parchment paper set aside. In a bowl mix flour, baking soda, salt, baking powder, set aside. Cream butter, acai, and sugars until combined. Beat in eggs and vanilla until fluffy. Mix the cream in the dry ingredients until combined. Add the chocolate chips and mix well. Roll 23 tablespoon of dough at a time into balls and place them evenly spaced on your prepared cookie sheets. Bake in preheated oven for approximately 8-10 minutes. Take them out when they start to turn brown. Let them sit on the baking pan for 2 minutes before removing it to a cooling rack.

Homemade Beet-Licorice Twizzles

Ingredients

75g	Wheat flour for all-purpose	5g	Licorice extract
1 pinch	Himalayan Pink Salt	5g	Beetroot juice
114g	Butter	-	Corn Starch to powder the twist
85g	Honey	180g	Condensed Milk ((sweetened)
200g	Cane Sugar	-	-

Preparations

Combine the dry licorice recipe ingredients in a mixing bowl. Set aside. In a saucepan, combine the sugar, honey, condensed milk, and butter. Bring to a boil, stirring occasionally. Continue to heat until the temperature reaches 240°F. This is the softball stage.

Check the temperature with a candy thermometer. Reach into the water and try to form a ball from the syrup with fingers. It if stays together for a few seconds, it's ready. Remove from the heat right away and pour over the flour mixture.

Mix well. Add the beetroot juice for color and the licorice extract for flavor. Mix these in well too.

Pour the mixture in a pan covered with a sheet of parchment paper and set in the refrigerator for about an hour, or until set and well chilled.

When chilled cut into strips with a pizza cutter, keeping the strips about ⅓ to ½inch wide and twist them. Dust with corn starch to keep from sticking and store in an airtight container.

Beet-Licorice Ice Cream

Ingredients

100g	Beet-Licorice Twizzles
250 ml	Milk (whole)
125 ml	Double crème (48-60% Fat Milk cream)
2	Egg Yolk
50 g	Sugar
	Licorice (ornament optional)

Preparation

Heat in a pot 80ml of water, add the licorice and stir until dissolved. Slowly heat the milk together with the cream in a saucepan without boiling. Meanwhile, beat the yolks together with the sugar. Gradually pour the milk and hot cream over the mixture of eggs and sugar and continue beating. Put everything again in the pot together with the dissolved licorice and heat slowly, continuously moving the mixture with a wooden spoon until a thin layer is created on the back of it. Remove from heat and let sit for about 30 minutes, until reaching room temperature. Put the mixture in the freezer for 50 minutes. Take it out of the freezer and beat it to remove any possible crystals that have formed. Then put it back in the freezer and take it out every 30 minutes and beat it again. Do this operation 5-6 times, for 3 more hours, to reach the ice cream quite creamy. After the last beat operation add small pieces of licorice to decorate. Finally, leave it in the freezer for at least 2 hours so that it freezes completely. Take it out a few minutes before serving from the freezer so that it is at the right serving temperature for the ice cream.

Note: Feel free to skip the simmer step and simply whisk everything together, then pour directly into the ice cream maker. The ice cream is delicious this way, as well as when simmered and chilled first.

CONSENT FOR PUBLICATION

Not Applicable.

CONFLICT OF INTEREST

The author confirms that this chapter contents have no conflict of interest.

ACKNOWLEDGEMENT

Declared none.

REFERENCES

[1]   WHO. 2003. https://www.who.int/csr/sars/en/ea56r29.pdf?ua=1

[2]   Law S, Leung AW, Xu C. Severe acute respiratory syndrome (SARS) and coronavirus disease-2019 (COVID-19): From causes to preventions in Hong Kong. Int J Infect Dis 2020; 94: 156-63.
[http://dx.doi.org/10.1016/j.ijid.2020.03.059] [PMID: 32251790]

[3]   Hernández G. SARS: epidemiología y mecanismos de transmisión SARS: epidemiology and mechanisms of transmission. Med Intensiva 2003; 27(10): 686-91.
[http://dx.doi.org/10.1016/S0210-5691(03)79993-8]

[4]   Peiris JS, Yuen KY, Osterhaus AD, Stöhr K. The severe acute respiratory syndrome. N Engl J Med 2003; 349(25): 2431-41.
[http://dx.doi.org/10.1056/NEJMra032498] [PMID: 14681510]

[5]   Poon LL, Chan KH, Wong OK, *et al.* Early diagnosis of SARS coronavirus infection by real time RT-PCR. J Clin Virol 2003; 28(3): 233-8.
[http://dx.doi.org/10.1016/j.jcv.2003.08.004] [PMID: 14522060]

[6]   Vaqué Rafart J. Síndrome respiratorio agudo grave (SARS). In: Mesa redonda. Patología respiratoria importada. An Pediatr (Barc) 2005; 62(Supl 1):6-11.

[7]   Astuti I, Ysrafil . Severe Acute Respiratory Syndrome Coronavirus 2 (SARS-CoV-2): An overview of viral structure and host response. Diabetes Metab Syndr 2020; 14(4): 407-12.
[http://dx.doi.org/10.1016/j.dsx.2020.04.020] [PMID: 32335367]

[8]   Kim J. Director-general of the International Vaccine Institute 2020. https://www.cnbc.com

[9]   Sanjuán R, Domingo-Calap P. Mechanisms of viral mutation. Cell Mol Life Sci 2016; 73(23): 4433-48.
[http://dx.doi.org/10.1007/s00018-016-2299-6] [PMID: 27392606]

[10]   Koche D, Shirsat R, Kawale M. An overview of major classes of phytochemicals: their types and role in disease prevention. Hislopia J 2016; 9(1/2): 1-11.

[11]   Edeoga HO, Okwu DE, Mbaebie BO. Phytochemical constituents of some Nigerian medicinal plants. Afr J Biotechnol 2005; 4(7): 685-8.
[http://dx.doi.org/10.5897/AJB2005.000-3127]

[12]   Webb D. Role in Good Health. 2020. Available from: http://www.todaysdietitian.com

[13]   Hahn NI. Is phytoestrogens nature's cure for what ails us? A look at the research. J Am Dent Assoc 1998; 98: 974-6.
[http://dx.doi.org/10.1016/S0002-8223(98)00223-5] [PMID: 9739795]

[14]   Ramawat KG, Dass S, Mathur M. The chemical diversity of bioactive molecules and Therapeutic potential of medicinal plants.Herbal drugs: Ethnomedicine to modern medicine; Verlag Berlin Heidelberg. Springer 2009.
[http://dx.doi.org/10.1007/978-3-540-79116-4_2]

[15]   Lai ST. Treatment of severe acute respiratory syndrome. Eur J Clin Microbiol Infect Dis 2005; 24(9): 583-91.
[http://dx.doi.org/10.1007/s10096-005-0004-z] [PMID: 16172857]

[16]   Stadler K, Masignani V, Eickmann M, *et al*. SARS--beginning to understand a new virus. Nat Rev Microbiol 2003; 1(3): 209-18.
[http://dx.doi.org/10.1038/nrmicro775] [PMID: 15035025]

[17]   Zhang L, Liu Y. Potential interventions for novel coronavirus in China: A systematic review. J Med Virol 2020; 92(5): 479-90.
[http://dx.doi.org/10.1002/jmv.25707] [PMID: 32052466]

[18]   Wen C-C, Shyur L-F, Jan J-T, *et al*. Traditional Chinese medicine herbal extracts of Cibotium barometz, Gentiana scabra, Dioscorea batatas, Cassia tora, and Taxillus chinensis inhibit SARS-CoV replication. J Tradit Complement Med 2011; 1(1): 41-50.
[http://dx.doi.org/10.1016/S2225-4110(16)30055-4] [PMID: 24716104]

[19]   European Drugs Encyclopedia Gentiana (Gentianae radix). 2009. Available from: https://theodora.com

[20]   Prakash O, Singh R, Kumar S, Srivastava S, Ved A. *Gentiana lutea* Linn. (Yellow Gentian): A comprehensive review. Journal of Ayurvedic and Herbal Medicine 2017; 3(3): 175-81.

[21]   Park E, Lee CG, Kim J, *et al*. Antiobesity effects of *Gentiana lutea* extract on 3t3-l1 preadipocytes and a high-fat diet-induced mouse model. Molecules 2020; 25(10): 2453.
[http://dx.doi.org/10.3390/molecules25102453] [PMID: 32466183]

[22]   Kunkel G. Plants for Human Consumption. Koeltz Scientific Books 1984.

[23]   Useful Tropical Plants Database. 2004. http://tropical.theferns.info

[24]   Kim M, Gu MJ, Lee JG, Chin J, Bae J-S, Hahn D. Quantitative analysis of bioactive phenanthrenes in *Dioscorea batatas* decne peel, a discarded biomass from postharvest processing. Antioxidants 2019; 8(11): 541.
[http://dx.doi.org/10.3390/antiox8110541] [PMID: 31717654]

[25]   Database Plant Search Page. Plant for a Future 2020. https://pfaf.org/user/plant.aspx?LatinName=Dioscorea+batatas

[26]   Pérez EE, Faks J, Cira LE, Schroeder M, Diez N. Estimation of the dioscorin extracted from cultivars of yams (Dioscorea genus) growing in the Venezuelan Amazonas. Acta Hortic 2014; (1016): 53-60. [ISHS].
[http://dx.doi.org/10.17660/ActaHortic.2014.1016.5]

[27]   Rakib M, Ansari VA, Arif M, Ahmad A. A review of phytochemical and biological studies on Cassia obtusifolia Linn. 2018.

[28]   Glória MBA. Intense sweeteners and synthetic colorants.Food analysis by HPLC. New York: Marcer Dekker, Inc 1997; pp. 523-74.

[29]   Glória MBA. Sweeteners.Encyclopedia of Food Sciences and Nutrition. 2nd ed. New York: Academic Press 2003; pp. 42-7.
[http://dx.doi.org/10.1016/B0-12-227055-X/01404-8]

[30]   Modi SV, Borges VJ. Artificial sweeteners: boon or bane? Int J Diabetes Dev Ctries 2005; 25: 1-8. [Review].
        [http://dx.doi.org/10.4103/0973-3930.26753]

[31]   Lee KW, Kim YJ, Lee HJ, Lee CY. Cocoa has more phenolic phytochemicals and a higher antioxidant capacity than teas and red wine. J Agric Food Chem 2003; 51(25): 7292-5.
        [http://dx.doi.org/10.1021/jf0344385] [PMID: 14640573]

[32]   Pérez EE, Álvarez C, Medina O. Cocoa phytochemicals: Chemical structure, changes during processing and uses.The uses of cocoa and cupuaçu byproducts in industry, health, and gastrony. NOVA Science Publisher 2018; pp. 47-89.

[33]   Neida S, Elba S. [Characterization of the acai or manaca (*Euterpe oleracea* Mart.): a fruit of the Amazon]. Arch Latinoam Nutr 2007; 57(1): 94-8.
        [PMID: 17824205]

[34]   Brondízio E, Safar C, Siqueira A. The urban market of Açai fruit (*Euterpe oleracea* Mart.) and rural land use change: ethnographic insights into the role of price and land tenure constraining agricultural choices in the Amazon estuary. Urban Ecosyst 2002; 6: 67-97.
        [http://dx.doi.org/10.1023/A:1025966613562]

[35]   Shanley P, Cymerys M, González G. Productos forestales no madereros, frutales y plantas útiles en la vida amazónica 2012. http://ebookcentral.proquest.com

[36]   Radujkovic A, Hippchen T, Tiwari-Heckler S, Dreher S, Boxberger M, Merle U. Vitamin D deficiency and outcome of covid-19 patients. Nutrients 2020; 12: 2757.
        [http://dx.doi.org/10.3390/nu12092757]

SUBJECT INDEX

A

Acceptable daily intake (ADI) 118, 122, 123
Acid(s) 9, 10, 11, 12, 19, 35, 39, 63, 91, 107,
　　110, 117, 129, 130, 153, 160, 181, 185,
　　188, 208, 214, 215, 216, 217, 218, 220,
　　221, 223, 226, 227
　alpha-linolenic (ALA) 9, 214, 215, 217,
　　218, 223
　bile 208, 227
　caffeic 129
　citric 19
　docosahexaenoic 214, 215, 216
　folic 12, 35, 188
　gallic 129
　glutamic 11, 181
　lactic 91
　linoleic 10, 39, 214, 215, 217, 220, 221
　maleyacetoacetic 160
　nicotinic 12
　oleanolic 130
　oleic 220, 223
　palmitoleic 220
　pantothenic 12, 188
　phenolic 107
　phenylacetic 153
　tannic 129
Agricultural research service (ARS) 228
Allium sativum 127
Amino acid 87, 152, 163
　metabolism 152
　profile 87, 163
Anosmia 62, 63, 64, 69
Antigen-presenting cells (APCs) 181, 182,
　183
Antioxidant properties 107, 108, 114, 192
Aromatic amino acids (AAA) 156, 161, 162
Asperger's syndrome 175
Aspergillum oryzae 163
Autism 174, 175, 176, 177
　disorder 175

spectrum disorders (ASDs) 174, 175, 176,
　177
Autoimmune diseases 188
Autonomous thyrocytes 67

B

Bacterial glycosidases 119
Bone mineral 67, 81
　content (BMC) 81
　density (BMD) 67
Bowel movement 29, 68

C

Carbohydrate intake 87
Carcinogenesis 29
Cardiovascular 3, 30, 59, 101, 108, 115, 116,
　211, 212, 215, 227, 228
　disease 30, 59, 101, 108, 115, 116, 211,
　212, 215, 227, 228
　sickness 3
Catabolic pathway 152
Celiac 173, 174, 175, 176, 177, 178, 179, 180,
　181, 182, 183, 184, 188, 189, 194
　and autism disease 173
　disease (CD) 173, 174, 175, 176, 177, 178,
　179, 180, 181, 182, 183, 184, 188, 189,
　194
Chemokine receptor 180
Cholesterol 91, 207, 208, 209, 227
　circulating 208
　elevated 207
　free 209
　synthesis 91, 227
Cholesteryl ester transfer protein (CETP) 209
Chylomicronemia syndrome 211
Coeliac diseases 177
Coronary heart disease (CHD) 10, 28, 30, 210,
　211, 212, 214, 216, 220, 224
Creatinine supplementation 90
Crohn's disease 226

D

Deficiency 5, 36, 37, 63, 64, 67, 130, 153,
      160, 193, 195, 206, 217
   folate 193
   lipoprotein 206
   melanin 160
   micronutrient 193
de novo lipogenesis (DNL) 229
Dental 59, 60
   disease 59
   remineralization 60
Diabetes mellitus (DM) 100, 101, 102, 103,
      106, 107, 109, 110, 114, 125, 129, 130,
      132, 211, 212
   gestational 101, 103
Diet 27, 29, 39, 80, 125, 175, 176, 177, 210,
      226
   carbohydrate-controlled 210
   casein-free 176, 177
   celiac 175
   diabetic 125
   gluten-restricted 175
   low-fat 80, 226
   omnivorous 27
   plant-based 39
   vegetable-rich 29
Dietary 8, 29, 33, 88, 89, 104, 108, 110, 112,
      113, 131, 183, 184, 209, 226, 227, 228
   education program 183
   fiber 8, 29, 104, 110, 112, 131, 184, 226,
      227, 228
   intake 33, 113, 209
   supplements 88, 89, 108
Digestion 12, 60, 61, 131, 177, 179, 180, 185,
      189, 194
   gastrointestinal 180
   intestinal proteolytic 177
   rice starch 185
Digestive system function 13
Dihydropteridine reductase 153
Disorders 2, 3, 4, 61, 64, 65, 102, 103, 122,
      152, 174, 176, 178, 206, 207, 210, 211,
      229
   autistic spectrum 176
   autoimmune 174, 178
   endocrine 103
   genetic 122, 152, 211
   idiopathic 102
   lipid 210

   mental 4
   neurological 61
   sarcopenic 65
Dysfunction 103, 130, 175
   endothelial 103
   metabolic 130
Dyslipidemia 4, 103, 108, 206, 211, 212, 213,
      229
   atherogenic 103
   disease 213
Dyslipidemia-related diseases 229
Dysphagia 61, 62, 65
   disease-related 65
   rehabilitation 65

E

Effects 108, 109, 127, 215
   anti-diabetic 127
   antihyperglycemic 109
   hypoglycemic 108
   hypolipidemic 215
Elastase 179
Electrophoresis 206
Electrophoretic mobility 179
Energy metabolism 88
Environmental hazards 106, 241
Enzymes 33, 34, 88, 89, 106, 111, 113, 126,
      128, 130, 152, 153, 163, 174, 181, 192,
      194, 195, 242
   digestive 225
   endopeptidase 194
   glucokinase 126
   hepatic 153
   phenylalanine hydroxylase 152
   protease 163
   tissue transglutaminase 174, 181
Essential fatty acids (EFAs) 10, 28, 38, 156,
      160, 206, 214, 215, 216, 223
European vegetarian union (EVU) 33, 34
Exercise 91, 210
   lactic-anaerobic 91
   regular aerobic 210
Eye damages 106

F

Facial trauma 64
Failure, heart 119, 244

Fasting plasma glucose 112
Fat-free mass (FFM) 81
Fatigue 85, 173, 178
Fats 9, 10, 80, 81, 82, 83, 87, 125, 159, 213, 214, 217, 218, 219, 221, 222, 223, 224, 225, 226, 229, 231, 249
  dietary 213
  healthy 80, 222
  mass (FM) 81
  milk cream 249
  natural 10
  polyunsaturated 159, 213, 218, 223
  solid 224
  stored 83
  unsaturated 9, 213, 214, 223
Fatty acids 9, 10, 35, 38, 39, 104, 106, 177, 206, 213, 214, 215, 216, 217, 218, 219, 220, 221, 223
  monounsaturated 9, 104, 220, 221
  polyunsaturated 9, 35, 177, 213, 214, 217, 220, 223
  saturated 9, 213, 214, 219
Fiber 7, 8, 14, 29, 35, 37, 67, 68, 69, 191, 195, 207, 226, 227
  crude 8, 226
  fermented 227
  insoluble 227
  nerve 207
Fish 161, 213, 215, 216
  oils 213, 215, 216
  proteins 161
Food(s) 1, 4, 6, 12, 16, 17, 31, 33, 37, 41, 59, 89, 119, 122, 124, 131, 154, 155, 156, 159, 160, 161, 173, 174, 184, 188, 190, 193, 244
  and agriculture organization (FAO) 59, 193
  and drug administration (FDA) 119, 122, 156, 160, 184
  based dietary guidelines 31
  conventional 4, 89
  fermented 131
  for celiac consumers 173, 190
  for medical purpose (FMP) 124
  for special dietary uses (FSDU) 4, 124
  gluten-containing 173, 174
  information regulation 17, 33
  intolerance 16, 17
  medical 1, 154, 155, 159, 160, 161
  noncariogenic 244
  nutritious 6, 41, 188

  processing methods 37
  protein 12, 161
  protein-free 161
  staple 184
  technologists 161
Fuel 11, 85
  mix-matching 85
  respiratory 11
Functionality, technological 8

G

Gastric ulcer 30
Gastritis 119, 243
Gastrointestinal proteolysis 187, 188
Genetic 103, 190
  diversity 190
  syndromes 103
Glucocorticoids 211
Glucose 103, 116, 117, 125, 126, 129, 130
  homeostasis 125, 130
  intolerance 103
  syrups 116, 117
  transporter 126, 129
Gluten 175, 176, 177, 179, 182, 184, 189
  and casein-free diet 176, 177
  degradation 179
  epitopes 182
  intolerances 189
  sensitivity 175, 176
  test methods 184
Gluten-free 2, 173, 175, 176, 178, 179, 183, 184, 187, 189, 190, 193, 195
  bakery products 173, 195
  diet 173, 175, 176, 178, 179, 183, 184, 187, 190, 193, 195
  foods 2, 173, 183, 184, 187, 189, 193, 195
  products 195
Gluten peptides 180, 181, 194
  intact 181
Glycemic Index (GI) 100, 106, 130, 131, 132, 184, 192
Glycogenesis 117
Glycogenolysis 114, 117
Gustatory dysfunctions 58, 59

H

Health 1, 2, 4, 6, 10, 12, 27, 29, 30, 32, 39, 58,
    61, 68, 69, 101, 112, 121, 124, 161, 215
  bone 39
  cardiovascular 30
  care professionals 61
  gastric 121
  gastrointestinal 30
  mental 161, 215
  system implications 101
Health problems 60, 153, 189
  diabetesrelated 189
Hemicelluloses 224, 227
Hemoglobin 101, 117, 132
  glycated 101, 132
  glycosylated 117
Hepatic de novo lipogenesis 229
Herbal medicine 109
High 37, 64, 112, 117, 211, 212
    density lipoproteins (HDL) 112, 211, 212
    fructose corn syrup (HFCS) 117
    magnesium levels 37
    risk geriatric syndrome 64
Hormones 8, 9, 27, 67, 83, 91, 125, 191, 208
  metabolic 125
  sex 191
  thyroid-stimulating 67
Human 174, 179, 181
    leukocyte antigen (HLA) 174, 179, 181
    tissue transglutaminase 181
Hypercholesterolemia 207, 210, 212
Hyperchylomicronemia 206
Hyperglycemia 100, 101, 102, 103, 108, 113,
  125
Hyperlipidemia 113, 132, 206, 207, 210, 212
Hyperlipoproteinemia 207, 212
Hypersensitivity reaction 174
Hyperthyroidism 67
Hypertriglyceridemia 207, 210, 212
Hypoalbuminemia 178
Hypocholesterolemia 108, 114

I

Immune 177, 181, 182, 189
  mediated alteration 189
  reactions, adverse 177
  system, adaptive 181, 182

Immune response 59, 102, 174, 175, 179, 180,
    182, 185, 194, 241
  adaptive 174, 179, 182
  innate 179, 180, 182
Immunity, activating human anti-leukemia
  186
Impaired glucose tolerance (IGT) 101
Infections 5, 59, 101, 211, 216, 239, 242
  cholestatic liver diseases HIV 211
  lung 242
Infectious diseases 100, 239
Inflammation, adipose tissue 130
Inflammatory 186, 226
  bowel diseases 226
  diseases 186
Insulin 80, 102, 104, 105, 125, 126, 129, 227
  deficiency 102
  hormone 102, 129
  receptor 125
Insulin resistance 65, 102, 103, 108, 109, 114,
    128, 130, 212
  hepatic 130
  diseases 212
Insulin secretion 114, 127, 128, 131
  glucose-induced 128
International 101, 123
  agency for research on cancer (IARC) 123
  diabetes federation (IDF) 101
Intraepithelial lymphocytosis 174, 178
Iodine 66, 67
  absorption 67
  deficiencies 66
Iron absorption 36
Islet cell antigen (ICA) 102

K

Ketoacidosis 102
Ketones, urinary 82
Kidney diseases 108

L

Lactobacillus acidophilus 53
Linum usitatissimum 223
Lipoprotein 209, 211
  lipase 209, 211
  metabolism 209
Loss of chewing capacity 60

Low 112, 206, 207, 208, 209, 211, 212, 229
    calorie sweeteners (LCSs) 121
    density lipoprotein (LDL) 112, 206, 207,
        208, 209, 211, 212, 229

M

Malnutrition 5, 110
MAP- kinase pathway 126
Medical foods industry 160
Menstrual function 82
Mental retardation 156
Metabolic 2, 3, 83, 100, 103, 108, 125
    disorders 2, 3, 100, 125
    function 83
    pathway 117, 160
    syndrome 103, 108
Microbial transferase 120
Milk 10, 15, 17, 32, 34, 36, 37, 38, 40, 72, 74,
        91, 92, 93, 164, 167, 223, 224, 248, 249
    almond 93
    breast 38, 91
    by-products 40
    casein 40
    condensed 248
    fermented 32
    non-fat 223
    sesame 72, 74
    skim 223
    whole-fat 224
Minerals, dietary 37, 190
Mucosal damage 181
Multisensory interactions 62
Multi-stimulus programs 68
Muscle(s) 10, 11, 65, 86, 90
    athlete's 86
    atrophy 10
    protein synthesis 11, 90
    weakness 65

N

Nausea 91, 104
Neonatal screening program 155
Nephropathy 100
Nerve function 88
Neurodegenerative diseases 61
Neutral-flavored oil 47
Nigella sativa 127, 223

Non-celiac gluten sensitivity (NCGS) 173,
    174
Non-communicable diseases (NCDs) 3
Nutrients 5, 6, 7, 14, 15, 30, 31, 32, 37, 39, 69,
        79, 82, 85, 106, 116, 124, 130, 158, 160,
        208, 214
    deficiencies 37
    essential 116, 208, 214
    losses 14, 15
    requirements 79, 158
Nutritional deficiencies 66, 124, 175, 184, 195

O

Obesity 4, 7, 59, 64, 65, 100, 105, 106, 108,
        115, 124, 224, 226, 229
    sarcopenic 64, 65
    upper-body 105
Oils 9, 41, 43, 44, 45, 50, 104, 114, 133, 159,
        210, 213, 214, 215, 218, 219, 223, 224,
        230
    canola 43
    essential 114
    frying 214, 219
    hydrogenated 213, 224
    polyunsaturated 104
    seed 215
    sesame 41, 133
    soybean 218
    virgin 218
    walnut 215
Olfactory dysfunction 63
Olive oil 46, 47, 48, 49, 51, 132, 133, 165,
        232, 247
    extra-virgin 49
Orange juice, calcium-fortified 28
Organic matter 12
Origanium vulgare 127
Osteopenia 67
Osteoporosis 4, 59, 67, 124, 174, 188, 215
Oxygen oxidoreductase 153

P

Pancreatitis 210, 211
Parkinson's diseases 63
Pathways 12, 29, 129, 130, 179, 182, 215
    biochemical 215
    cell signaling 29

critical transduction 130
immunological 182
transcriptional regulation 129
Peptides 162, 174, 177, 179, 180, 181, 182,
    187, 189, 194
deamidated gliadin 181
immunodominant 180
immunodominant gluten 179
present antigenic 174
wheat gluten immunodominant 187
Peroxisome proliferator-activated receptors
    (PPARs) 129
Phenylalanine 10, 11, 121, 122, 152, 153, 154,
    155, 156, 157, 159, 160, 161, 162, 163
hydroxylase 156, 157
pathway 160
Phenylketonuria 122, 152, 157, 158
Physical activity (PA) 80, 81, 83, 86, 158, 160
regime 81
Physical therapy program 67
Physiological development 6
Phytochemicals, phenolic 244
Poly-unsaturated fatty acids (PUFAs) 9, 214,
    215, 217, 218, 219, 220
Process 1, 9, 13, 14, 33, 40, 59, 67, 83, 88,
    102, 129, 153, 179, 209, 210, 215, 219
atherosclerotic 210
autonomization 67
cheese-making 40
immune-mediated 102
metabolic 83
technological 1, 13
thermal 14
vascular 129
Processed 2, 27, 32, 35, 40, 41, 193, 213, 224
foods 2, 27, 32, 35, 40, 41, 193, 213, 224
oils 40
Processing 13, 14, 35, 111, 120, 153, 213
industrial juice 111
methods 14
phenylalanine 153
Products 2, 7, 15, 16, 17, 18, 29, 34, 35, 38,
    40, 68, 69, 88, 89, 113, 128, 162, 176,
    180, 195, 191, 208, 210, 213, 217, 227,
    228, 244
animal 29, 38, 208, 210, 213, 217
bacterial 227
baked 210, 228
baking 191
confectionary 244

dietary 113
gelatin 40
gluten-containing 176
gluten-degraded 180
Properties 106, 108, 110, 114, 119, 120, 1164,
    78, 185, 186, 216, 227, 239, 242, 244
anti-diabetic 110, 114
anti-inflammatory 216, 244
anti-obesity 242
hypoallergenic 186
hypocholesterolemic 120, 227
immunomodulatory 108
metabolic 185
organoleptic 164
Proteases 161, 177, 179, 192
Protein(s) 2, 4, 10, 11, 12, 14, 27, 28, 39, 66,
    80, 82, 86, 87, 88, 93, 94, 153, 159, 161,
    163, 164, 177, 178, 186, 187, 188, 190,
    192
animal 2, 28, 159
cereal 186
corn 188
dietary 87
egg 14
metabolism 100
monomeric 177
natural whey 163
pea 94
peanut 4
potato 190
reservoirs 86
soy 93
synthesis 28, 66, 153
vegetable 28
Protein intake 66, 86, 87
insufficient 66

Q

Quantitative ingredient declaration (QUID) 16

R

Rash, eczematous 153
Reactive oxygen species (ROS) 29, 106
Receptor tyrosine kinase (RTK) 125
Renal disease 216
Resistant starch (RS) 8, 130, 227
Retinopathy 100

Reverse cholesterol transport pathway 209
Rheumatoid arthritis 30, 216
Rice protein (RP) 185, 186

S

Saccharina japonica 114
Salivary gland function 60
Saliva secretion 60
SARS-associated coronavirus 240
Sensations 62, 63
  olfactory 62
  somatosensory 63
Severe acute respiratory syndrome (SARS)
    239, 240
Short-chain fatty acids (SCFAs) 226
Skimmed milk 223
Small intestinal glycosidases 120
Soluble dietary fiber (SDFs) 227, 228
Sorghum proteins 189
Starch 8, 116
  fermented 8
  hydrolysates 116
Steroids, anabolic 211
Stroke 30, 61, 103, 106, 211, 212, 223 224
  ischaemic 224
Sugars 7, 11, 45, 50, 71, 72, 73, 94, 115, 117,
    166, 167, 197, 228, 229, 245, 246, 247,
    248, 249
  amino 11
  brown 73, 247
  colored 197
  consumption 228
  fruit 117
  raw 228
Symptoms 60, 61, 104, 152, 158, 173, 174,
    175, 176, 178, 189, 193, 195, 217
  dysphagic 61
  gastrointestinal 175
  non-gastrointestinal 189, 193
  respiratory 174
Syrup 7, 109, 116, 117, 118, 184, 248
  high-fructose 116
  malt 184
  maple 7
Systemic autoimmune disease 174

T

Thyroid 66, 67
  dysfunctions 66, 67
  stimulating hormone (TSH) 67
Total cholesterol (TC) 211
Tran fatty acids (TFA) 9, 10, 224
Transglutaminase 194
Trigeminal system (TS) 62
Triglycerides concentrations 185
Tyrosine kinase activity 125

U

Ulcerative colitis 216, 226

V

Vegetarian(s) 31, 32, 33, 38
  nutrition 32, 33
  pregnancy 38
  food guides (VFGs) 31
Veggie meatballs 50, 51
Venezuelan Amazons 243, 244
Vitamin(s) 15, 106, 178
  antioxidant 106
  deficiencies 178
  loss 15

W

Wheat 173, 174, 187, 218
  allergy 173, 174
  germ oils 218
  gluten proteins 187
Whey protein 92, 93, 163
Wine vinegar 46, 47
  white 46, 47
Woman's nutritional health 38
World health organization (WHO) 6, 58, 59,
    193, 239, 240

X

Xerostomia 60

www.ingramcontent.com/pod-product-compliance
Lightning Source LLC
Chambersburg PA
CBHW050820220326
41598CB00006B/265